THIRD EDITION

AF713707

LANGE Q&A™

MAMMOGRAPHY EXAMINATION

Olive Peart, MS, RT(R)(M)
Program Director
Harlem Hospital School of Radiography
New York, New York

Mc Graw Hill Education

New York Chicago San Francisco Athens London Madrid Mexico City
Milan New Delhi Singapore Sydney Toronto

Lange Q&A™: Mammography Examination, Third Edition

Copyright © 2015 by McGraw-Hill Education. All rights reserved. Printed in the United States of America. Except as permitted under the United States Copyright Act of 1976, no part of this publication may be reproduced or distributed in any form or by any means, or stored in a database or retrieval system, without the prior written permission of the publisher.

Previous edition copyright © 2009, 2003 by The McGraw-Hill Companies.

Lange Q&A™ is a trademark of McGraw-Hill Education.

1 2 3 4 5 6 7 8 9 0 QVS/QVS 19 18 17 16 15

ISBN 978-0-07-183392-9
MHID 0-07-183392-7

Notice

Medicine is an ever-changing science. As new research and clinical experience broaden our knowledge, changes in treatment and drug therapy are required. The author and the publisher of this work have checked with sources believed to be reliable in their efforts to provide information that is complete and generally in accord with the standards accepted at the time of publication. However, in view of the possibility of human error or changes in medical sciences, neither the author nor the publisher nor any other party who has been involved in the preparation or publication of this work warrants that the information contained herein is in every respect accurate or complete, and they disclaim all responsibility for any errors or omissions or for the results obtained from use of the information contained in this work. Readers are encouraged to confirm the information contained herein with other sources. For example and in particular, readers are advised to check the product information sheet included in the package of each drug they plan to administer to be certain that the information contained in this work is accurate and that changes have not been made in the recommended dose or in the contraindications for administration. This recommendation is of particular importance in connection with new or infrequently used drugs.

This book was set in Palatino by Cenveo® Publisher Services.
The editors were Andrew Moyer and Christina M. Thomas.
The production supervisor was Catherine Saggese.
Project management was provided by Tanya Punj, Cenveo Publisher Services.
The printer was Quad Graphics.

This book was printed on acid-free paper.

Library of Congress Cataloging-in-Publication Data

Peart, O. J. (Olive J.), author.
Lange Q & A. Mammography examination / Olive Peart—Third edition.
p. ; cm.
Lange Q and A. Mammography examination
Mammography examination
Includes bibliographical references and index.
ISBN 978-0-07-183392-9 (pbk. : alk. paper)—ISBN 0-07-183392-7 (pbk. : alk. paper)
I. Title. II. Title: Lange Q and A. Mammography examination. III. Title: Mammography examination.
[DNLM: 1. Mammography—Examination Questions. 2. Breast Neoplasms—radiography—Examination Questions. WP 18.2]
RG493.5.R33
618.1'907572—dc23 2014031867

McGraw-Hill Education books are available at special quantity discounts to use as premiums and sales promotions, or for use in corporate training programs. To contact a representative please visit the Contact Us pages at www.mhprofessional.com

Contents

Preface

This third edition of the mammography review and self-assessment is primarily geared to help those with a basic knowledge of breast imaging who are considering the American Registry of Radiologic Technologists (ARRT) advanced level mammography certification. However, with the new online instructor resources including objectives, PowerPoint slides, and test questions, this review can now be a valuable teaching tool for educators, managers, and others interested in enhancing their skills and knowledge of mammography and breast imaging. For access to online instructor resources, go to http://mhradiography.com, click on the book's page, then the 'Instructor Ancillaries' tab at the left, and provide your program/institution and course information, and an access code will be promptly emailed to you.

Lange Q&A Mammography Examination is not intended as a comprehensive mammography book on breast imaging. It includes a summary of the important points in the categories identified by the ARRT in the advanced level mammography certification. For a comprehensive study of mammography and breast imaging, this book is best used with the companion text, Mammography and Breast Imaging PREP: Program Review and Exam Prep (Copyright (C)2012 by The McGraw-Hill Companies, ISBN: 978-0071749329.

The first five chapters review the content category guidelines: (1) **Patient Education, Assessment, and Diagnostic Options,** (2) **Instrumentation and Quality Assurance,** (3) **Anatomy, Physiology, and Pathology of the Breast,** (4) **Mammographic Technique and Image Evaluation,** and (5) **Diagnostic, Interventional, and Treatment Procedures**. Each chapter provides a brief summary, highlighting the major points and important information in each content category, followed by test questions and answers. The book assumes that the reader already has some knowledge of mammography and breast imaging therefore the test questions can include material not covered in the chapter summaries. However, the answers for the test questions are fully explained and referenced and cover all the information required by the ARRT mammography examination. Chapters 6 and 7 each contain a complete practice mammography examination. The simulated examinations, also available online at http://mhradiography.com, have been designed to reduce examination jitters by providing a simulation of the actual certification examination. The online practice exams will also allow the user to self-test in the subject area of choice. When completing the simulated examinations, the examinee should plan to spend up to 2½ hours in a distraction-free environment to practice pacing and the economical use of time.

For the actual mammography examination, the ARRT allots 2½ hours to complete 115 questions and 25 unscored or pilot questions, broken down as follows: 12 questions in category A (Patient Care: Education and Assessment); 27 questions in category B (Instrumentation and Quality Assurance); 23 questions in category C (Anatomy, Physiology, and Pathology; 22 questions in category D (Mammographic technique and Image Evaluation); and 31 questions in category E (Breast Imaging Procedures). With built-in time to compete the tutorial and survey, the total examination time is actually 3 hours.

Eligibility requirements for the ARRT mammography certification can be found at https://www.arrt.org/Certification/Mammography. Candidates must meet three important requirements: ethics, education, and examination. The new education requirements, in effect after January 1, 2016, require candidates for the mammography examination to complete 16 hours of structured education in the form of CE credits or a college or university course.

The last few years have seen a rapid crossover to digital technology. In recognition of this change, this text focuses on digital imaging with only brief summaries or reference to analog technology. Breast imaging can be a rewarding and fulfilling profession and it is my hope that readers will be able to utilize the information and resources of this text to advance their career options or perhaps even more importantly, use the technical skills and the knowledge gained to provide meaningful help to patients.

For questions or comments please visit my web site at http://www.opeart.com or email me at olive@opeart.com.

Good luck!

Olive Peart, MS, RT(R)(M)
Program Director
Harlem Hospital School of Radiography
New York

Acknowledgments

In preparing for this edition, I am indebted to the many users of the previous editions. Many readers gave me valuable insight and practical suggestions on the review questions. Indeed, your questions, suggestions, criticisms, corrections, comments, and compliments were greatly appreciated and many have been incorporated into this edition. I especially wish to thank Cheryl Joseph, technologist with the Stamford Hospital, Mobile Wellness Program and Aileen Veliz for taking the time to assist me with images for this text.

I am particularly grateful for the help and suggestions that I received from Dorothy Saia, program director with the Radiography Program at Stamford Hospital, Teresa Whiteside, clinical instructor with the Radiography Program at Stamford Hospital, and Elizabeth Dwyer, mammography supervisor, at Hudson Valley Hospital Center.

This text would certainly not be possible without the care and commitment of my reviewers and my editors at McGraw-Hill. Indeed, the entire production team and other professionals at McGraw-Hill deserve special thanks for their attention to detail when preparing the final manuscript.

Finally, I wish to acknowledge the steady support from my husband, George Peart and the encouragement and help given by my children—Dione, Nadine, and George.

Reviewers

Kathy DeGelder, BS
Director of Women's Imaging Education
Medical Technology Management Institute (MTMI)
A Continuing Education Division of HERZING UNIVERSITY
Waukesha, Wisconsin

Karen Foster, MS, RT(R)(ARRT)
Assistant Professor of Radiography/Clinical Coordinator
St. Mary's Medical Center
School of Medical Imaging
Huntington, West Virginia

Alicia Giaimo, MHS, RT(R)(M)(BD)(ARRT), ROT
Clinical Assistant Professor-Diagnostic Imaging Program
Academic Coordinator-Diagnostic Imaging Department
Clinical Coordinator-Mammography
Quinnipiac University
Hamden, Connecticut

Caren E. Greenstein, MD
Director of Breast Imaging
White Plains Hospital Medical Center
White Plains, New York

Wendy J. Marshall, RT(R)(M)(QM)
Mammography Quality Management Technologist
The Dean Health Systems,
Madison, Wisconsin

Deborah Rayburn Moore, MS, RT(R)(CT)(ARRT)
Assistant Professor of Radiography, Didactic/Clinical Instructor
St. Mary's Medical Center
School of Medical Imaging
Huntington, West Virginia

Eugene Rodda, AB, RT(R)
X-ray Technologist
The Tully Imaging Center
Stamford, Connecticut

Beth Siegelbaum, BA, RT(R)(M)(BD), CBDT
X-ray Technologist
Darien Imaging Center
Darien, Connecticut

CHAPTER 1

Patient Education, Assessment, and Diagnostic Options

Summary of Important Points

PATIENT EDUCATION AND ASSESSMENT

Reasons for Patient Communication

- Helps to relax the patient
- Helps to identify patients with unusually sensitive breast
- Helps to educate the patient and combat misconception or fear of mammography
- Helps to identify concerns and answer questions before the patient leaves the facility
- Helps to ensure compliance with request for follow-ups

Factors that can Influence the Patient Compliance or Noncompliance

Influencing Compliance

- Pleasant experience
- Understanding mammographer

Influencing Noncompliance

- Painful experience
- Unsympathetic mammographer

The Role of the Mammographer

Link between patient and radiologist

- Provide appropriate clinical and didactic education
- Obtain patient's medical information
- Conducts physical assessment of the patient's breast
  - Performs visual inspection
  - Performs manual palpation
- Documents assessment findings

The Informed Consent

- Consent given by the patient before any invasive procedure or a procedure of significant risk
  - Patient must be of legal age and mentally competent.
  - Patient must offer consent voluntarily.
  - Patient must be adequately informed about the medical care being given.

Types of Consent

- **Written consent**—consent given in writing. It should include the name of the health-care professional who discussed the proposed treatment with the patient, the name of the health-care provider who is to perform the procedure, and the date, time, and location where the consent was signed.
- **Oral consent**—consent given verbally.
- **General consent or authorization for treatment**—consent signed at the time of admission to a hospital or health-care setting. It authorizes general treatment and excludes invasive procedures.
- **Expressed consent**—assumed by nonverbal cues such as nodding or lifting the arm when told that an injection is required or oral.
- **Implied consent**—assumed in an emergency situation where the patient is unable to make a decision. Generally, additional documentation is required.

Objective and Subjective Data

- Objective data defines information collected from the patient that can be seen, heard, or felt, e.g., a lump in the breast.

- Subjective data is perceived by the affected individual only (e.g., pain in the breast). Subjective data should never be disregarded. However, it should be clearly defined.

Method of Questioning

- **Listening** (rather than asking questions) will allow the patients to tell their stories unasked. Listening is used to assess the patient's life experience and educational background and can help in determining whether the patient will understand medical or technical terms for future questions.
- **Open-ended questions** use nondirected or nonleading methods to avoid leading the patient and to allow an unbiased input.
- **Facilitation** uses gestures such as a nod or saying "yes," "okay," or "go on" to encourage elaboration.
- **Silence** is used to give the patient time to remember and ensure accuracy.
- **Probing questions** are used to get more detail of the problem.
- **Repetition** will reword the question to clarify information and can be used to verify that the patient has not changed his/her mind.
- **Summarization** is used to verify the accuracy of the information.

Medical or Clinical History Documentation

- Used to document information on symptoms or any abnormalities of the breast
- Serves as a guide for the radiologist

Documentation Using the Medical or Clinical History

- Imaging history and patient limitations
  - Previous mammogram—when and where it was obtained.
    - The previous mammograms are vital for comparison.
  - The mammographer should document any limitation (mental or physical) that will affect the imaging, e.g., the placement of a pacemaker could limit the imaging of the pectoral muscle on the mediolateral oblique (MLO).
- Signs or symptoms—palpable or visible abnormalities of the breast
  - Changes in nipple or areola
    - Nipple discharge
    - Inverted nipple
  - Dimpling or puckering of skin
    - Skin thickening
  - Accessory breast tissue or nipples can develop along the milk line. Examples include congenital abnormalities such as asymmetry in breast size, shape, or position.
    - Accessory tissue must be documented.
    - Imaging will depend on the policy of the facility.
  - Persistent skin conditions such as swelling, eczema, itchiness, or redness.
  - Lump/s in breast or axilla.
    - Trauma to the breast especially recent trauma should be documented.
  - Skin lesions or scars.
    - Skin lesions or palpable lumps should be identified.
    - Schematic diagram can be used to localize scars.
- Personal and family history of breast cancer
  - Documentation of first-degree relatives with breast cancer and include the age cancer was detected.
  - Major and/or minor risks factors.
- Surgical history related to the breast
  - History of augmentation or reduction including type and date of surgery
  - Type of breast biopsies with results and date of surgeries
  - History of lumpectomy or mastectomy including dates of surgeries
  - Autologous reconstruction—surgical flap procedures
- Childbearing or gynecological history
  - Patient's age at birth of first child
  - Patient's age at menarche
  - Date of patient's last menstrual period
  - Patient's age at menopause, hysterectomy, or oophorectomy
- Hormonal history including status of menstrual cycle
  - Types of hormone taken including start date and duration

The Breast Self-Examination

The breast self-examination (BSE) can serve as an important tool in the detection of breast cancer. Often the woman herself is the first to notice abnormal changes in the breasts. The American Cancer Society suggests that women aged 20 and older should perform a BSE every month.

- The best time to conduct a BSE is a few days after the menstrual period ends when the breasts are least tender or swollen or 5-10 days after the start of the period.
- For women not having regular menstruation the BSE should be done on the same day every month.

The Clinical Breast Examination

The clinical breast examination (CBE) is a check of the breast by a qualified health-care professional. The examination is performed to locate any lumps or suspicious areas and to examine the texture, size, and shape of the breast.

- The CBE takes the same format as the BSE—looking and feeling for changes in the breast.
- In a CBE special attention is paid to lymph nodes in the axilla and around the clavicle because breast cancer leaves the breast via the lymph nodes.
- Both breasts should be examined in the upright and the supine positions because a cancer in the upper half of the breast is easier felt when the woman is upright whereas a cancer in the lower breast is best felt when the woman is supine.

Two Main Criteria in any Breast Examination

- **Looking for changes**
    - The woman should check for indentations, retracted nipples, dimpling, or prolonged skin conditions such as eczema.
- **Feeling for changes**
    - While feeling for changes the woman should examine her breast in both the upright and the supine positions.

Breast Screening Guidelines Approved by the ACR

- Women aged 20-39
    - CBE every 3 years
    - Monthly BSE
- Women older than 40 years
    - Annual screening mammogram
        - Magnetic resonance imaging (MRI) or ultrasound screening only for women with high-risk factors or very dense breast
    - Annual CBE
    - Monthly BSE

Advantages and Disadvantages of Mammography Screening

Advantages

- The mammogram is the single most effective tool in early breast cancer detection.

Disadvantages

- The sensitivity of the mammogram will be dependent on breast density, plus the age and hormone status of the patient.
    - Cancer is generally visualized as a white area within the background density of the breast. If the background density is black (as in fatty tissue), the cancer will be easily seen. If the background density is "white" (as in dense breast tissue), the cancer will be harder to detect.
- The mammogram is not 100% effective.
    - Mammography screening is generally acknowledged to have a 10%-15% miss rate. As the patient ages the density of the breast generally decreases, thus the sensitivity of the mammogram will increase.
- Mammography tends to understate the multifocality of a lesion.
- The positioning skills of the mammographer can affect the outcome.
    - Cancer can be missed due to inadequate compression or missed breast tissue due to poor positioning.
- The interpretation skills of the radiologist can affect patient outcome.

Dose Calculations in Mammography

- Most patient dose reports in radiology is a fact check of the ESE (entrance-skin-dose) only. However, the biological effect of a mammogram is assumed to be more closely associated with the total energy absorbed by the glandular tissue of the breast.
- The *glandular dose* is therefore the dose of choice when calculating radiation doses associated with mammography. In mammography screening, when compared to the skin dose, the glandular dose is very low because the dose falls off

rapidly as the low photon energy beam penetrates the breast.

- **The average glandular dose for a typical mammogram:** The American College of Radiology (ACR) recommends that the average glandular dose on a single mammogram projection should not be greater than 3 mGy (0.3 rad or 300 mrad) with a grid or 1 mGy (0.1 rad or 100 mrad) without a grid.

Risk Factors for Breast Cancer

Risk factors are anything that increases a person's chance of getting a disease. The risk for breast cancer is not the same for all women at a given age. Some women have an increased chance of developing breast cancer.

Increased Breast Cancer Risks

Major risk factors are often those outside of a woman's control. These are factors that cannot be changed. Minor risks are often those within a woman's control or do not significantly increase a woman's chance of developing the disease. They may be cancer-causing factors in the environment or may be related to personal choices.

Major Risk Factors for Breast Cancer

- **Gender:** Although men can develop breast cancer this disease is much more common among women than men. The biggest risk factor for breast cancer is therefore gender, i.e., being female.
- **Age:** Age is an important risk factor because as a woman ages, the incidence of cancer increases.
- **Genetic risk factors:** About 5%-10% of breast cancer cases are hereditary. A woman with a hereditary risk for breast cancer may carry a harmful mutation of the BRCA1 or BRCA2 genes which are the most common. These are mutated genes that can be inherited from either parent. The genes help to control the rate of cell growth and division and are regarded as tumor suppressors. Women with a normal gene have a protective effect because the genes make proteins that keep cells from growing abnormally. Therefore with the mutated gene there is an increase susceptibility to breast cancer. It is estimated that women with the BRCA1 mutation have a 55%-65% risk of developing breast cancer before age 70, and often at a younger age. Women with a BRCA2 mutation have a 45% risk. Another gene, PALB2 (partner and localizer of BRCA2) provides instructions for making a protein that works with the BRCA2 gene to repair strands of DNA and control the rate of cell growth and division. Individuals with a defective PALB2 have a 33% chance of developing breast cancer by the age of 70. Molecular tests are available to identify the BRCA and PALB2 mutations in individuals.
- **Family history of breast cancer:** Breast cancer risk is higher among women whose close blood relatives (mother, sister, and/or daughter) have this disease. A blood relative can be from either the mother's or father's side of the family, but the closer the relative, the higher the risk factor. Women are also at a higher risk if the breast cancer occurs in a relative before age 50.
- **Personal history of cancer or breast cancer:** A woman with cancer in one breast has a greater risk of developing a new cancer in the other breast.
- **Abnormal breast biopsy:** A biopsy of atypical hyperplasia, lobular carcinoma in situ (LCIS) or ductal carcinoma in situ (DCIS), are associated with increased risks. Because some cases of DCIS will eventually become cancer, this type of breast change is actively treated. Women with atypical hyperplasia or LCIS are usually monitored carefully and not actively treated.
- **Radiation therapy:** Radiation therapy to the chest and breast before age 30 carry an increased risk. The younger a woman was when she received treatment, the higher is her risk of developing breast cancer later in life. Also, women who have had the chest area radiated because of a previous cancer treatment such as for Hodgkin disease (or non-Hodgkin lymphoma) are at a slightly increased risk for breast cancer.

Other Risk Factors for Breast Cancer

- **Menstrual history:** Starting menstruation at an early age (before age 12) or menopause at a later age (after age 55) are both considered increased risks for breast cancer. The greater the amount of menstrual cycles in the woman's lifetime, the greater then would be the risk of breast cancer.
- **Reproductive history:** Pregnancy is thought to have a protective effect against having breast

cancer because during the pregnancy the woman is not menstruating. It therefore follows that the longer a woman goes without getting pregnant the greater are her risks for breast cancer. Also, women who had their first full-term pregnancy after age 30 or who have never had a full-term pregnancy are at increased risk of breast cancer. Breast-feeding at any age has a protective effect.

- **Hormone:** The use is thought to influence breast cancer risk, but does not actually cause breast cancer. Women who used combined estrogen and progestin menopausal hormone therapy for more than 5 years have an increased chance of developing breast cancer.
- All factors that affect the reproductive hormones in a woman's body increase risks for breast cancer.
- **Diethylstilbestrol (DES):** It was used by pregnant women in the United States during 1940-1971. It was used to prevent miscarriage and studies show that women who took DES during pregnancy have a slightly increased risk of breast cancer. Also, women who were exposed to DES in utero, whose mothers took DES while they were pregnant, may also have a slightly increased risk of breast cancer after age 40.

Purpose of Hormone Replacement Therapy

- Relieves symptoms of perimenopause:
  - Hot flushes
  - Sleep disturbance
  - Insomnia
- Side effects can include fatigue, slower involution process, reduces osteoporosis.

Dangers of Hormone Replacement Therapy

- The combination estrogen and progesterone in hormone replacement therapy (HRT) may increase the risk of developing cancer in the breast and uterus.
- The administration of hormones generally increases the proliferation of glandular tissue, fibroadenomas, and breast cysts.
- Use of HRT increases the incidence of asthma, dementia, heart attacks, strokes, and blood clots.
- Cancers can be harder to detect in dense breast tissue, therefore the increase in glandular tissue caused by the HRT can reduce the effectiveness of the mammogram. However, other modalities can be very effective when imaging dense breast tissue.

BREAST IMAGING MODALITIES

Analog Imaging

- Analog imaging produces the images in a purely mechanical way with a final hard copy that cannot be modified.
- In analog imaging a film is used to acquire the diagnostic information, to display the information, and to store the information.

Disadvantages of Films

- Films can be costly.
- Storage costs are high and a large storage area is needed.
- Films are easily lost or stolen.
- Rigid techniques are required to produce optimum exposures and there is no adjusting for over or under exposure.
- The final image has a narrow dynamic range and the fixed gradient or contrast can be a challenge for the mammographer to optimize and for the radiologist to interpret.

Full-Field Digital Mammography and Computed Mammography

- Full-field digital mammography (FFDM) utilizes a totally cassetteless flat-panel detector system whereas computed mammography (CM) combines an analog imaging x-ray unit with digital technology using photostimulable phosphor (PSP) technology.
- Both are considered digital technologies and have the capability of providing high-quality mammography images.

Monitors—AWS versus RWS

Most modern mammography imaging uses a liquid crystal display (LCD) monitor.

- Acquisition workstation monitors (AWS) are the technologist monitors.
  - Low-resolution monitor
  - Allows rapid viewing of the image

    - The mammographer can determine whether to repeat the examination immediately after the exposure.
  - Allows postprocessing of an image while viewing the changes being made
    - Images can be magnified, rotated, flipped, or inverted as needed.
    - Patient's demographic information can be modified or corrected and retransmitted.
    - Images can be sent to multiple destinations.
- Review workstation monitors (RWS) are the radiologist monitors.
  - The only monitor approved for interpreting the mammogram
  - High-resolution monitor

Advantages of Digital Mammography

The biggest advantage of digital and computed systems is associated with the wide latitude of the digital signals.

- The higher sensitivity of the detectors demonstrates a linear response (input to output) to the intensity of x-ray exposure over a broad range. This allows better penetration of denser breast tissue, plus, because the response to exposure is linear, optimum contrast can be obtained for both fibroglandular and fatty regions of the breast.
- Improves an institution's workflow by reducing the number of repeated examinations due to improper exposures.
- Reduces repeats, therefore reduces the cost associated with repeats.
- Offers an efficient imaging system, reducing the overall time needed to complete the examination.
- Reduces the possibility of lost images.
- Offers an easier and more efficient means of managing images or finding previous records.
- Eliminates poor copies because every copy is as exact as the original.
- Reduces the medicolegal risks and expenses associated with lost films.
- Offers multiple archival systems allowing a variety of storage and retrieval options.
- Allows picture archiving and communication system (PACS).
  - Images from one modality can be linked with images from other modalities.
  - Images from multiple modalities can be viewed quickly and easily from any monitor within the facility.
- Allows teleradiography.
  - Images can be transmitted to workstations outside the facility.

Disadvantages of Digital Imaging

- High start-up cost
- Reduced awareness of manipulating individual technical factors
- Lack of awareness of radiation safety and patient protection
- Outsourcing of reporting with possible elimination of on-site radiologist
- Possibility of backup system failure, corruption, or loss of digital records

Digital and Patient Positioning

- Patient position in digital imaging is the same as with analog. However, because of the fixed size of the digital detector, modifications are sometimes needed especially when imaging the small breast.

Image Storage Devices

- Redundant array of independent (inexpensive) disk (RAID) can store 6-12 months of patient data and can transfer image files to the monitor in 2 minutes.
- Digital linear tape (DLT) is not recommended for high capacity storage. They can wear out with heavy use.
- Jukebox storage is used for long-term storage. They hold image data in digital tapes, disks, or other media and typically have a retrieval time of 2-5 minutes.
- Optical disk or magneto-optical disk (MOD) is similar to compact disk (CD) or digital versatile disk (DVD). They are more reliable and robust and are faster than jukebox storage.
- Ultra density optical (UDO) is the newest type of high capacity optical disk system that utilizes blue violet laser technology.

Digital Imaging and Communications in Medicine

- DICOM is a set of computer software standards that permit a wide range of digital imaging programs to understand each other.

Picture Archiving Communications System

- PACS is a computer network that allows images from multiple modalities to be viewed at a single monitor, transmitted or stored.
- The images can be accessed over the Internet, over the telephone, via satellite communication, or from a cable modem. This allows images to be sent from multiple modalities to remote locations across the nation or even across the world.
- All equipment used must be Digital Imaging and Communications in Medicine (DICOM)-compliant.

Teleradiography

- Teleradiography is the remote transmission and viewing of images. Transmission can be Internet, cable, or telephone based. The interface format of transmission is called DICOM.

Computer-Aided Detection

- The use of computers to preread the mammograms, by scanning every part of the radiograph and reporting any suspicious area.
  - The computer will display or analyze suspicious areas to make the interpretation consistent from patient to patient.
  - The computer system must be programmed to act as a second reader.

DIGITAL BREAST TOMOSYNTHESIS

Digital breast tomosynthesis (DBT) uses a high-resolution cross-section 3-dimensional imaging to eliminate tissue overlap.

Advantages and Potential Use of Tomosynthesis

- Detection and screening especially for women with dense breasts.
- Diagnostic workup or problem solving.
- Help to reduce recall rate.

The Hologic tomosynthesis unit does not use a grid and the number of reconstructed images is based on the breast thickness in millimeters. Reconstruction is always in 1-mm-thick slices with the first slice starting at the detector. The x-ray tube rotates in an arc around the breast taking 15 exposures in 4 seconds, and sweeping from –7 to 0 to +7 degrees with no movement of the patient. A typical tomosynthesis unit can image in 2D, 3D, or a combination of 2D and 3D (COMBO).

Hologic also offers *synthesized 2D imaging*

- This technique offers a reconstructed 2D image of the breast without the additional radiation. After taking a 3D projection, the computer will synthesize and reconstruct the tomosynthesis slices of the breast and create a 2D image without added radiation to the patient. The technology is called the *C-view* imaging by Hologic.

Disadvantages of Hologic Tomosynthesis

- Greater risks of motion due to the longer acquisition time.
  - Long total exposure time of 12 seconds for COMBO.
- Motion artifacts hard to detect on the reconstruction images at the radiologist workstation.
- Large number of images.
- Degraded imaging of calcifications.
  - Thin slicing may mask calcification. However, slabbing of the slices help with calcification visualization.
- Tomosynthesis is not possible for the From-Below (FB) projection, magnification and if the breast tissue is more than 24.5 cm.
- Higher overall radiation dose.
  - 2D imaging gives approximately 1.2 mGy of radiation per projection.
  - 3D tomosynthesis gives approximately 1.45 mGy of radiation per projection.
  - COMBO imaging (2D + 3D) will give approximately 2.65 mGy per projection.
  - Imaging implants in 3D gives even more radiation to patient because lower peak kilovoltage (kVp) is used.

Motion Checks in the Hologic System

- In the Hologic system the mammographer must review the projection dataset at the AWS. Because motion can occur at any point of the imaging, motion is best appreciated in the cine mode and a motion check must be made before submitting the images. Motion can be caused by inadequate compression, movement, or heavy breathing during the exposure. The long exposure time leading to patient motion is also a contributing factor.

- Motion is best visualized on the projection dataset of images at the AWS.
  - Motion is seen as anterior/posterior movement of the breast tissue or of structures in the breast such as calcification or lymph nodes.
  - Medial to lateral movement of breast tissue or structures on the tomosynthesis projection images is normal and does not indicate motion.

The GE SenoClaire 3D Breast Tomosynthesis takes 9 exposures and utilizes only one 3D projection, the MLO. The craniocaudal (CC) projection is imaged in 2D. The tube makes a complete stop after each exposure in a technology called step-and-shoot tube motion. This system reduces image blur. The GE system uses a grid. However, radiation dose is kept low because only 1 projection is taken in 3D. The GE system offers reconstructed 2D images called V-Preview. The disadvantage of the system is the higher recall rates when compared when compared to other screening systems.

The MicroDose Photon-Counting Tomosynthesis System uses a slot-scanning design. The detector consists of an array of parallel crystalline silicon strips combined with photon-counting electronics, designed to absorb 90% of the incident x-rays. The x-ray tube, collimator and detector pivot about the breast taking up to 21 images. Imaging uses high kVp—up to 40 kVp with a tungsten target and aluminum filtration. However, the dose is 1/20 the dose of 2D mammography imaging. As the tube moves laterally across the breasts, the images produced are reconstructed and sent for viewing. The disadvantage of the system is the higher recall rates when compared to other screening systems.

CONTRAST DIGITAL MAMMOGRAPHY

- This involves injecting a contrast while the breast is under compression. Precontrast and postcontrast images are taken.
- Dual-energy subtraction can be performed to assess the contrast in tumors. Dual-energy subtraction is used to subtract high- and low-energy images to separate soft tissue from contrast or calcium deposits. The technology can also be used to enhance masses and eliminate obscuring structures.

ULTRASOUND IMAGING OF THE BREAST

- Ultrasound uses the piezoelectric principle to generate high-frequency sound waves that are used to create images of the organs and blood vessels in the body.
- The patient can rest comfortably on a bed during the ultrasound examination of the breast.
- Higher frequency transducers provide greater resolution but have less penetrating power. Mammography imaging can use frequencies up to 16 MHz.

Ultrasound Transducer

The diagnostic ultrasound transducers serve 2 functions:

- Converts electric energy to acoustic pulses that are sent into the patient.
- Receives the reflected echoes and converts their weak pressure changes into electrical signals so the computer can process them.

Breast Imaging with Ultrasound

- Ultrasound does not use ionizing radiation.
- Ultrasound cannot image microcalcifications.
- No documented risks or harmful bioeffects have been reported.
- Sound cannot travel through a vacuum and will not travel easily through air. To eliminate the air gap between the skin and the transducer a water-based gel is always applied. This gel acts as a conducting medium to transmit sound from the transducer the skin surface.

COLOR DOPPLER ULTRASOUND

This technology can be used to provide an anatomic display of blood flow and can therefore be used to outline the vascularity of a lesion. The technology is based on the fact that highly vascular lesions are often malignant.

MAGNETIC RESONANCE IMAGING OF THE BREAST

- MRI uses very complex magnetic properties to create detailed images of the breast. There is no ionizing radiation and no documented side effects from an MRI examination. The MRI system is able to switch magnetic fields and radio waves to take images in any plane and from any orientation.

- MRI is performed with the contrast material, Gadolinium diethylenetriamine penta-acetic acid (DTPA). Gadolinium (Gd) is a paramagnetic metal which by itself is toxic. A complex solution of Gd and DTPA is stable with very little toxicity. This can be injected into a vein of the arm before the MRI examination to enhance image contrast.
- MRI of the breast has been approved by the FDA since 1991 as a supplemental tool in addition to the mammogram.

Risks and Potential Complications of MRI of the Breast

- All the major risks of MRI are associated with the magnetic properties of the MRI machine.
  - During an MRI, the patient is placed within a powerful magnetic field. Patients are required to provide the technologist with a detailed medical history before the MRI examination because any ferromagnetic metal object can potentially be extremely dangerous inside the magnet of the MRI unit.
- The MRI cannot be used on patients with some pacemakers, aneurysm clips in the brain, nerurostimulators, shrapnel, surgical clips or plates, prostheses, metal implants, cochlear implants or if the patient has been exposed to metallic flakes or slivers as a result of working around metal finishing, welding, or grinding equipment.
- Patients must remove all metals from their bodies or clothing including metal piercings, coins, watches, keys, bobby pins, credit cards, pocketknives, and clothing with metal zippers, buttons, belts, or fasteners.

Disadvantages of MRI of the Breast

- Poor visualization of the axillary nodes mainly because contrast enhancement occurs for both normal and pathological nodes.
- MRI is unable to image microcalcifications—which is often associated with early-stage DCIS.
- MRI is expensive and not always an available option.
- The MRI examination is longer than the mammogram and the patient needs to lie prone/very still during the examination for 30-60 minutes.
- MRI is extremely sensitive and has a higher false-positive rate than mammography and often results in unnecessary biopsies.
- Patients can experience claustrophobia when placed in the bore of the MRI unit.
- Any contrast injection has associated risks and breast MR imaging must be done with contrast.

NUCLEAR IMAGING

Nuclear imaging represents the emerging molecular imaging technologies where the function of the organ can be assessed and not just the anatomy. In nuclear imaging a radioactive substance, called a tracer or radiopharmaceutical is injected into the vein. Nuclear imaging technologies include:

- Positron emission tomography (PET) imaging
- Breast scintigraphy or scintimammography
- Lymphoscintigraphy—sentinel node mapping

Positron Emission Tomography

- PET imaging is usually performed using fluorodeoxyglucose (FDG), which is the most common radioactive tracer. This tracer—(fluorodeoxyglucose, methionine, tyrosine, fluoro-estradiol, nor-progesterone), 2-deoxy-2-fluoro-D-glucose labeled with fluorine—also has a half-life of 109.8 minutes. It is used because the breast cancer has a particular affinity to it.
- Typically, 10-20 mCi of the radioactive substance is injected into an arm vein then a special gamma scanner is used to detect the radiation emitted.
- The technology works on the principle that most cancerous tissue uses vast amounts of sugar. The FDG is metabolized in the body like sugar. It will therefore go to the tissues that are most active. PET imaging is a valuable tool in detecting the metastatic spread of breast cancer.
- PET imaging can be modified using a special breast gamma camera in a technology called positron emission mammography (PEM). In PEM imaging, the breast can be position similar to the CC and MLO mammographic projections for easier comparisons.

Breast Scintigraphy or Scintimammography or Breast-Specific Gamma Imaging

- With scintigraphy, the radiopharmaceutical is injected into the arm vein of the patient.
- The radiopharmaceutical used is technetium-99m (Tc-99m) sestamibi which is sometimes marketed under the trade name of Miraluma. The radiopharmaceutical will accumulate only in malignant lesions in the breast. A benign lesion does not take up the radioactive isotope.
- In BSGI the patient is imaged with a special gamma camera which images the breast in the same positions and projections as the mammography unit.

Lymphoscintigraphy or Sentinel Node Mapping

- In this technique, the radiopharmaceutical is injected into subareola lymphatic plexus of the affected breast. The radioactive material is then taken up by the lymph system and travels to the lymph nodes under the arm. At surgery, the surgeon uses a Geiger counter to locate the radioactive lymph nodes. Surgery should follow 1-9 hours after the radiopharmaceutical injection.
- Often a blue dye is also injected into the region of the tumor and the dye is also then carried to the sentinel node.
- The first nodes picked up by the radiopharmaceutical can be removed for biopsy. If the nodes test negative for cancer then axillary node dissection is not needed.
- The procedure can provide prognostic information based on the presence or absence of regional lymph node metastases. And because the cancerous node is identified, fewer lymph nodes are removed.

Questions

1. The biggest risk factor for breast cancer is

   (A) a family history of breast cancer
   (B) a personal history of breast cancer
   (C) gender
   (D) not breast-feeding

2. One of the minor risk factors for breast cancer could include

   (A) gender
   (B) aging
   (C) genetic risk factors
   (D) not breast-feeding

3. What is the approximate risk of developing breast cancer for a woman whose sister has the disease?

   (A) higher than normal risk
   (B) no significant change in risk
   (C) lower than normal risk
   (D) none of the above

4. A woman with the greatest risk of developing breast cancer is

   (A) age 30 or below
   (B) above age 50
   (C) between ages 30 and 40
   (D) above age 20 but below age 30

5. Symptoms of a possible breast disease that will not be demonstrated on the mammogram can include

   (A) nipple discharge
   (B) skin thickening
   (C) circumscribed tumors
   (D) stellate lesions

6. Symptoms of a very early DCIS can include

   (A) skin thickening
   (B) nipple discharge
   (C) macrocalcifications
   (D) none of the above

7. Skin thickening can be malignant but could also be caused by nonmalignant factors such as

   (A) esophageal metastases
   (B) bronchial cancer
   (C) Hodgkin disease
   (D) sarcoidosis

8. MRI could be used

   1. as a primary breast cancer detection tool
   2. to image patients with breast implants to evaluate ruptures
   3. to determine tumor margins and the extent of tumor spread

   (A) 1 only
   (B) 1 and 2 only
   (C) 2 and 3 only
   (D) 1 and 3 only

9. The ACS recommends that

   (A) women older than 40 years should have a yearly MRI
   (B) women younger than 40 years should have a screening mammogram every year
   (C) new masses or lumps in the breast should be checked by a health-care provider
   (D) women between ages 20 and 39 should have a CBE every year

10. A health-care provider should evaluate which of the following breast changes?
    1. lumps or swellings
    2. skin irritation or dimpling
    3. milky discharge from the nipple
    (A) 1 only
    (B) 1 and 2 only
    (C) 2 and 3 only
    (D) 1, 2, and 3

11. A CBE should be performed every
    1. year after age 40
    2. 3 years between ages 20 and 39
    3. month after age 50
    (A) 1 only
    (B) 2 only
    (C) 1 and 2 only
    (D) 2 and 3 only

12. A CBE can be performed by which of the following?
    1. the radiologist
    2. the patient
    3. a health-care professional
    (A) 1 only
    (B) 2 only
    (C) 2 and 3 only
    (D) 1 and 3 only

13. A BSE should be done regularly by
    1. the radiologist
    2. the patient
    3. a health-care professional
    (A) 1 only
    (B) 2 only
    (C) 2 and 3 only
    (D) 1 and 3 only

14. All women above the age of _______ should perform a BSE regularly.
    (A) 20
    (B) 30
    (C) 40
    (D) 50

15. The 2-step method of BSE is to
    (A) look and feel for changes in the breast
    (B) examine your breasts and have a regular mammogram
    (C) check for lumps in the breast and keep a journal of changes in the breast
    (D) examine your breasts and nipples

16. When visually inspecting the breast, the changes that should be recorded include
    1. changes in breast size and shape
    2. changes in texture or color of the breast
    3. indentations on the skin of the breast
    (A) 1 and 2 only
    (B) 2 and 3 only
    (C) 1 and 3 only
    (D) 1, 2, and 3

17. The patient's medical history and documentation will
    1. provide the radiologist with information on the patient's risk factors for breast cancer
    2. give the radiologist information about general symptoms of breast cancer
    3. provide information about possible benign breast conditions of the patient
    (A) 1 and 2 only
    (B) 2 and 3 only
    (C) 1 and 3 only
    (D) 1, 2, and 3

18. Stressing the importance of the BSE can be controversial because
    (A) the BSE tends to detect only benign breast cancer
    (B) the BSE will help in the detection of malignant breast conditions
    (C) a mammogram is not 100% effective
    (D) the BSE can cause unnecessary anxiety in women

19. Which of the following are methods used in BSE?
    1. using the pads of the 3 middle fingers to palpate the entire breast
    2. palpating around the breast in a vertical pattern
    3. using varying degrees of pressure while palpating of the breast

    (A) 1 only
    (B) 1 and 2 only
    (C) 1 and 3 only
    (D) 1, 2, and 3

20. For a menstruating woman, when is the best time of the month to perform a BSE?

    (A) 1 week before the start of menstruation
    (B) on the first day of the month
    (C) on the last day of the month
    (D) when the breast is least tender

21. Which of the following statements is true?
    1. Breast cancer death rates in United States are going down.
    2. Breast cancer is the leading cause of cancer death in women in United States.
    3. The second leading cause of cancer death in women in United States is breast cancer.

    (A) 1 and 2 only
    (B) 2 and 3 only
    (C) 1 and 3 only
    (D) 1, 2, and 3

22. Postmenopausal obesity is associated with

    (A) a relatively high risk of developing breast cancer
    (B) overall reduction in breast cancer risks
    (C) circulating estrogen that is produced in fatty tissue
    (D) a lower overall estrogen level

23. In routine mammography, the glandular dose per projection is generally about

    (A) 1-2 mGy (0.1-0.2 rad)
    (B) 10-20 mGy (1.0-2.0 rad)
    (C) 0.1-0.2 mGy (0.01-0.02 rad)
    (D) 2-3 mGy (0.2-0.3 rad)

24. Which age group is likely to get the most radiation dose from a mammogram?

    (A) between 20 and 35
    (B) between 40 and 50
    (C) between 55 and 60
    (D) above 70

25. The 5-year survival rate for a patient with a stage 0 breast cancer is about

    (A) 22%
    (B) 72%
    (C) 93%
    (D) 100%

26. During a mammogram, which of the following will affect the average glandular dose per breast?
    1. degree of breast compression
    2. the half-value layer (HVL) of the x-ray beam
    3. breast size and composition

    (A) 1 only
    (B) 2 only
    (C) 3 only
    (D) 1, 2, and 3

27. Patients who are allowed to play an active role in applying the compression are usually
    1. less likely to tolerate the compression
    2. more likely to tolerate the compression
    3. more relaxed during the compression

    (A) 1 only
    (B) 2 only
    (C) 1 and 3 only
    (D) 2 and 3 only

28. With its high sensitivity, MRI is ideal as
    (A) a routine screen tool for breast cancer
    (B) a replacement for mammography screening in detecting breast cancers
    (C) an adjunctive tool in detecting breast cancer
    (D) a screening tool for older women

29. MRI imaging involves the use of
    (A) radiation to detect breast lesions
    (B) sound waves in the imaging of the breast
    (C) magnetic properties plus radio waves to image the breast
    (D) strong sound and radio waves in imaging the breast

30. Ultrasound uses
    (A) high-frequency sound waves to image the breast
    (B) low-frequency sound waves to image the breast
    (C) longitudinal microwaves to image the breast
    (D) radio-frequency waves to image the breast

31. MRI can be used to
    1. map the extent of a tumor
    2. image patients with implants
    3. evaluate patients with dense breast
       (A) 1 and 2 only
       (B) 2 and 3 only
       (C) 1 and 3 only
       (D) 1, 2, and 3

32. Ultrasound imaging of the breast is often used to
    (A) map the extent of a breast tumor
    (B) verify that a lesion seen on the mammogram is solid or fluid filled
    (C) verify the presence of microcalcifications
    (D) biopsy a lesion seen only on MRI

33. All of the following are forms of subjective patient data *except:*
    (A) patient has a palpable lump in the right breast
    (B) patient complains of severe pain during breast compression
    (C) the mood or demeanor of the patient
    (D) patient's complaints of pain and tenderness in the left breast

34. When questioning patients to obtain an accurate patient history:
    (A) keep your questions general in nature so as not to offend the patient
    (B) start with open-ended questions and then follow up with more direct inquiries
    (C) do not let the patient talk too much, in order to keep the examination moving
    (D) use medical "jargon" to impress the patient with your expertise

35. Which of the following are positive questioning skills that the radiographer can use when verifying the accuracy of the patient information?
    (A) leading questions
    (B) open-ended question
    (C) repeating information
    (D) facilitation

36. What is the purpose of "probing" questions used when interviewing patients?
    (A) clarifies information by asking for specific details
    (B) gives the patient time to remember
    (C) allows the patient time to tell their story
    (D) summarizes the accuracy of the information

37. In gathering more information on a patient's complaint of pain, a good probing question to ask would be

(A) "How would you describe the pain?"
(B) "When did the pain first happen?"
(C) "If the pain comes and goes, how often does it occur and what is the time span between occurrences?"
(D) all of the above are good questions to ask

38. There are 2 types of data collection processes. If your patient says, he/she has a bruise on her left breast, this data is regarded as

(A) objective
(B) subjective
(C) open-ended scenario
(D) probing

39. When questioning your patient, what is the purpose of repetition?

(A) to give the patient time to remember
(B) to get more detail
(C) to summarize
(D) to allow the patient to tell their story

40. "Where is your pain?" Is an example of

(A) a probing question
(B) repetition
(C) summarization
(D) an open-ended question

41. Which of the following will not result in increased breast cancer risks?

(A) having mother who took DES while pregnant
(B) having a first child before age 30
(C) a history of Hodgkin lymphoma
(D) menarche at age 10

42. An informed consent is required before performing which of the following examination?

(A) ultrasound
(B) mammogram
(C) fine-needle biopsy (FNB)
(D) MRI

43. Phone consent is an example of

(A) written consent
(B) oral consent
(C) implied consent
(D) expressed consent

44. The patient has to sign an informed consent

1. when there are significant risks associated with the procedure
2. for all procedures in the imaging department
3. if the procedure is invasive

(A) 1 and 2 only
(B) 1 and 3 only
(C) 2 and 3 only
(D) 1, 2, and 3

45. Which kind of consent is binding but difficult to prove?

(A) oral
(B) written
(C) implied
(D) printed

46. Which of the following is not required information that must be included on any informed consent?

(A) name of the procedure
(B) risks and benefits of the procedure
(C) patient height and weight
(D) possible alternative procedure

47. The monitor used to interpret the mammograms is the

(A) acquisition workstation monitor
(B) LCD monitor
(C) AWS monitor
(D) RWS monitor

48. A system used to store 6-12 months of image data that can be retrieved within a few minutes is the

(A) jukebox
(B) RAID
(C) DLT
(D) CD

49. A computer network system that allows images to be viewed at various monitors or transmitted or stored is termed

(A) PACS
(B) LAN
(C) WAN
(D) DICOM

50. The remote transmission of images is

(A) RAID
(B) DICOM
(C) PACS
(D) teleradiography

51. All the following statements, referencing the Hologic digital tomosynthesis unit, are true EXCEPT

(A) tomosynthesis does not use grid
(B) highest slice number is closest to the detector
(C) reconstruction is always in 1-mm-thick slices
(D) slices can be slabbed together to visualize calcifications

52. Disadvantages of the Hologic digital tomography system include

(A) it does not use a grid resulting in lower resolution images
(B) greater risks of motion due to the longer acquisition time
(C) the technology can be used to reduce the recall rate
(D) it can be used to remove overlapping tissue when imaging dense breast

53. Motion on images with the Hologic DBT unit are better appreciated on

(A) the projection images at the radiologist workstation
(B) the projection images at the technologist workstation
(C) the reconstruction images at the radiologist workstation
(D) the reconstruction images at the technologist workstation

54. The C-view imaging offered by Hologic is a

(A) 2D reconstruction of the 3D image
(B) 3D reconstruction of the 2D image
(C) 2D imaging with tomosynthesis
(D) 3D tomosynthesis imaging

55. CAD is used to

(A) visually enhance an image for viewing
(B) modify the contrast and brightness of an image
(C) analyze or preread the image
(D) provide accurate diagnostic information about the image

56. The results from one of the following techniques is often used to reduce the amount of lymph nodes removed during a check for breast cancer spread

    (A) sentinel node mapping
    (B) scintimammography
    (C) PEM
    (D) MRI

57. What technique is used to eliminate scatter in the photon-counting digital systems?

    (A) tomographic image reconstruction
    (B) 3D imaging
    (C) slit scanning and double collimation
    (D) computer-aided detection

Answers and Explanations

1. **(C)** Risk factors increase a woman's risk for breast cancer. These are divided into major and minor. Major risks are those outside of a woman's control, such as gender and age. Minor factors are linked to cancer-causing factors in the environment or may be related to personal choices, such as using HRT. Simply being a woman is the main risk factor for developing breast cancer. Breast cancer can affect men, but this disease is much more common among women than men.[1,2]

2. **(D)** A risk factor is anything that increases a person's chance of getting a disease. Major risk factors cannot be changed. Minor factors are linked to cancer-causing factors in the environment or may be related to personal choices, such as breast-feeding.[1,2]

3. **(A)** Higher than normal or major risk factors carry a significantly higher risk for breast cancer than minor risk factors. Breast cancer risk is higher among women whose close blood relatives have the disease. Blood relatives can be either from the mother's or father's side of the family.[1,2]

4. **(B)** A woman's risk of developing breast cancer increases with age. Older women have the greatest risk. At age 30 a woman has a 0.44% (or 1 in 227) chance of developing breast cancer. At age 40 the woman has a 47% (or 1 in 68) chance of developing breast cancer. At age 50 the change increases to 2.38% (or 1 in 42). At age 60 the change increases to 3.56% (or 1 in 28). At age 70 the chance is 3.82% (or 1 in 26).[1,2]

5. **(A)** Whereas skin thickening or tumors and lesions will be seen on a mammogram, nipple discharge is not seen mammographically. Although a nipple discharge can indicate a malignancy, most nipple discharges or secretions are not cancerous. In general, if the secretion appears clear or milky, yellow or green, cancer is very unlikely. Further testing using high-frequency ultrasound techniques or tests such as a ductogram or galactogram help in determining the cause of nipple discharge.[3,4]

6. **(D)** Unfortunately, breast cancer in its early states is symptomless. Early DCIS can show on the mammogram as clusters of microcalcifications. As the cancer grows, some symptoms may appear. These symptoms can include lumps in the breast, thickening of the breast skin, puckering or dimpling of the breast, inverted nipples, or a discharge from the nipples.[5,6]

7. **(D)** Skin thickening or lymphedema of the breast can indicate breast cancer, but may also be because of a breast abscess located behind the nipple, severe infection involving the axillary nodes, mediastinal blockage owing to advanced stage of sarcoidosis (an inflammatory disease). Malignant skin thickening can be cause by Hodgkin disease (cancer of the lymphocytes), lung cancer, bronchial cancer with mediastinal metastases, esophageal cancer with mediastinal metastases, right heart failure, advanced gynecologic malignancy, or postoperative or postradiation lymphedema.[5,6]

8. **(C)** There is no evidence at this time that magnetic resonance imaging (MRI) will be an effective screening tool for women at average risk for breast cancer. If MRI is used, it should be in addition to, not instead of a screening mammogram. Although MRI is more sensitive than mammograms, it

also has a higher false-positive rate, which would result in unnecessary biopsies, and it still misses some cancers that a mammogram would detect. The ACS recommends that women at high risk (> 20% lifetime risk) should get an MRI and a mammogram every year. Women at moderately increased risk (15%-20% lifetime risk) should talk with their doctors about the benefits and limitations of adding MRI screening to their yearly mammogram. Yearly MRI screening is not recommended for women whose lifetime risk of breast cancer is less than 15%. MRI, however, is useful for evaluating ruptures, leaks, free silicone in the surrounding breast tissue, or the formation of silicone granulomas. Also, the tumor margins and the extent of tumor spread are often better defined on the MRI than on mammography.

Recommendations for breast MRI

- Women with a lifetime risk greater than 20%.
- Women with BRCA1 or BRCA2 gene mutation or a first-degree relative (parent, brother, sister, or child) with a BRCA1 or BRCA2 gene mutation.
- Women who had radiation therapy to the chest between the ages of 10 and 30 years.
- Women with Li-Fraumeni syndrome, Cowden syndrome, or Bannayan-Riley-Ruvalcaba syndrome, or have first-degree relatives with one of these syndromes.[5,6]

9. **(C)** The guidelines as suggested by the ACS are
   - Women aged 40 and older should have a screening mammogram and CBE every year.
   - Women between ages 20 and 39 should have a CBE every 3 years.
   - Women aged 20 and older should perform a BSE every month.
   - All lumps or suspicious areas and any changes in the nipple or skin of the breast should be reported to a health-care provider.[1,2]

10. **(B)** Changes such as a lump or swelling, tenderness, skin irritation or dimpling, or nipple pain or retraction should be evaluated as soon as possible. In general, if the nipple discharge is clear or milky, yellow or green, a cancer is unlikely. If the discharge is red or red-brown, suggesting blood, it could be caused by either a malignant or a benign condition and should be evaluated.[1,2]

11. **(C)** A CBE is an examination of the breast by a health-care professional such as a physician, nurse practitioner, nurse, or physician assistant. Between ages 20 and 39, women should have a CBE every 3 years. After age 40, women should have a CBE every year.[1,2]

12. **(D)** A CBE is an examination of the breast by a health-care professional such as a radiologist, physician, nurse practitioner, nurse, or physician assistant. A similar examination, performed by the patient on herself, is referred to as the BSE.[1,2]

13. **(B)** A BSE should be done by the patient, 5-10 days after the start of the menstrual period, or when the breasts are not tender or swollen. For women not having regular menstruation, the BSE should be done on the same day every month.[1,2]

14. **(A)** The ACS recommends that the BSE should be performed monthly beginning at age 20. After age 40 the BSE should be 1 part of a 3-part program: BSE, CBE, and mammogram. BSE is useful before age 40 to help woman learn both the appearance and feel of their breast. After age 40 the BSE provides a safety net, detecting cancers that may not be seen on the mammogram.[1,2]

15. **(A)** For BSE, the first step is to look for changes, either while standing or sitting. A check should be made for indentations, retracted nipples, dimpling, or prolonged skin conditions such as eczema. Other visual changes can include the development of unequal breasts; changes in texture, color, or contour; redness or scaliness. Moles and scars should also be noted and recorded. The next step is feeling for changes. While feeling for changes, the woman should examine her breast in both the upright and the supine

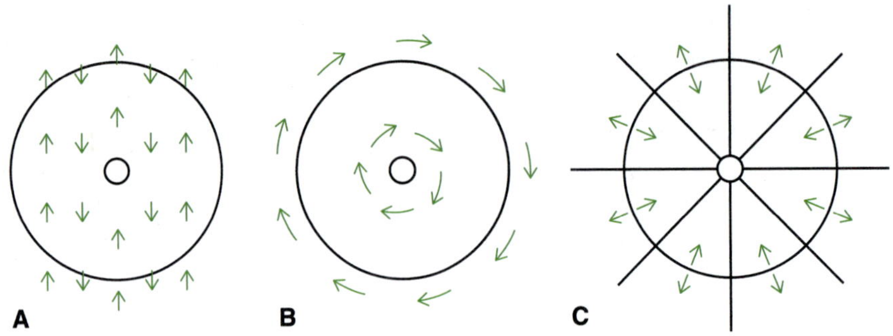

Figure 1-1. Using the pads of finger, the breast must be checked with firm pressure for deep lesion, medium pressure of intermediate depth lesions, and light pressure for lesions below the skin surface. Patterns that can be used (A) up-and-down pattern, (B) circular pattern, or (C) wedge pattern. (Reproduced with permission from Peart O: Mammography and Breast Imaging PREP: Program Review and Exam Prep. New York, NY: McGraw-Hill Education; 2012.)

positions by using the pads of 3 or more fingers to apply varying degrees of pressure—firm pressure to assess deep lesions, medium pressure for intermediate depth lesions, and light pressure to assess lesions below the skin surface. The entire breast must be checked. In any examination, lotion or powder can be used to help the fingers glide across the breast. Some women also prefer to examine their breasts in the shower where wet fingers will glide easily over the breast (Figure 1-1).[1,2]

16. **(D)** The visual stage of a BSE is a check for signs of breast cancer. These signs can include changes in size, texture, or color of the breast; prolonged skin irritation; redness or scaliness; dimpling; or nipple retraction.[1,2]

17. **(C)** The first step in evaluating a woman with suspected breast cancer is a complete medical history and physical or clinical examination. The medical history will provide information about the patient's symptoms and any other health problems and risk factors for benign or malignant breast conditions. A clinical examination will be done to locate any lump or suspicious areas and examine the texture, size, and shape of the breast. Any changes in the nipples or skin of the breast will also be noted. Once the medical and clinical examinations are completed, biopsies or imaging tests such as mammography can be performed.[1,2]

18. **(D)** Some studies have called for an end to routine BSE for women age 40-69. The theory is that BSE and BSE education do not reduce deaths, and will increase unnecessary biopsies and anxiety. However, although the BSE and the CBE cannot detect all malignant breast conditions, they are primarily important as complimentary tests. The ACS suggests that both the BSE and CBE will complement the mammogram and help in the detection of breast cancers. Unfortunately, the mammogram is not foolproof. Even under ideal conditions, the mammogram will not find all breast cancers 100% of the time.[1,2]

19. **(D)** The ACS suggests examining the breast with 3 different levels of pressure: light pressure to feel the tissues closest to the skin; medium pressure to feel a little deeper; and firm pressure to feel the tissue closest to the chest and ribs. The up and down pattern (sometimes called the vertical pattern) is the most effective pattern for covering the entire breast without missing any breast tissue, and the pads of the 3 middle fingers (not the fingertips) are most sensitive to palpate for abnormalities. The patient should use small dime-sized circular motions to examine the entire breast.[1,2]

20. **(D)** The patient should perform a BSE 5-10 days after the start of menstrual period, or when the breasts are not tender or swollen.[1,2]

21. **(C)** Breast cancer is the second most common cancer in women in the United States. The most common is certain types of skin cancer. Breast cancer is also the second most common cause of death from cancer among

women. Lung cancer is the leading cause of cancer death in women in the United States. In 2013, approximately 39,620 women were expected to die from breast cancer. Breast cancer incidence and death rates generally increase with age. The death rates from breast cancer have been decreasing since 1989—with larger decreases in women younger than 50 years. Seventy-nine percent of new cases and 88% of breast cancer deaths occurred in women aged 50 years and older. The decrease in the incidence of breast cancer is thought to be related to the reduced use of hormone replacement therapy (HRT) after the published study by the Women's Health Initiative in 2002 which linked HRT with breast cancer risks. The decrease in breast cancer death is thought to be the result of advanced treatment options, earlier detection, and increased awareness.[1,2]

22. **(C)** Circulating estrogen is mostly produced in fatty tissue, therefore in postmenopausal women, having more fatty tissue can lead to increased estrogen levels. Weight gain is therefore associated with increased estrogen levels and increased likelihood of developing breast cancer.[1,2]

23. **(A)** With modern mammography equipment, the patient will usually receive only about 1-2 mGy (0.1-0.2 rads) per projection. The ACR recommends that the average glandular dose on the mammogram be no greater than 3 mGy (0.3 rads or 300 mrad) with a grid or 1 mGy (0.1 rad or 100 mrad) without a grid.[7]

24. **(A)** Although breast tissue composition is affected by menarche, hormonal fluctuation—both normal and synthetic, pregnancy, lactation, menopause, and weight gain or loss, in general the breasts of young women are denser than those of older women. Younger breasts will therefore require more radiation to penetrate and will absorb more radiation than those of older women. Fortunately, the incidence of breast cancer in this age group is very low.[1,2]

25. **(D)** A stage 0 carcinoma refers to carcinoma in situ, cancer that is still contained within the duct or lobule. The prognosis for this type of cancer is 100% survival after 5 years. Five-year survival rate refers to the percent of patients who live at least 5 years after their cancer is diagnosed. Many of these patients live much longer than 5 years after diagnosis, but 5-year rates are used to produce a standard way of discussing prognosis. Five-year rates will exclude from the calculations patients dying of other diseases and is considered to be a more accurate way to describe the prognosis for patients with a particular type and stage of cancer (Table 1-1).[1,2]

Table 1-1. **BREAST CANCER SURVIVAL BY STAGE**

Stage and Grouping		5-Year Relative Survival Rate
O	Carcinoma in situ	**100%**
IA	Tumor ≤ 2 cm; axillary node negative	**100%***
IB	Tumor ≤ 2 cm; axillary node negative with cancer cell in lymph node ≤ 2 cm	
IIA	Tumor 2-5 cm with 1-3 positive nodes or tumor > 5 cm without positive lymph nodes	**93%***
IIB	Tumor 2-5 cm with positive nodes 0.2-2 mm	
IIIA	Tumor > 5 cm or no tumor with 1-3 positive nodes or any size tumor with 4-9 positive nodes	**72%***
IIIB	Any size tumor with cancer spread to chest wall and/or skin of breast and up to 9 lymph nodes	
IIIC	Any size tumor with cancer spread to chest wall and/or skin of breast and up to 10 axillary or clavicular lymph nodes	
IV	Cancer has spread to other organs, i.e., there is distant metastasis (e.g., to bone, lungs)	**22%**

*Survival rates for the subgroups are close to the rate for the overall stage. For example, rate for stage IA is closer to the given rate while IB is slightly lower.

26. **(D)** The major factors affecting dose are

- *The imaging chain*—the imaging conditions including type of mammography unit.
- *The x-ray beam energy*—the higher the kVp and HVL, the lower the patient dose.

- *The compression*—greater compression will result in decreased exposure and therefore decreased dose.
- *The patient's breast* tissue type (composition) and thickness—denser glandular breast requires more exposure than fatter breast.[2]

27. **(D)** Studies have shown that if a patient plays an active role in applying the compression that patient will be able to tolerate the compression better and will be more relaxed during the compression. The more the patient knows about compression and understands the procedure, the more she will be relaxed. To give the patient an active role in compression, the mammographer can allow the patient to apply the compression or constantly monitor the patient, stopping the compression when the patient indicates. If the sensitivity is extreme and/or hormone related, the mammogram could be rescheduled.[8]

28. **(C)** The ACS now recommends contrast-enhanced MRI in conjunction with a mammogram for women with approximately 20%-25% or greater lifetime risk of breast cancer. The technology is not however recommended as a screening tool because of the high cost and the modality's lack of specificity, which often results in a high false-positive rate of biopsies. Also, there is not enough evidence to support MRI screening for women with a lifetime risk of 15%-20% according to risk assessment tools that are based mainly on family history.

    Recommendations for breast MRI

    - Women with a lifetime risk greater than 20%
    - Women with BRCA1 or BRCA2 gene mutation or a first-degree relative (parent, brother, sister, or child) with a BRCA1 or BRCA2 gene mutation
    - Women who had radiation therapy to the chest between the ages of 10 and 30 years
    - Women with Li-Fraumeni syndrome, Cowden syndrome, or Bannayan-Riley-Ruvalcaba syndrome, or have first-degree relatives with one of these syndromes.[9]

29. **(C)** MRI technology uses a powerful magnetic field, radio waves, and a computer to produce highly detailed images of the breast. The technology is based on the magnetic properties of hydrogen atoms in the body. MRI technology is extremely sensitive and is now recommended as an adjunctive screening tool for high-risk women. Ultrasound uses high-frequency sound waves to image the breast and mammography uses x-radiation to image the breast[9,10] (Figure 1-2).

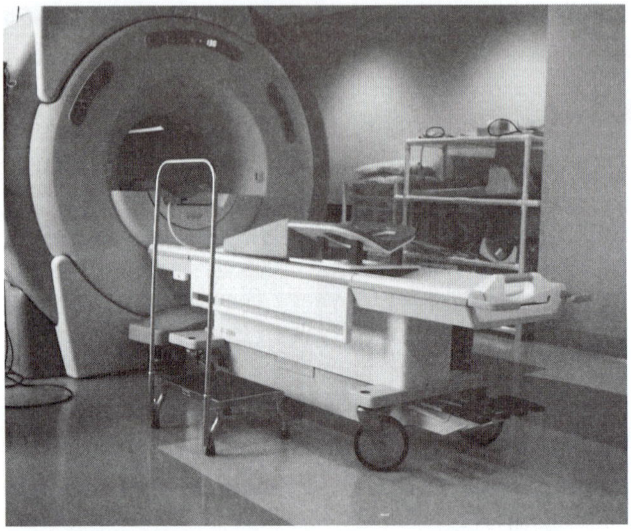

Figure 1-2. MRI unit with MRI breast coils. (Reproduced with permission from Peart O: Mammography and Breast Imaging PREP: Program Review and Exam Prep. New York, NY: McGraw-Hill Education; 2012.)

30. **(A)** Sound is a mechanical, longitudinal wave that needs a medium to travel. Breast imaging with ultrasound uses high frequencies, sometimes above 20,000 Hz, which are beyond human hearing. Microwaves are electromagnetic waves with a short radio frequency[9,10] (Figure 1-3).

31. **(D)** MRI is an imaging test that uses strong magnets and radio waves to create very detailed breast images. Because of its sensitivity, it can find tumors even in very dense breasts, and can find very small tumors. It can be used to stage cancers, map the extent of the tumor, evaluate the effectiveness of chemotherapy, and distinguish postoperative or postradiation scarring from recurrent cancer. MRI can also be used to image implants for leakage or ruptures.[9,10]

32. **(B)** Ultrasound is an adjunctive modality and is useful in determining whether the

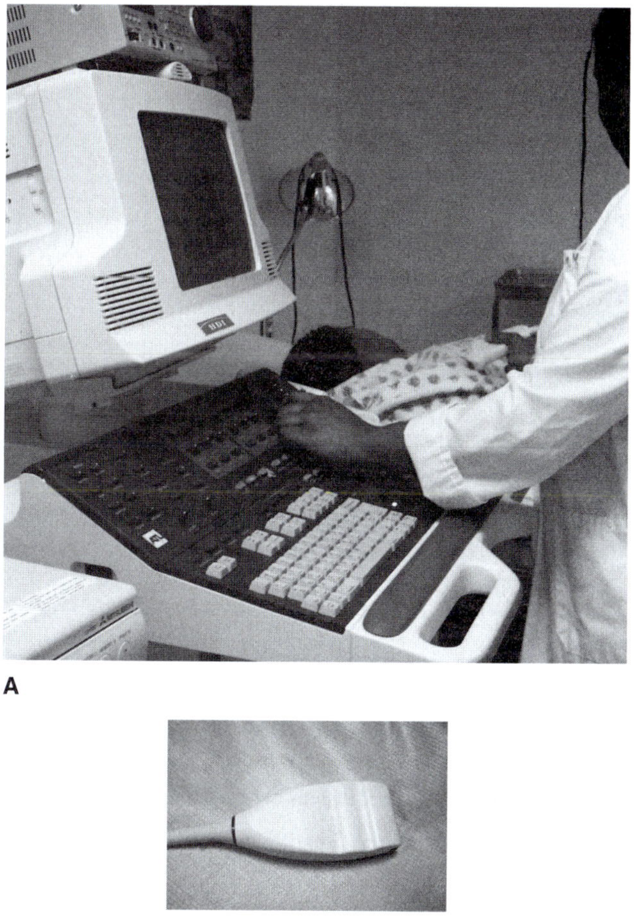

A

B

Figure 1-3. (A) Ultrasound unit. (B) Ultrasound transducer.

mass seen on the mammogram is solid versus cystic (malignant vs. benign). Ultrasound is close to 100% accurate in diagnosing cysts (fluid-filled lesions), but the technology does not image calcifications well. Although ultrasound can be used to image dense breast tissue and to detect cancers missed on the mammogram, the technology is not sensitive enough to map the extent of a tumor. Lesions must be biopsied in the modality in which they are visualized; therefore a lesion seen *only* on MRI can only be biopsied using MR technology.[9,10]

33. **(A)** Objective data are signs that can be seen, heard, or felt and such things as laboratory reports. Subjective data includes things that are perceived by the affected individual only, e.g., pain. Both objective and subjective data are equally important and the mammographer should never disregard anything the patient says, even if it does not fit with standard opinions or the patient's symptoms.[11]

34. **(B)** The best approach to clinical history documentation is to start with open-ended questions. This avoids leading the patient and inserting your opinions or views. Example of a leading question: "Is the pain in your right breast?" Example of a nonleading question: "Where is the pain?" Also listening rather than asking questions will allow the patient to tell you their stories unasked. From listening you can assess the patient's life experience and educational background. This will determine whether you can use medical or technical terms or overly simplified words for future questions[11] (Figure 1-4).

35. **(C)** Repeating or rewording the question will help to clarify the information and verify that the patient has not changed his/her mind. Open-ended questions are used at the start of the medical history documentation to avoid leading the patient. Leading questions should never be used at the start of any assessment because its use can insert a personal bias into the patient's answers. Facilitation can encourage elaboration.[11]

36. **(A)** Probing questions are used to get more detail. Listening rather than asking questions will allow the patient time to tell you their stories unasked. Silence will also give the patient time to remember. Repetition of rewording or summarization of the question can be used to review the information and verify accuracy.[11]

37. **(C)** "A" and "B" are good open-ended questions that can be used to start the clinical history documentation. This avoids leading the patient and inserting your opinions or views. "C" is a probing question that could be used to get more details.[11]

38. **(A)** Objective data are signs that can be seen, heard, or felt and such things as reports or visible injuries. Subjective data includes

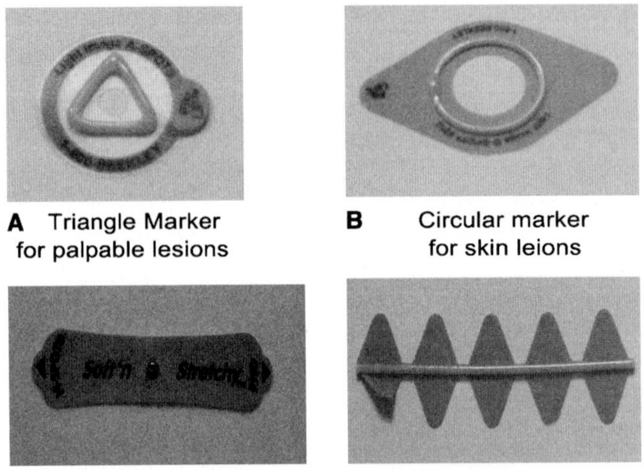

A Triangle Marker for palpable lesions

B Circular marker for skin leions

C 'BB' marker pinpoints the nipple

D Scar marker for surgical sites

Figure 1-4. Radiopaque markers can be used to locate areas of interest on the mammogram A, B, C, D are some of the markers used.

things that are perceived by the affected individual only, e.g., pain. Both objective and subjective data are equally important and the mammographer should never disregard anything the patient says, even if it does not fit with standard opinions or the patient's symptoms. Open-ended questions are questions that can be used to start the clinical history documentation. This avoids leading the patient and inserting your opinions or views. A probing question is used to get more details.[11]

39. **(C)** Repetition of rewording or summarization of the question can be used to review the information and verify accuracy or clarify the information. In repeating information always use precise and clear words because words do not always mean the same thing to patients as they do to the mammographer, e.g., lumpectomy for a patient can refer to the removal of any lump from the breast yet the medical meaning is the removal of a cancerous lump. Probing questions are used to get more detail. Listening rather than asking questions will allow the patient time to tell you their stories unasked. Silence will also give the patient time to remember.[11]

40. **(D)** This is an open-ended question that can be used to start the clinical history documentation. This avoids leading the patient and inserting your opinions or views. A probing question is used to get more details. Repetition of, rewording or summarization of the question can be used to review the information and verify accuracy or clarify the information.[11]

41. **(B)** Pregnancy is thought to have a protective effect against breast cancer and the longer a woman goes without getting pregnant, the greater the risks. An early pregnancy is therefore beneficial. Starting menstruation early (before age 12) is considered an increased risk because it increases the amount of menstrual cycles in a woman's lifetime. Treatment for Hodgkin lymphoma can often require radiation to the chest area which can result in increased breast cancer risks in later years. DES was used to prevent miscarriages during the period 1940-1971. Women who took DES and children whose mothers took DES have an increased risk for breast cancer.[2]

42. **(C)** An informed consent is required for any invasive procedure which involves risks. Although the risks are minor, a fine-needle biopsy (FNB) is considered an invasive procedure because the skin is penetrated by a needle and cell samples removed. The mammogram, ultrasound and MRI are not considered invasive. The term ***informed consent*** implies that the patient has been informed of the procedures or operation to be performed, of the risks involved, of the possible consequences and any alternative options. By signing the consent form, the patient or the patient's representative indicates that he or she has been informed of and consents to the procedure or treatment.[12]

43. (B) Consents can be written or oral. Written consents offers some tangible proof, but is subject to scrutiny and disbelief if other facts relevant to the situation indicate the patient did not fully understand what affixing of his/her signature meant in relation to his/her medical care. Oral consent is verbal. It is binding but difficult to prove. Expressed consent can be nonverbal, such as nodding or lifting the arm when told that an injection is required, or oral. Implied consent is usually assumed in an emergency situation where the patient is unable to make a decision.[12]

44. (B) An informed consent is required for any invasive procedure which involves risks. Not all procedures in the imaging department are considered invasive. The term *informed consent* implies that the patient has been informed of the procedures or operation to be performed, of the risks involved, of the possible consequences and any alternative options. By signing the consent form, the patient or the patient's representative indicates that he or she has been informed of and consents to the procedure or treatment.[12]

45. (A) Oral consent is verbal. It is binding but difficult to prove. Written or printed consents offers some tangible proof, but is subject to scrutiny and disbelief if other facts relevant to the situation indicate the patient did not fully understand what affixing of his signature meant in relation to his medical care, e.g., a Russian speaking patient signing a consent form written in English. Implied consent is usually assumed in an emergency situation where the patient is unable to make a decision.[12]

46. (C) Although height and weight are needed for some examinations this type of data is not considered essential information. Any consent must include the patient demographic information, name, date of birth or other identifier, and the current date. The consent should also include an authorization clause allowing the physician to perform the examination; a disclosure clause to explain the procedure, its risks and benefits and possible alternative to the procedure; an anesthesia clause if required; a no-guarantee clause for therapeutic procedures; a tissue disposal clause if removal of tissue may be necessary; a patient understanding clause—stating that the patient has received an explanation and understands the explanation; a signature clause—including the signature of patient. An informed consent must be explained by a qualified clinician, such as a physician, but can be witnessed by a technologist.[12]

47. (D) The radiologist's monitor at the review workstation (RWS) is a high-resolution monitor and the only monitor approved for breast interpretation. The monitor resolution can be written as the width and height of the image or as the total number of pixels in the image. For example a monitor that is 2560 pixels wide and 2048 pixels high (2560 x 2048) contains (multiply) 5,242,880 pixels (or is a 5 megapixel monitor). Most digital monitors are liquid crystal display (LCD). Typically the technologist's monitor at the acquisition workstation monitor (AWS) has lower resolution and is therefore not recommended for use when interpreting the images (Figure 1-5).[8]

48. (B) Redundant array of independent (inexpensive) disk (RAID) uses several hard drives and are connected with the data stored on multiple devices which serve as a backup if 1 drive fails. RAID can store 6-12 months of patient data and can transfer image files to the monitor in 2 minutes. Digital linear tape (DLT) is not recommended for high capacity storage. The can wear out with heavy use. Jukebox storage is used as a long-term storage option. The jukebox holds image data in digital tapes, disks or other

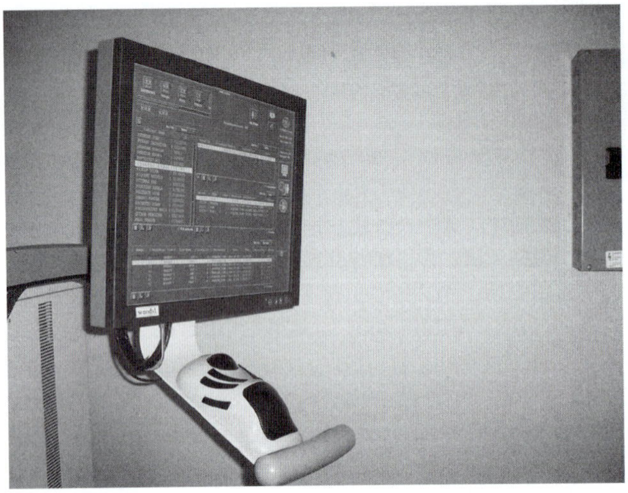

A

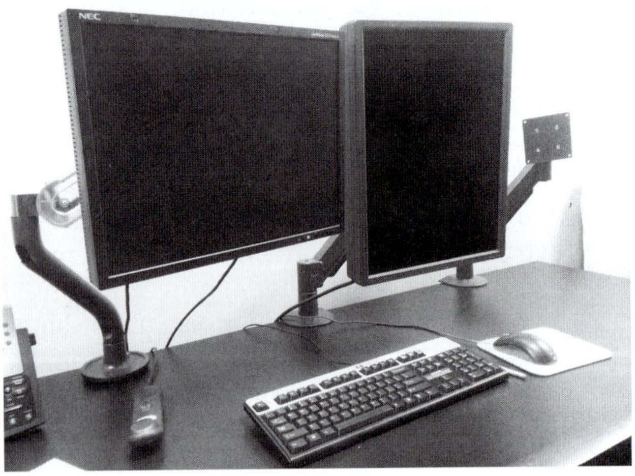

B

Figure 1-5. (A) Low-resolution technologist monitor, (B) high-resolution LCD monitor used for image interpretation.

media, and typically has a retrieval time of 2-5 minutes. Optical Disk or magneto-optical disk (MOD) is similar to a compact disk (CD) or digital versatile disk (DVD). They are more reliable and robust and are faster than jukebox storage but are not intended as a high capacity storage option.[13]

49. **(A)** PACS (picture archiving and communication system) is a system that allows images from multiple modalities to be viewed at a single location, or sent from multiple modalities to remote locations across the nation or even across the world. Images can be sent over the Internet, over the telephone, via satellite communication or from a cable modem. All equipment used in a PACS system must be DICOM-compliant (Digital Imaging and Communications in Medicine). The PACS system can include, reading station with processing capabilities (e.g., radiologists can reconstruct tomosynthesis image or stitch images), physician review stations, web access, technologist quality control station, administrative stations, an archive system and an interface to various hospital and radiology systems. DICOM is a set of computer software standards that permit a wide range of digital imaging programs to understand each other. LAN is local area network limited to a small geographical area (e.g., can be interhospital). WAN is a wide area network that covers a large geographical area.[13]

50. **(D)** Teleradiography is the remote transmission and viewing of images. Transmission can be Internet, cable, or telephone based. Images are compressed before transmission. There is *lossy* and *lossless* compression. Lossy is acceptable in general radiography but not acceptable for mammography. The interface format of transmission is called Digital Imaging and Communications in Medicine or DICOM. DICOM is a set of computer software standards that permit a wide range of digital imaging programs to understand each other. RAID uses several connected hard drives to store digital data. PACS is a computer network that allows images from multiply modalities to be viewed at a single location at various monitors, transmitted or stored.[13]

51. **(B)** Digital breast tomosynthesis (DBT) uses high-resolution cross-section 3-dimensional imaging to eliminate tissue overlap. In the Hologic DBT unit, the x-ray tube rotates in an arc around the breast taking 15 exposures in 4 seconds, and sweeping from –7 to 0 to +7 degrees with no movement of the patient. Features of the Hologic tomosynthesis unit (Figure 1-6):

- A typical tomosynthesis unit can image in 2D, 3D, or a combination of 2D and 3D (COMBO).

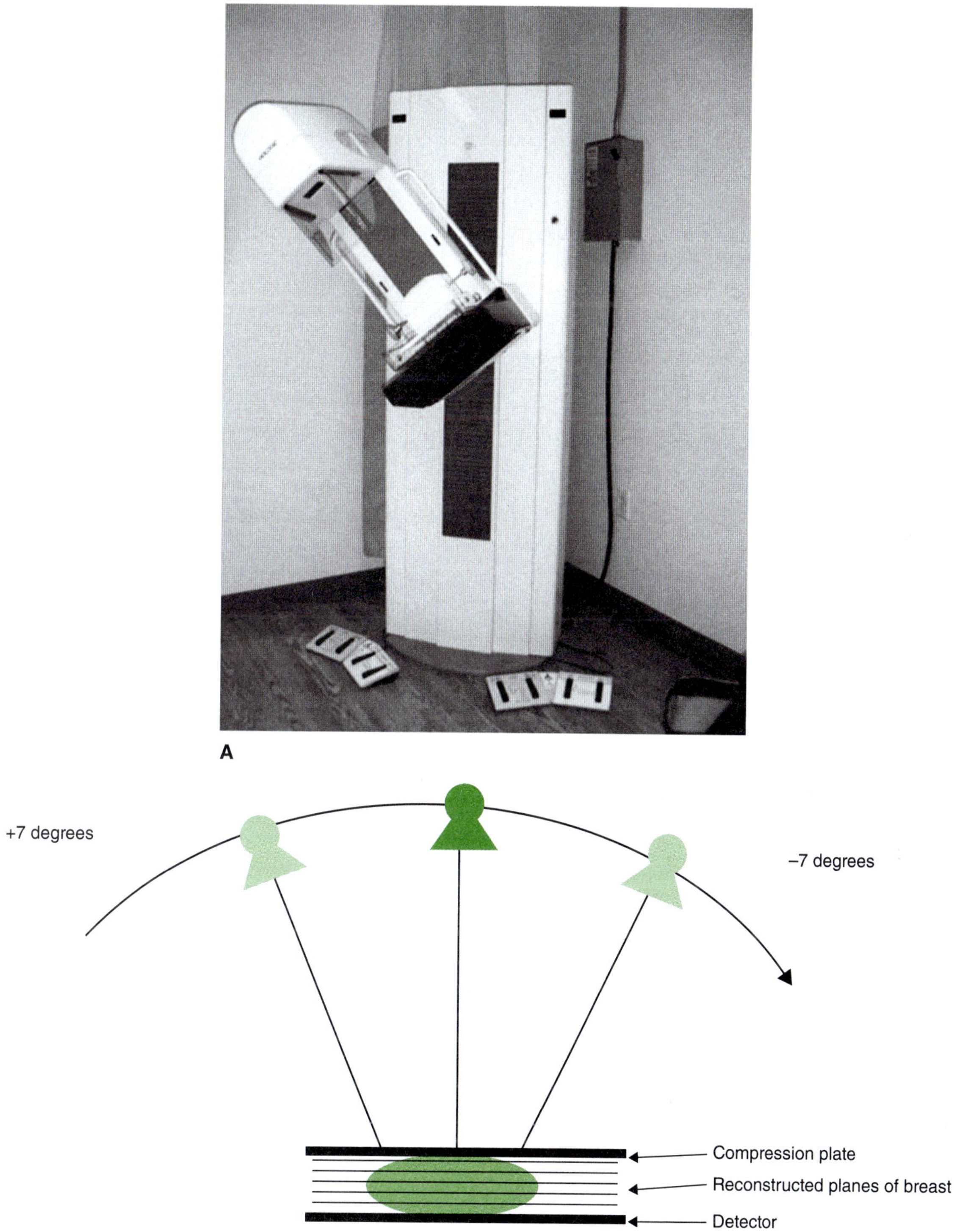

Figure 1-6. (A) Hologic digital breast tomosynthesis (DBT) unit, (B) Tomo travel on DBT.

- Tomosynthesis does not use grid.
- The number of reconstruction images based on the breast thickness in millimeters.
- Slice number 1 is closest to the detector.
- Highest slice number is closest to compression paddle.
- Reconstruction is always in 1-mm-thick slices.

  - A breast 4-cm-thick equals 40 mm therefore 40 + 6 slices = 46 slices
  - A breast 5-cm-thick equals 50 mm, therefore 50 + 6 slices = 56 slices
- Slices can be slabbed together to visualize calcifications.[14]

52. **(B)** Although the system does not use a grid the tomography feature allows high contrast, high-resolution imaging.

    Advantages of the DBT unit by Hologic include:

    - Detection and screening, especially women with dense breasts
    - Diagnostic work-up or problem solving
    - Possible reduction in the recall rate

    Disadvantages of the system can include:

    - Long total exposure time of 12 seconds for COMBO
    - Motion artifacts that can be hard to detect at radiologist workstation
      - Motion is easier appreciated at the AWS where the mammographer can view the projection dataset of images.
      - Motion is harder to appreciate on the reconstruction images at the radiologist workstation.
    - Large number of images
    - Degraded imaging of calcifications
    - Higher radiation dose when imaging implants in 3D because a lower kVp is used[13,14]

53. **(B)** Motion can occur at 1 point, multiple points, or throughout the duration of the entire imaging series. Motion can affect the sharpness of image detail. In the Hologic system motion is best visualized on the projection dataset of images at the AWS. It is seen as anterior/posterior movement of the breast tissue or structures in the breast. On the Hologic system, the mammographer must review the projection dataset in the cine mode to check for motion before submitting the imaging. Medial to lateral movement of breast tissue and structures is normal and does not indicate motion. Motion is much harder to detect on reconstruction images at the RWS because the reconstructed image incorporates the motion. Projection images are not available at the RWS and reconstruction images are not available at the AWS.[13,14]

54. **(A)** C-view offers a reconstructed 2D image of the breast without the additional radiation. After 3D imaging, the computer will reconstruct the tomosynthesis slices and create a synthesized 2D image (Figure 1-7).[14]

55. **(C)** CAD combines digital technology with computers to preread the mammograms. The computer will then display suspicious areas, in effect acting as a second reader. CAD works by first mapping the breast for a normal reference. The normal mapping is stored and all images are compared and analyzed based on the normal mapping. Microcalcifications and abnormalities are enhanced while normal structures are de-emphasized. CAD technology works with both digital mammography and analog imaging. CAD is also available for breast ultrasound and breast MR.[2]

56. **(A)** Lymphoscintigraphy or sentinel node mapping injects the radioactive isotope directly into the subareola lymphatic plexus of the affected area. The isotope travels to the lymph nodes in the axilla and the sentinel node can be identified and removed. This process of lymphatic mapping can eliminate most of the pain and discomfort of breast surgery for a majority of women with early breast cancer. Lymph node removal causes various side effects including extreme swelling of the arm and hand (lymphedema). By identifying the sentinel node, patients are spared an extensive node dissection surgery with its resultant side effects. PEM and scintimammography injects the radioactive isotope in the arm vein and uses a gamma camera to image the uptake in the breast. MRI images the breast based on the magnetic properties of elements.[6,10]

57. **(C)** Grids are not used with magnification mammography, Hologic 3D tomosynthesis—a flat-panel detector system—and photon-counting systems. In the photon-counting system x-rays leaving the tube passes through

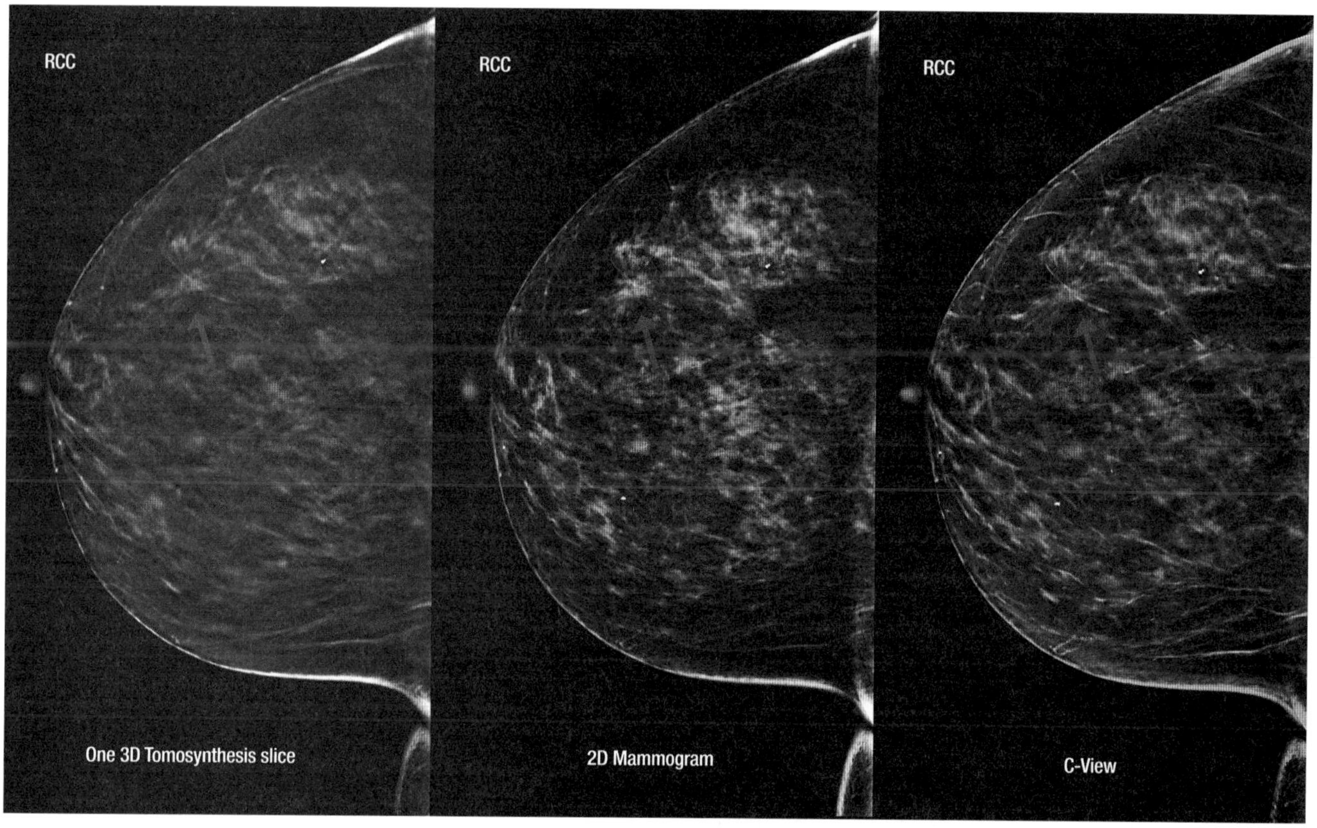

Figure 1-7. (A) A digital mammogram, (B) digital breast tomosynthesis, (C) C-view from the hologic tomosynthesis unit. (Used with permission of Hologic.)

a slot collimator before entering the breast. After leaving the breast, the beam again passes through a slot collimator before the individual rays are collected by the detector. The overall effect of the double collimation is a 97% reduction in scatter. By virtually eliminating scatter, a grid is not necessary, allowing a further reduction in patient dose. In the Hologic digital tomosynthesis system, the image contrast is provided by the tomographic image reconstruction processes. Magnification mammography utilizes the air gap which effectively removes scatter. Computer-aided detection is the use of computers to preread the mammograms, by scanning every part of the radiograph and reporting any suspicious area. The computer will display or analyze suspicious areas to make the interpretation consistent from patient to patient (Figure 1-8).[2,15,16]

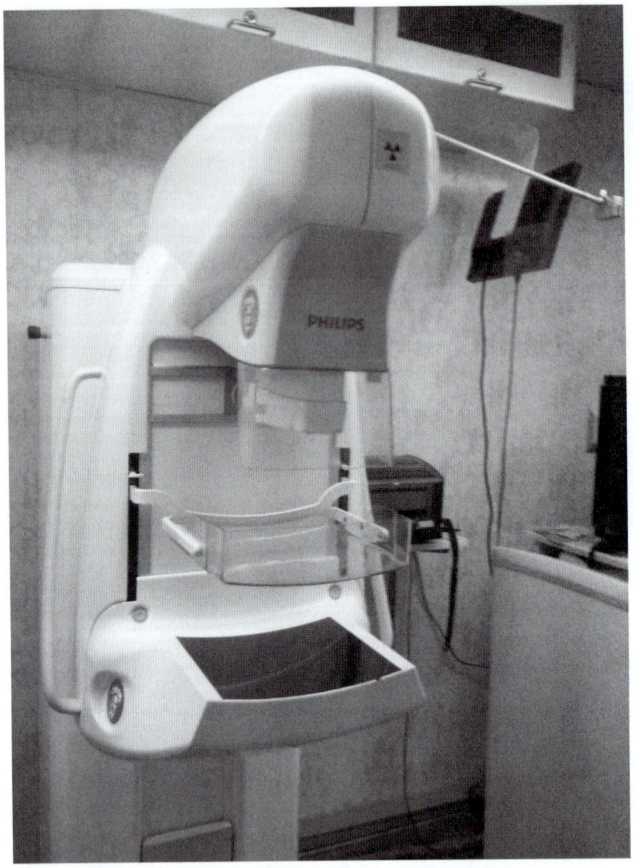

Figure 1-8. Photon-counting Microdose mammography system.

References

1. American Cancer Society: Causes, Risk Factors and Prevention. What are the risk factors for breast cancer? http://www.cancer.org/cancer/breastcancer/detailedguide/breast-cancer-risk-factors. Last Medical Review: 01/14/2014. Accessed March 14, 2014.
2. Peart O. Patient education and assessment. In: *Mammography and Breast Imaging: Prep*. New York, NY: McGraw-Hill; 2012:23-61.
3. American Cancer Society: Non-Cancerous Breast Conditions. http://www.cancer.org/healthy/findcancerearly/womenshealth/non-cancerousbreastconditions/index. Last Review: 01/14/2014. Accessed March 14, 2014.
4. Tabár L, Dean PB. Skin thickening syndrome of the breast. In: *Teaching Atlas of Mammography*. 4th ed. New York, NY: Thieme; 2011:239-247.
5. Peart O. Physiology and pathology of the breast. In: *Mammography and Breast Imaging: Prep*. New York, NY: McGraw-Hill; 2012:65-85.
6. American Cancer Society: Early Detection, Diagnosis, and Staging. Can breast cancer be found early? http://www.cancer.org/cancer/breastcancer/detailedguide/breast-cancer-detection. Last Review: 01/31/2014. Accessed March 14, 2014.
7. American College of Radiology (ACR). Mammography Accreditation Program Requirements. http://www.acr.org/Quality-Safety/Accreditation/Mammography. http://www.cancer.org/healthy/findcancerearly/cancerscreeningguidelines/american-cancer-society-guidelines-for-the-early-detection-of-cancer. Last Reviewed: 01/15/14. Accessed March 24, 2014.
8. Peart O. Breast imaging mammography. In: *Mammography and Breast Imaging: Prep*. New York, NY: McGraw-Hill; 2012:213-262.
9. American Cancer Society: Early Detection, Diagnosis, and Staging. Can breast cancer be found early? http://www.cancer.org/cancer/breastcancer/detailedguide/breast-cancer-detection. Last Review: 01/31/2014. Accessed March 14, 2014.
10. Peart O. Breast imaging emerging modalities. In: *Mammography and Breast Imaging: Prep*. New York, NY: McGraw-Hill; 2012:333-396.
11. Adler A, Carlton R. History taking. In: *Introduction to Radiologic Science and Patient Care*. 5th ed. St. Louis, MO: Elsevier Saunders; 2012:141-145.
12. Adler A, Carlton R. Health records and health information management. In: Galocy LC, Skurka MA, eds. *Introduction to Radiologic Science and Patient Care*. 5th ed. St. Louis, MO: Elsevier Saunders; 2012:317-328.
13. Bushong SC. The digital radiographic image. In: *Radiologic Science for Technologists—Physics, Biology and Protection*. 10th ed. St. Louis, MO: Mosby; 2004:265-332.
14. Hologic Inc. Selenia Dimensions with acquisition workstation 8000. Product and Clinical Education Training manuals. Courtesy of Hologic Inc. www.hologic.com. Accessed December 2013.
15. Weigel S, Berkemeyer S, Girnus R, et al. Digital mammography screening with photon-counting technique: can a high diagnostic performance be realized at low mean glandular dose? In: *Radiology* 2014; 271:345-355.
16. Schmitzberger FF, Fallenberg EM, Lawaczeck R, et al. Development of low-dose photon-counting contrast-enhanced tomosynthesis with spectral imaging. In: *Radiology* 2011; 259:259-564.

CHAPTER 2

Instrumentation and Quality Assurance

Summary of Important Points

DESIGN CHARACTERISTICS OF MAMMOGRAPHY UNITS

All mammography units are designed to image the soft tissue of the breast while displaying the necessary subtle contrast differences. All modern generators are high-frequency generators. Like the older units, these rectify the input to produce a direct current (DC) voltage waveform, but the modern high-frequency generators essentially provide a constant potential with about 1% ripple. The high frequency allows more efficient x-ray production and therefore produces a higher effective energy x-ray beam. The result is higher x-ray output for a given peak kilovoltage (kVp) and milliamperes (mA) setting.

Dedicated Mammography Unit

The breast consists of all soft tissue structure with very similar mass densities and atomic numbers. Because of the similarity in tissue, general radiography tubes cannot be used to image the breast tissue. In order to maximize the contrast at the highest possible resolution yet keeping radiation doses low, the general radiography systems had to be modified for mammography imaging.

Target Materials in Analog and Digital Mammography Units

- Breast tissue consists mostly of adipose, fibrous, and glandular tissue which all have relatively low atomic number. The energy of the x-ray produced must be just high enough to penetrate the tissue without overpenetration. The x-ray range found most useful in maximizing contrast in breast tissue is in the 17-24 keV range.
- Molybdenum targets produce characteristic x-rays in the 17-19 keV range after a photoelectric interaction. These are ideal when imaging fatty breast.
- The characteristic x-ray produced using rhodium targets are similar to that from molybdenum, but because rhodium has a slightly higher atomic number, more Bremsstrahlung x-rays are produced and the K-characteristic x-rays will be in the 20-23 keV range, which provides a better penetration of dense breast.
- With tungsten targets, Bremsstrahlung x-rays will predominate at energies above and below the 17-24 keV range. Although tungsten emits "harder" spectrum rays, the wider dynamic range can be utilized in digital imaging.

Common Target Material—Analog Units

- Molybdenum
- Rhodium

Common Target Material—Digital Units

- Rhodium
- Tungsten
  - Some digital systems have a single anode target made of tungsten.
  - Single track tubes can sometimes be more reliable and less expensive to manufacture.
  - Single track x-ray tubes can support a higher anode heat loading therefore allowing for shorter exposure times when compared to dual track x-ray tubes. This is especially useful when imaging large breasts.
  - Single track tungsten tubes can support 2-3 times the maximum anode load when compared to dual track tubes.

Beam Filtration

- Filtration is defined by the half-value layer (HVL). In mammography added filtration shapes the emission spectrums of the x-ray beam and makes it compatible with the image receptor and breast characteristics of each patient.
- Filtration will also improve the energy-distribution x-ray spectrum by selectively removing the very low energies that will be absorbed in the superficial layers of the skin and contribute to skin dose. Also, filtration will remove the higher energies outside of the desired range. With proper filtration, the x-ray beam entering the breast will have very few photons above or below the preferred mammographic energy range.
- In digital imaging, filtration will also help to reduce exposure time, eliminating potential motion artifacts.
- Minimum HVL is specified by regulations and should not measure less than 0.30 mm Al at 30 kVp or 0.25 mm at 25 kVp to ensure that the patient will not receive excessive radiation dose. The HVL also should not exceed 0.40 mm Al at 30 kVp to avoid excessive filtration that would reduce contrast by filtering out the low-energy photons necessary to penetrate the breast tissue.
- Any HVL assessment must include an assessment of both the *inherent* and *added* filtration.

Inherent or Added Filtration

As the x-ray beam leaves the target of the anode, it is filtered in 2 ways.

- Inherent filtration includes the glass or metal window of the x-ray tube, oil in the tube housing, the mirror of the collimation assembly and the compression paddle.
- Added filtration is usually an aluminum (Al) equivalent material, positioned in the path of the emerging beam thus affecting its penetrating power which is defined by HVL.

Compression Plate

The compression plate is made of a radiolucent material that will not attenuate the low photons necessary for breast imaging. The Mammography Quality Standard Act (MQSA) has specific standards regulating the shape of the compression device and semiannual tests are required to ensure that the compression device is working properly. MQSA standards:

- Minimum automatic compression should not be less than 25 lbs (111 N).
- Automatic compression should never exceed 45 lbs (200 N) on the initial power drive.
- All units should have a manual, hand-controlled compression device, controlled by the mammographer.

Material of the Exit Port

Beryllium (Be) is most often used because a regular glass or metallic window would harden the emerging beam by eliminating the low photons needed for breast imaging.

Common Target/Filtration Combinations

- In analog units, the filters used are often the same element as the x-ray tube target. Matching the filter to the same element as the x-ray tube target will allow the K-characteristic x-rays to pass while blocking the higher and lower energy Bremsstrahlung x-rays. Therefore with molybdenum and rhodium targets, the filtration is generally the same element.
- If the tube target is tungsten, rhodium (Rh) can be used for fatty breast and silver (Ag) for large or dense breast.
- Some tungsten targets use molybdenum (Mo) for fatty breast and rhodium (Rh) for dense breast.
- Aluminum (Al) is used as the filtration in the Hologic digital tomosynthesis units and low dose photon-counting imaging systems.

The Line-Focus Principle

- The focal spot is the area that electrons strike on the target.
- As the size of the focal spot decreases, the heating of the target is concentrated into a smaller and smaller area.
- In the design known as the line-focus principle, the target is angled to allow a larger area for the electrons to strike while maintaining a small effective focal spot.
  - A large effective focal spot area on the target is therefore matched with a much smaller actual focal spot size.

Anode Heel Effect

- Portions of the x-ray beam at the anode side of the tube will pass through the anode, resulting in a lower intensity beam.
- To increase the chances of an even intensity beam across the breast, the thickest part of the breast (nearest the chest wall) is positioned at the cathode and the nipple area of the breast is positioned to the anode. This reduces the anode heel effect and allows more equal x-ray intensity across the detector.

Anode Angle and Tube Tilt

- Mammography tubes have anode angles ranging from 0-16 degrees depending on the manufacturer. A common tube tilt is 6 degrees.
- Tubes are positioned with a source to image-receptor distance (SID) of about 60-75 cm (24-30 in). Therefore, in order to achieve adequate field coverage for a field of view of 24 × 30 cm, and also to allow the central axis of the x-ray beam to run perpendicular to the plane of the detector at the chest wall, the tube must be tilted. Half-field geometry ensures that the x-ray beam does not extend beyond the edge of the detector especially at the chest wall.
- Decreasing the target angle will further decrease the effective focal spot.

Advantages of Tube Tilt

- Allows smaller target angle
- Allows greater anode heating capacity
- Reduces anode heel effect

Factors Affecting Focal Spot Size in Mammography

The size and shape of the focal spot can be affected by

- Size and shape of electron beam hitting anode
- Design and relationship of the filament coil to the focusing cup
- Angle of the anode

Focal Spot Sizes in Mammography

Most mammography units are dual focus, i.e., they have 2 focal spot sizes.

- The larger focal spot may be 0.4 but is generally 0.3 mm.
- The small focal spot ranges from 0.15-0.1 mm. The most common size is 0.1 mm.

Routine work utilizes the large focal spot size while the small focal spot size is used for magnification work.

Grids

- Grids are used to improve radiographic contrast by decreasing the amount of scattered radiation that reaches the image receptor.
- Modern mammography units utilize a moving grid to improve contrast.
- Grids are not used with magnification mammography, Hologic tomosynthesis, and photon-counting systems.

Grids and Exposure

All grids result in increased exposure and patient dose but will improve contrast. Because grid use necessitates an increase in radiation exposure and will therefore significantly increase the radiation dose to the patient, mammography grids are thinner than general x-ray grids. They also have a lower grid ratio than general radiography grids.

- The grid ratio of mammography grids usually varies from 3:1 to 5:1 (average of 4:1), focused to the SID for increased contrast. Grid frequencies of 30-50 lines per centimeter are common.
- The interspace material of the grid may be carbon fiber, wood, or other low-attenuation interspacing instead of the aluminum that is used in general radiography grids.
- High transmission cellular (HTC) grid is a specialized grid used in some mammography units. It has the characteristics of a crossed-grid capable of reducing scatter in 2 directions rather than 1. Copper is used instead of lead for the grid strip and air is used as the interspace material. This combination maintains a low radiation dose to the patient.

SYSTEM GEOMETRY (SID, OID, SOD, AND MAGNIFICATION)

SID is the source to image-receptor distance and refers to the distance from the x-ray source to the image receptor.

- SID is one of the many factors affecting recorded detail. The image loses recorded detail at short

SID. In imaging, the aim is to have the smallest focal spot coupled with longest SID. In mammography the units have very low kVp coupled with very small focal spots, in order to reduce unsharpness. The units generally have relatively short SID of 60-75 cm (24-30 in).

OID is the object to image-receptor distance (OID) and refers to the distance the object (or body part) is from the image receptor.

- The OID should be as small as possible to minimize magnification.
- The only exception is the microfocus magnification techniques used in mammography imaging.

SOD is the source to object distance and refers to the distance of the source to the object or body part.

- The SOD should be as long as possible to reduce skin dose.
- The only exception is the microfocus magnification techniques used in mammography imaging.

Magnification

- Magnification is used in mammography to assess small lesions or microcalcifications.
- To magnify the breast, the OID is increased.
- Without modification, magnification will reduce the resolution of the image because of geometric unsharpness. To compensate for the loss of resolution when using magnification, a very small focal spot is utilized.
- Magnification factor = SID/SOD or image size/object size. The magnification factor or degree in which the image is magnified will vary. The standard is 1.5 times and 1.8 times but some manufacturers offer 2 magnification factors with one as high as 2.0 times.
- Magnification mammography should not use a grid. The scattered radiation is significantly reduced as a result of the large OID or air-gap and a grid will only contribute to increase radiation dose to the patient.
  - Radiation dose to the patient is of concern because with magnification the radiation to the breast can double for just a single exposure because the breast is closer to the radiation source where the radiation intensity is greater.
  - The greater the magnification factor the greater the skin dose to the patient.

Density Compensation Circuit

- The density compensation circuit allows the selection of at least 2 steps above and 2 steps below the normal setting. Each step translates to a 12%-15% increase or decrease in the mAs or a 0.15 change in the optical density.

Beam-Restricting Devices

- In general radiography the beam-restricting devices are cones, collimators, or diaphragms used to limit or collimate the size of the x-ray field to the area of interest. Collimating or decreasing field reduces scatter and therefore improves the contrast but decreasing the x-ray field will therefore require an increase in exposure to maintain constant density.
- Despite the benefits of collimation, no collimation is used in routine mammography imaging and the entire detector—not just the area of the breast—is therefore exposed.
- The main reason is to prevent extraneous light from compromising the perception of fine detail when the radiograph is viewed. Under MQSA standards the collimation should not extend beyond any edge of the image receptor by more than 1% of the SID.

Analog Mammography Cassettes

In analog imaging the cassette holds and stores the film during exposure. The newer, thinner cassettes are designed for both daylight and regular systems and have an identification system slot, capable of recording patient information on the radiograph.

- All cassettes are easy to open, durable, and have low absorption characteristics relative to the kVp.
- Mammography cassettes are designed for used with a single emulsion film and are therefore matched with a single intensifying screen.

Effects of Exposure Time, mA and mAs

- Low mAs reduce radiation dose to the patient in both analog and digital systems.
- Short exposure times minimize motion blur due to patient motion.

- In analog imaging the mAs will affect image density and patient dose.
- In digital imaging mAs selection will affect patient dose; however, the mAs has little effect on image brightness (the term brightness replaces density in digital imaging).
  - Image acquisition and display are separated in digital imaging.
  - In digital imaging the user can alter the image brightness after the exposure.
  - In digital imaging the controlling factor of brightness includes not only the mA, but also the processing software and digital algorithm.

Effects of kVp in Analog and Digital Imaging

- The kVp controls the contrast in analog imaging. However, in digital imaging the image acquisition and display are separated.
  - In digital imaging the user can alter the image contrast after the exposure.
  - In digital imaging the controlling factor of contrast includes kV, processing software and digital algorithms.
  - The wide latitude in digital allows visualization of the skin and penetration of dense breast tissue.
  - The kVp selection on mammography generators can range from 20-40 kVp. However, the normal clinical practice use in the United States is 25-28 kVp.

Automatic Exposure Control in Analog Imaging

- Automatic exposure control (AEC) is used to control the length of the exposure and will therefore determine the density of the final image. The AEC allows the unit to respond to different breast compositions and various breast sizes.
- Units can have up to 10 AEC detector positions, which can be activated depending on the breast placement and size.

AEC Failure in Analog Imaging

- Commonly caused by activating the wrong detector relative to breast placement.
- If the activated detector is located under fatty breast tissue, the glandular tissue will be underexposed.

Exposure Control in Digital Imaging

- The surface that the breast rests on is the detector. The entire surface functions to monitor and control the exposure.

Back-Up Timer

- The back-up timer is used to prevent gross overexposure.
  - The back-up timer for grid techniques is set at 600 mAs and for nongrid at 300 mAs.
- The back-up timer is reached during an exposure when the selected exposure is too low. This will occur if there are low-energy photons that cannot penetrate the breast because the breast is too dense or too large.

Avoiding Back-Up Timer During an Exposure

- Select a high kVp value, since the maximum mAs was reached and increasing the mAs is no longer an option.
- The back-up timer is also reached whenever imaging implants, using AEC. Implants should be imaged using manual techniques unless sufficient breast tissue covers the AEC cell or detector.

DIGITAL IMAGING

Bit

- A single binary digit of data such as "0" or "1."
- The computer can only understand binary language which is "0" or "1"; however, the computer can use as many bits as necessary to express a decimal digit.
- A bunch of 8 bits is called a *byte*.

Bit Depth

- Number of gray shades that a pixel can produce. Represented by the formula 2*n*, where *n* = bit depth.
- Number of bits per pixel determines the bit depth or shades of gray demonstrated.
- The greater the bit depth the more accurate is the digital signal. It will have more shades of gray and therefore the image has greater detail.
- If the pixel has a bit depth of 8. Number of shades of gray that the pixel can produce = 2^8 or 256.

Matrix

- A digital image is a matrix of picture elements (*pixels*). Each cell corresponds to a specific location in the image. The matrix is therefore a box of cells with numeric values arranged in rows and columns.
- The size of the image matrix is determined by the number of pixels in the rows and columns. It is expressed by listing the number of pixels in each dimension (length and width).
  - Common sizes: 256 × 256, 512 × 512, and 1024 × 1024

Pixel (Picture Element)

- One individual cell in a matrix

Recorded Detail or Resolution

- Controlled by the digital acquisition, i.e., pixel size and display matrix and the capabilities of the monitor.
- *Spatial resolution* of the imaging system is the minimum separation between 2 objects at which they can be distinguished as 2 separate objects in the image.
  - The smaller the pixels, the greater the spatial resolution.
- The *image resolution* of the system is controlled by the number of pixels.
  - The greater the number of pixels, the greater the image resolution.

Digital Printers

- Any printer used for full-field digital mammography (FFDM) must meet Food and Drug Administration (FDA) 510(k) clearance for digital mammography. Most digital printers offer daylight film loading features and use a photothermographic dry laser system.
- After exposure to an ultraprecise laser, the photosensitive film is then uniformly heated using a unique thermal element technology.

Preprocessing

- In digital imaging, preprocessing is automatic and occurs before the image is visualized at the acquisition workstation monitors (AWS). Preprocessing involves:
  - *Automatic rescaling* to correct the raw data.
  - Enhancing of contrast and image sharpness.
  - Correction of artifacts due to bad detector elements or bad pixels.
  - Application of processing algorithms to generate a histogram.

Postprocessing

- Image brightness is controlled mainly by the processing software and the algorithms that can be applied.
  - Brightness can be altered after the exposure, independent of the mAs used to acquire the image.
- Image contrast is controlled by processing software and the algorithms that can be applied.
  - Contrast can be altered after the exposure, independent of the kVp used to acquire the image.
- Windowing
  - Changing the brightness and/or contrast.
  - Window width controls the ratio of black to white displayed, therefore the contrast. Increased window width equals decreased contrast.
  - Window level controls the brightness displayed. Increased window level equals increased brightness.
- Noise reduction or suppression removes digital signals that do not provide useful image data. Noise suppression tends to blur the image which reduces the visibility of fine details and can result in loss of contrast.
- Edge enhancement, frequency processing, or spatial frequency filtering is the averaging of the signal strength of 1 pixel with the strength of adjacent pixel or neighboring pixels. The more pixels involved in the averaging, the smoother the image appears.
- Smoothing is the averaging of each pixel's frequency with surrounding pixels' values to remove high-frequency noise. Smoothing reduces noise and contrast.

Film Digitizers

- Film digitizers are used to convert a hard copy x-ray film produced with an analog imaging system to a digital version that can be electronically transmitted, viewed, analyzed, and stored.

- In some of the film digitizers, a precalibrated light source is used to scan the image and a photodetector (PD) then measures the intensity of light passing through the film.
- Output from the PD is converted to a digital signal.

DETECTOR TECHNOLOGY IN DIGITAL MAMMOGRAPHY SYSTEMS

- Computed mammography (CM)
  - CM adapts an analog imaging system to digital. It uses an imaging plate (IP) instead of a cassette.
  - Mammography unit with IP plus a computer reader. The IP is physically removed from the unit and inserted into the computer reader.
- FFDM or DM uses a cassetteless system
  - Built-in flat panel detector technology
- Photon-counting MicroDose
  - A multislot scanning technology eliminates the scattered radiation.

COMPUTED MAMMOGRAPHY

Components of a Computed Mammography System

- IP or CM cassette which contain a photostimulable phosphor (PSP)
- Processing reader
- Computer
- Display monitor

The Imaging Plate

- A rigid cassette device with a radiolucent front, made of a hard plastic or similar radiolucent material to allow x-rays to enter and expose the PSP.
- Contains a PSP that is sometimes called a storage phosphor screen (SPS). The phosphor is the site of latent image formation.

Layers of the PSP

Protective Layer

- A thin tough layer of plastic that protects the phosphor layer from damage.

Phosphor Layer

- Common phosphor is europium-doped barium fluorohalide (BaFl: Eu). Europium (Eu) acts as an activator and is responsible for the storage properties of the PSP.

Conductive Layer

- This layer holds and traps excited electrons at higher energy levels.
- The conductive layer also grounds the plate to reduce static electricity problems and absorbs light to increase sharpness.

Support Layer

- Semirigid material provides the imaging sheet with strength and is a base for the other layers.

Light Shield Layer

- Prevents light from erasing the data on the image recorder or striking through the backing layer.

Backing Layer

- A soft polymer that protects the back of the IP.

Phosphor Characteristics

- Turbid phosphors have crystals distributed throughout the phosphor level. They produce lateral spreading of light which reduces the spatial resolution of the image. For example, barium fluorobromide and europium, barium fluorobromide iodide with europium, barium fluoroiodide with europium, barium strontium-fluoride bromide-iodide, gadolinium oxysulfide, and rubidium chloride.
- Needle phosphors have crystals growing in columns. They have less lateral spread of light and better spatial resolution. For example, cesium iodide.

Process of PSP Image Capture

- When x-rays strike the atoms of barium fluorobromide the outer shell electrons become excited (due to Compton and photoelectric x-ray interactions) and gain energy. These excited electrons are called *metastable* electrons.
- The metastable electrons in the crystals move from their normal orbital location to conductive

layer. The electrons are then move to the *F-Trap* where they are held. This process represents the *latent* image formation.

- The number of electrons captured in the F-Trap is directly proportional to the amount of energy absorbed by the PSP.
- The latent image can last for several hours but loses 25% of its energy in 8 hours. *Fading* is the term used to describe the time it takes for the latent image to disappear.
- Some but not all electrons raised to a higher energy level will spontaneously return to their resting state.

The Computer Processing or PSP Reader

- The computer reader device opens the IP and removes the PSP. It scans, reads, and erases the exposed PSP.
- The entire process can take up to 60 seconds and depends on the manufacturer.
- After scanning, the PSP is returned to the IP and the IP is ejected from the computer reader.

Image Extraction Process

- The IP is taken to a computer processing reader and the PSP is extracted.
- The conductive layer of the PSP has the excited electrons trapped at higher energy levels.
- A finely focused beam of infrared light scans the PSP in a transverse raster pattern.
- The light provides energy to the electrons trapped in the conductive layer. This causes electrons to release the energy that they absorbed from the x-ray beam and to return to their lower energy resting state.
- The energy released from the metastable is in the form of a bluish-purple light.
- The bluish-purple light released by the metastable electrons is collected by light guides of a *photomultiplier tube* (PMT), *photodetector* (PD), *or charge-coupled device* (CCD) and used to record the image.
    - *Photostimulable luminescence* (PSL) is the emission of the bluish-purple light from electrons as they transition from higher energy to a lower energy state.
    - The amount of light (photostimulable luminescence or PSL) emitted by the PSP during the reading process, related to the level of exposure received by the receptor, is termed the *speed class*. The technical factors (exposure received by the PSP) will determine the speed class of the system.
- The PSP must undergo a final erasure by a high-intensity light source to ensure that all the electrons are back at their ground state.
- The laser light is red while the PSP emits a bluish-purple light. This allows the PD to differentiate between the light used for PSP scanning versus the light emitted for image formation.

Types of Computer Reader–Processing Technology

- **Point-scan reader (flying-spot scanner)** is an older method of reading the PSP. The laser beam scans the entire PSP.
- **Line-scan reader** have several lasers in a row. The PSP is pulled under the linear scanner or the PSP remains stationary and the scanner moves across the plate. This method is capable of processing an entire line of the PSP at one time so is faster than the point-scan readers.
- **Dual-sided readers (dual-head flying-spot scanner)** scan both sides of the PSP which allows the collection of more image data with less image noise.

The Photomultiplier Tube, Photodetector, or Charge-Coupled Device

- The PMT collects the bluish-purple light given off by the trapped electrons as they return to their normal neutral state.
- The light is transmitted to an analog-to-digital converter (ADC).
- The ADC converts the analog signal to into a digital signal (the binary language or numeric data) that can be read by a computer.
- The digital signal is sent to a computer for processing.
- After processing, the digital signal (binary data) must be converted back to an analog signal (various shades of gray) for viewing at the display monitor.

Function of the High-Intensity Light Source

- The high-intensity light erases the plate by releasing any remaining electron energy.

- Some excited electrons will always remain in the conductive layer and if they are not removed they will result in ghosting on subsequent IPs.
- Any residual latent image is removed by flooding the phosphor with very intense light. This allows the PSP to be reused many times.
- IPs must be erased every 48 hours to remove background radiation even if not used.
- The IPs must be erased before using if the last time of erasure is unknown.

Function of the Analog-to-Digital Converter

- The ADC converts analog (light or electronic) signals from the PMT/detector to a digital signal consisting of binary or numerical data.
- Binary language is the only language that the computer will understand therefore any electronic or light signals must be converted to binary language. The computer then manipulates, processes, and stores the data.

Function of the Computer in the CM Digital System

- The computer receives a digital signal from the PMT/detector; applies selected algorithms to the data received, processes the data, and sends the digital data to a digital-to-analog converter (DAC).
- The DAC converts the binary computer language back to an electronic signal (various shades of grays) to be sent to the display monitor.

Function of the Digital-to-Analog Converter

- The DAC converts digitally manipulated computer data to an analog (electronic) signal.
- The image will appear on the display monitor as various shades of gray. However, the computer outputs a signal in computer language. This digital signal must be converted to an analog signal for display.

Advantages of CM

- Wide latitude and dynamic range.
- CM is faster than analog imaging systems.
- Reduced repeat due to exposure errors.
- Reduced risk of lost films.
- Allows a more efficient and faster workflow.

Disadvantages of CM

- Lower spatial resolution (digital can manipulate the pixel value after the exposure which compensates for the lower spatial resolution).
- IPs can be easily damaged during transport.
- IPs are susceptible to scratches in computer reader.
- Noise images at low exposures.
- Increased image noise due to the sensitivity of the PSP to radiation.
- "Exposure creep" due to lack of awareness of radiation safety and patient dose.

FULL-FIELD DIGITAL MAMMOGRAPHY

There are a number of DM systems available including indirect capture flat-panel detector and direct capture flat-panel detector.

Flat-Panel Detector Systems

- Nonscintillator based. Direct: 2-step process.
  - The x-ray beam strikes a photoconductor, e.g., amorphous selenium (a-Se).
    - a-Se converts x-ray to electrons.
      - A high-voltage charge is applied to the a-Se after the x-ray exposure.
      - Electrons are released from the amorphous selenium as a result of the exposure.
  - Electrons migrate to the detector element (DEL) on a thin-film transistor (TFT).
    - The electron signal is sent to an ADC then to a computer for analysis.
    - Information from the computer is displayed on LCD monitor.
- Scintillator based. Indirect: 3-step process.
  - The x-ray beam strikes a scintillator, e.g., cesium iodide.
    - *Cesium iodide* converts x-ray to light.
  - Light strikes the photoconductive material, e.g., amorphous silicon (a-Si), i.e., photomultiplier, photodiode, or thin-film diodes (TFD).
    - TFD converts light to electrons.
  - Electrons migrate to the DEL on a TFT.
    - The electron signal is sent to an ADC then to a computer for analysis.
    - Information from the computer is displayed on LCD monitor.

Thin-Film Transistor

- The TFT is a device made of millions of detector elements, electrodes, photodiodes, storage capacitors, and other components that is used to accept and store electrons and to generate an electric charge from each stored electron.
- In the direct detection array, the components of the TFT are arranged on a-Se as the semiconductor material.
- In the indirect detection array the components of the TFT uses a-Si.
- A variation of the TFTs are used in high-quality flat-panel liquid-crystal displays (LCDs).

Detector Element (DEL or dexel)

- The detector elements (DELs or dexels) are located within rows and columns on the TFT and are part of the complex circuit device of the TFT.
- DEL is the sensitive component of the TFT that collects electrons emitted from either a-Se or a-Si, to represent individual components of a digital image.
- After the exposure, the DELs read those electrons in a sequential pattern that matches their location within the detector matrix.
- Once the DELs are read, the flat-panel detector automatically erases and is ready for another exposure.
  - DEL size controls the recorded detail, or spatial resolution, for the flat-panel device.
  - DEL size contributes to the image blur present in a flat-panel detector receptor.
  - The larger the DELs in a flat-panel detector, the more image blur.
  - DEL size is set by the manufacturer and is not under the technologist's control.

Fill Factor

- Each square in the TFT matrix has sensitive and nonsensitive areas. The sensitive area represents the DELs that collect the electron charge.
- The fill factor is the ratio of the sensitive area to the entire detector area and is usually expressed as a percentage.
- Fill factor will affect the spatial resolution and signal-to-noise (SNR) ratio. A typical fill factor is 80%.

Advantages of DM

- No plates to drop or damage.
- No plates to be transferred.
- Has increased DQE over CM systems (detective quantum efficiency or DQE describes how efficient the system is in converting x-ray input signals into a useful output image).

Disadvantage of DM

- Image lag or memory effect because the charge is trapped in the metastable band and is released slowly over time. Image lag time varies and is shorter for flat-panel digital detectors based on indirect conversion.

Photon-Counting Image Capture

- Photon-counting MicroDose mammography system detects and captures individual x-ray photons leaving the breast using a crystalline silicon detector and photon-counting electronics, therefore eliminating the signal loss which occurs in digital systems when analog-to-digital conversions are used.
- The system uses tungsten anode and aluminum as the added filter.
- The system uses a mulislot system that virtually eliminating scatter, therefore a grid is not necessary, allowing a further reduction in patient dose. Images are acquired with a resolution of 25 megapixels.

Advantages of the Photon-Counting System

- Ergonomic design
- Warm detector
- Lower radiation dose
  - 40% less than FFDM. Average glandular dose ranges from 0.4-0.8 mGy on the CC and 0.4-0.87 mGy on the MLO.
  - Robust and temperature tolerant.
    - 10-50°C (50-122°F)
  - No ADC needed—therefore no lost signals.
  - No ghost image—100% fill factor.

Disadvantages of the Photon-Counting System

- Higher recall rates

CONTINUOUS QUALITY IMPROVEMENT

Quality Assurance or Continuous Quality Improvement

- Quality assurance includes the total overall management of actions taken to consistently provide high image quality in the radiology department with the primary objective being to enhance patient care.
- Quality assurance is very important in mammography, both in meeting the MQSA standard and equally important in ensuring quality patient care. Every quality assurance program must include a quality control (QC) component which includes the collection and evaluation of data with a systematic and structured mechanism to control variables such as repeat radiographs, image quality, processing variations, patient technical factors, technical effectiveness, efficiency, and in-service education.

Mammography Quality Standard Act

- In mammography, concern about the poor quality mammograms available at some facilities in the United States led to the passage of the MQSA.
- It was enacted on October 27, 1992 after which the US Congress authorized the FDA to develop and implement the MQSA regulations. Interim regulation passed in Dec 1993, and became effective Feb 1994. In 1995 enforcement began.

Areas Subject to MQSA Inspection and Testing

- Policy and procedures manuals
- Mammography equipment testing
- Personnel records
  - Initial training requirements and continuing education (CE) requirements for radiologic technologist, physicist, and radiologist
- Medical records
  - Patient records and medical outcome audit

Advantages of MQSA

- Reduction of unnecessary radiation to patients by reducing repeats
- Improvement in overall efficiency of service
- Improved patient satisfaction
- Consistency of image production
- Cost-effectiveness

Analog QC Test and Frequencies (Performed by the Mammographer or Technologist)

- Daily tasks
  - Darkroom cleanliness
  - Processor quality control
- Weekly tasks
  - View box and viewing conditions
  - Phantom images
  - Screen cleaning
- Monthly tasks
  - Visual checklist
- Quarterly tasks
  - Repeat analysis
  - Analysis of fixer retention
- Semiannual tasks
  - Darkroom fog testing
  - Screen-film contact
    - Compression

Digital QC

- Specific digital quality control tests are determined by the manufacturer. They vary and can include varying schedules of daily, weekly, monthly, quarterly, and semiannually quality control duties

Common Digital QC Test and Test Frequencies (Performed by the Mammographer or Technologist)

- **Daily**
  - *Monitor cleaning*, overhead lights, and viewing conditions
- **Weekly or Monthly**
  - *Flat field test* is a check of the detector.
  - *SMPTE* is a test pattern that can be used to check the communication between detector to the printer or the detector to the monitor.
  - *Phantom image* is a check of the detector and communication between the detector and the AWS.
  - *CNR (contrast-to-noise ratio)* measures the ability of the digital system to demonstrate objects of different brightness separate from their surroundings. CNR compares the image contrast to the level of background noise.

Noise measures how much target is obscured by random signal variations.
- *MTF (modulation transfer function)* measurement is the ability of the detector system to transfer its spatial resolution characteristics to the image. The system should record the available spatial frequencies and produce an image exactly as the object. The ratio of image to object is expressed as a function of the spatial frequency.
- *SNR (signal-to-noise ratio)* compares the level of a desired signal to the level of background noise. It is defined as the ratio of signal power to the noise power. A ratio higher than 1:1 indicates more signal than noise. The signal represents the difference between x-rays transmitted to the detector and those absorbed. Sources of image noise can include scattered radiation, background radiation, or insufficient technical factors.
- *Dynamic range* is the receptor's ability to respond to different exposure levels. Quantum mottle will appear if the exposure is 50% below the ideal exposure. If the exposure is 200% higher than the idea, there is reduced contrast.
- Automatic optimization of parameters (AOP) check to ensure dose reduction.

- **Monthly**
  - *Visual checklist* surveys the room for cracks, missing lights or faulty equipment.
- **Quarterly**
  - *Repeat analysis* checks the repeat and reject rates.
- **Semiannually**
  - *Compression* checks the minimum and maximum compression force for automatic modes.

Quality Control Duties of the Radiologist

- The level of commitment by the radiologist is often reflected in the quality of a mammography program. General responsibilities include:
  - Signing and checking the medical auditing.
  - Patient communication.
  - Overseeing the activities of the mammographer and the medical physicist.

Quality Control Duties of the Medical Physicist

- The medical physicist is a good potential source to consult prior to contacting the equipment service personnel and before any inspection. Recommendations and reports from the physicist should be reviewed with the radiologist and mammographer incharge of quality control. At a MQSA inspection, the medical physicist's report is always checked. Most equipment failures allow a 30-day period to provide corrections. The exceptions are for excessive breast dose and phantom image quality, which must be immediately corrected. General responsibilities include:
  - Evaluations of the mammographic unit
  - Yearly reviews of all test procedures including records, charts, and mammography policies and procedures
  - Written report and any corrective recommendation on all equipment testing

COMMON MQSA REQUIREMENTS

Personnel Requirements for Radiologist, Technologist, and Physicists

- State license required for some states
- Mammography education and initial training
- Performing regular mammograms, interpretations, and inspections for the mammographer (technologist), radiologist, and physicists, respectively
- Annual CE requirements

FDA Certificate Placement

- The certificate must be prominently displayed where all patients can see.

Consumer Complaints Mechanism

- The facility must have a written policy system in place to collect and resolve all patients' complaints. Serious consumer complaints reports must be forwarded to the FDA or State certifying agency. The facility must have instructions on how to proceed with serious unresolved complaints and must maintain a record of each complaint for 3 years.

Infection Control

- Evidence of infection control, e.g., wipes, sink with soap, or hand sanitizer should be present.

Self-referrals

- A patient who comes for a mammogram but has no health-care provider is considered a self-referral. A facility can decide to accept or not to accept self-referrals. Facilities accepting self-referral must have a policy in place.

Medical Records

- Medical records must be kept for not less than 5 years in digital or hard copy format. If the patient has not had additional mammograms at the facility, records must be kept for not less than 10 years. Some state or local laws may require longer times. Originals, in hard copy or digital format, must be transferred at the request of the patient. Transferred records must be of interpretation quality.
- Medical records must contain the name of patient plus an additional patient identifier, e.g., medical record number, the date of examination, the name of radiologist interpreting the mammogram, and a final assessment of findings.

Assessment Categories

- These are categories recognized by all physicians and MQSA. They were designed to standardize breast interpretation.

BIRAD 0: Need additional imaging information and/or prior mammograms for comparison.
BIRAD 1: Negative
BIRAD 2: Benign finding
BIRAD 3: Probably benign finding—short-interval follow-up suggested
BIRAD 4: Suspicious abnormality—biopsy should be considered.
BIRAD 5: Highly suggestive of malignancy—appropriate action should be taken.
BIRAD 6: Known biopsy proven malignancy—appropriate action should be taken.

Communication of Results

- Results must be sent to the patient's physician and if it is a concerned finding, it should be sent within 3 days. A written result in lay terms must also be sent to the patient as soon as possible for concerned findings and within 30 days of the mammogram for normal findings. Most inspectors interpret a concerned finding to be BIRAD 0, 3, 4, 5, and 6.

Medical Audit

- The medical audit is used to follow positive interpretation and to correlate them with pathology results. At a minimum the medical audit must track BIRAD 4 and 5 and must be reviewed annually by the interpreting physician.

Questions

1. What target-filtration combination in analog imaging provides the best penetration for dense or thick breast?
   (A) molybdenum target with molybdenum filtration
   (B) rhodium target with rhodium filtration
   (C) tungsten target with tungsten filtration
   (D) molybdenum target with appropriate K-edge filtration

2. The material used for the exit port of the mammography tube is necessary because
   (A) the intensity of the beam is less on the anode side than on the cathode side
   (B) regular glass would harden the emerging beam
   (C) the intensity of the beam is more on the anode side than on the cathode side
   (D) regular glass would soften the emerging beam

3. The intensity of the x-ray beam from the cathode side of the tube is generally higher because
   (A) soft characteristic radiation emerges from the anode side
   (B) the cathode side is directed to the thickest part of the breast
   (C) the heel effect causes variation in the intensity of the x-ray beam
   (D) the heel effect increases the intensity of the beam at the anode side

4. The design of the lip of the compression paddle (both height and angle along the chest wall) affects all of the following *except* that it
   (A) prevents the posterior and axillary fat from overlapping the body of the breast
   (B) allows uniform compression of the posterior breast tissue
   (C) helps to increase structural strength of the compression paddle
   (D) ensures greater compression of the anterior breast tissue

5. The *primary* goal of compression is to
   (A) reduce the OID of the lesion
   (B) allow uniform penetration of structures within the breast
   (C) reduce the possibility of motion during the exposure
   (D) reduce the radiation dose to the breast

6. What features of the high-transmission cellular grid allow these grids to maintain equal or less radiation dose to the patient when compared to the linear grids?
   (A) These grids use lead as the strips and wood as the interspace material.
   (B) They have copper as the strips and air as the interspace material.
   (C) They use aluminum as the strips and air as the interspace material.
   (D) They use wood as the strips and copper as the interspace material.

7. The grid ratio can vary in modern mammography units. A common grid ratio used is

(A) 8:1
(B) 6:1
(C) 4:1
(D) 2:1

8. The chest wall edge of the compression paddle should be aligned just beyond the chest wall edge of the detector to

(A) avoid pushing the patient's chest away and losing breast tissue
(B) properly position and compress the breast
(C) permit uniform exposure and reduce patient discomfort
(D) avoid projecting the chest wall edge of the paddle on the mammogram

9. Which of the following affects focal spot size?

(A) angle of the anode
(B) a decrease in the SID
(C) decreasing the size of the collimated beam
(D) changing the relationship between the OID and the SID

10. In mammography, the commonly used focal spot size for routine work is

(A) 3 mm
(B) 0.3 mm
(C) 1 mm
(D) 0.1 mm

11. Which of the following mammographic quality control tests is performed quarterly?

(A) phantom images
(B) visual checklist
(C) repeat analysis
(D) CNR

12. The general criteria to pass the ACR Mammography Accreditation phantom imaging require a minimum of _______ masses.

(A) 2
(B) 3
(C) 4
(D) 5

13. One of the 2 reasons towels are used in the compression test is to

(A) protect the detector and compression plate
(B) ensure that the compression is adequate
(C) force slower application of compression
(D) simulate 4 cm of compressed breast

14. For the repeat analysis to be meaningful, a patient volume of at least _______ patients is needed.

(A) 50
(B) 100
(C) 250
(D) 300

15. If, after examining a phantom image, the number of visualized fibers or masses has changed significantly, the next step is to

(A) record the new values
(B) call the medical physicist
(C) call the equipment service personnel
(D) repeat the test

16. Repeats are

(A) images taken during a breast stereo localization
(B) images used for quality control
(C) images that involve exposure to the patient
(D) all discarded images

17. If the patient volume at a mammography site is 200 patients per week, the repeat/reject analysis could be performed every

(A) week
(B) 2 weeks
(C) 2 months
(D) 3 months

18. Mammography facilities can receive certification from

1. the ACR
2. the FDA
3. an SAC state

(A) 1 or 2 only
(B) 2 or 3 only
(C) 1 or 3 only
(D) 1, 2, or 3 only

19. Aluminum filtration is likely to be matched with _________ targets.

(A) molybdenum
(B) rhodium
(C) tungsten
(D) beryllium

20. If any of the visual checks fail, the first step is to

(A) correct or replace the item
(B) call the medical physicist
(C) consult with the radiologist
(D) ignore the defect if the equipment is functioning

21. Digital images can be viewed on a computer monitor or printed using

(A) dry laser technology
(B) single emulsion mammography film
(C) single emulsion laser film
(D) double emulsion film, sensitive to the red-light spectrum emitted by lasers

22. A single binary digit of data such as "0" or "1" is called a

(A) pixel
(B) matrix
(C) bit
(D) byte

23. In general, greater magnification will require the use of a

(A) larger focal spot size
(B) smaller OID
(C) smaller focal spot
(D) larger SID

24. A grid is not necessary during magnification because

(A) grid use decreases spatial resolution
(B) the small focal spot used will compensate for the loss of image detail
(C) the large OID produces the same effect as a grid
(D) magnification will magnify the normally invisible grid line

25. The air gap in magnification allows increase subject contrast by

(A) increasing scatter
(B) reducing scatter
(C) reducing motion
(D) increasing motion

26. If the magnification mammography is performed without using a small focal spot, the resulting image will be magnified

(A) and blurred
(B) and sharply outlined
(C) with increased subject contrast
(D) with increased detail

27. At higher magnification factors there is

1. higher skin dose
2. increased scatter
3. decrease source-to-object distance (SOD)

(A) 1 and 2 only
(B) 2 and 3 only
(C) 1 and 3 only
(D) 1, 2, and 3

28. Magnification is beneficial in all of the following situations *except*

(A) imaging the surgical site of a patient with a lumpectomy
(B) imaging a specimen radiograph
(C) evaluating microcalcifications in a lesion
(D) imaging the entire breast in a single exposure

29. Using a small focal spot size is recommended for magnification

(A) to compensate for the loss of image detail
(B) because of increased patient dose
(C) to compensate for the small OID
(D) to compensate for motion unsharpness

30. The greatest disadvantage of magnification is

(A) increased OID
(B) increased patient dose
(C) decreased subject contrast
(D) increased risk of motion unsharpness

31. If the back-up time stops a breast exposure, the mammographer can repeat the radiograph using a

(A) higher kVp setting
(B) greater density compensation
(C) higher mAs setting
(D) different AEC setting

32. The type of x-rays created from displacement of K-shell-binding electrons in the molybdenum atom are called

(A) coherent scattering
(B) characteristic radiation
(C) Compton effect
(D) Bremsstrahlung radiation

33. The function of the filter in mammography is to remove

(A) low-energy x-rays that would result in increase skin dose
(B) all low-energy photons
(C) low-energy x-rays needed to produce the breast image
(D) photon energies above and below the range needed for breast imaging

34. A recommended labeling for the mammographic image that is not required by the MQSA is

(A) technologist/mammographer identification
(B) date of service
(C) technical factors
(D) name of patient

35. Lack of breast compression is most likely to cause

(A) geometric unsharpness
(B) plate reader artifact
(C) motion unsharpness
(D) printer artifact

36. How long should a facility maintain records of serious complaints?

(A) 1 year
(B) 2 years
(C) 3 years
(D) 4 years

37. A digital imaging test of the printer could include the

(A) SMPTE test
(B) flat field test
(C) CNR
(D) SNR

38. Which of the following system is likely to have a slit collimator system instead of a grid?

(A) flat-panel detector tomosynthesis imaging systems
(B) PSP imaging systems
(C) any magnification mammography system
(D) Micro Dose photon-counting systems

39. Aluminum is used as the filtration in

(A) digital breast tomosynthesis tubes with tungsten targets
(B) tungsten target digital mammography tubes
(C) rhodium target digital mammography tubes
(D) analog mammography tubes

40. The detector element is located in the

(A) IP
(B) flat-panel detector
(C) thin-film transistor
(D) AEC

41. Which of the following statements on detector elements is *incorrect*?

(A) The detector element size controls the spatial resolution of the system.
(B) The size of the detector element can be controlled by the technologist.
(C) After reading the detector element the flat-panel detector automatically erases.
(D) The larger the detector element in a flat-panel detector, the more image blur.

42. To allow full coverage of the detector, a tube with a 16-degree anode angle requires a tube tilt of about _____ degrees to achieve an effective anode angle of 22 degrees.

(A) 2
(B) 4
(C) 6
(D) 8

Answers and Explanations

1. **(B)** All mammography units are manufactured with tungsten, molybdenum, or rhodium targets matched with the appropriate K-edge filters. *K-edge* describes a sudden increase in how quickly the x-ray beam is attenuated at photon energies just above the binding energy of the K-shell election of the atom (the electron shell that is closest to the nucleus).The varying targets have different atomic numbers and therefore different emission spectrums. The characteristic energies of molybdenum targets with molybdenum filtration are most effective for fatty breast tissue. The characteristic x-rays produced using rhodium targets with rhodium filtration are similar to those from molybdenum but, because rhodium has a slightly higher atomic number, more Bremsstrahlung x-rays are produced. However, the energy of the K-characteristic x-rays will be 3-4 keV higher, which provides a better penetration of dense breast although it generally results in lower contrast images. Tungsten targets with tungsten filtration are not used in analog mammography units because here Bremsstrahlung x-rays will predominate at energies above and below the 17-24 keV range. Tungsten targets with rhodium or silver filtration are used with digital units and silver (Ag) filtration is used in some digital tomosynthesis units. The x-rays most useful in maximizing contrast in breast tissue are in the 17-24 keV range.[1,2]

2. **(B)** Mammography uses very low-energy x-ray beams and it is important that the x-ray tube window does not attenuate the low-energy photons, therefore hardening the beam. The proper filter shapes the emission spectrum of the x-ray beam and makes it compatible with the detector and breast characteristics of each patient. In general, mammography units have beryllium as the port window. Borosilicate is another option that can be used.[3,4]

3. **(C)** The heel of the anode will reduce the intensity of the x-ray beam on the anode side only. When comparing the beam intensity on the cathode versus the anode side, the intensity on the cathode side will be higher. To compensate for this varying intensity, the mammography tube is turned to position the thickest portion of the breast (posterior) at the cathode end of the tube. In general, the smaller the anode angle, the larger the heel effect because there is an increased absorption of the rays (Figure 2-1).[3,5]

4. **(D)** Both the height and angle of the compression paddle make a difference in the final image and the overall design is considered to increase the structural strength of the compression paddle. A compression device with a rounded or gently sloping posterior edge would not allow uniform compression of the posterior area of the breast. The height of the compression reduces the chance of chest tissue overlapping on the mammogram. The design of the lip has a lesser effect on the anterior aspect of the breast[5] (Figure 2-2).

5. **(B)** Compression does all of these, but its *primary* goal is to reduce the breast thickness uniformly, separate breast structures and allow uniform penetration by the x-ray beam.[5]

6. **(B)** The high-transmission cellular (HTC) grid used in some units has the characteristics of

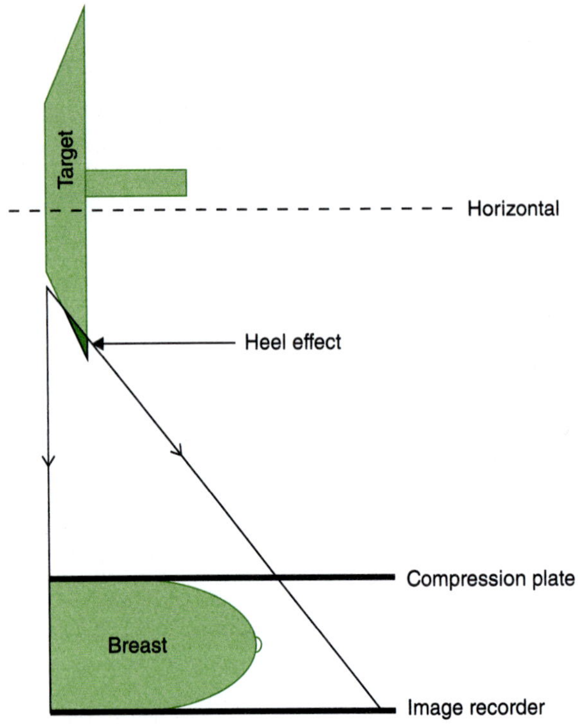

Figure 2-1. Heel effect. A portion of the beam is absorbed by the anode (target). This results in the lower energy beam at the anode end of the tube. This effect is minimized in mammography by tilting the tube and placing the anode toward the nipple (lower density) area of the breast. (Reproduced with permission from Peart O: Mammography and Breast Imaging PREP: Program Review and Exam Prep. New York, NY: McGraw-Hill Education; 2012.)

a crossed grid. It can reduce scattered radiation in 2 directions rather than the 1 direction of the linear or focused grid. These grids use copper rather than lead as the grid strip, and air rather than wood or aluminum as the interspace material. When compared to a similar ratio linear grid, the HTC grids result in equal or less radiation dose to the patient. All grids result in an increased exposure and patient dose, but improve contrast[5,6] (Figure 2-3).

7. **(C)** Higher grid ratios will require too large an increase in exposure. On an average, the mammography grids have a lower grid ratio than general radiography grids. The grid ratio of mammography grids ranges from 3:1 to 5:1 versus the 6:1 to 16:1 ratio of grids used in general radiography (grid ratio = height of the lead strips/the distance between the strips [h/d]), with frequencies of 30-50 lines per centimeter. A typical mammography grid may have a grid ratio of 4:1, and although such a grid will double the patient dose when compared to a nongrid exposure, the increased contrast will be significant[5,6] (Figure 2-4).

8. **(D)** The compression plate is specifically designed to properly position and compress the breast while reducing discomfort to the patient. The placement of the lip, just beyond the chest wall edge of the detector, prevents the projection of an image of the chest wall edge of the paddle on the mammogram.[5]

9. **(A)** The focal spot size is the area that electrons strike on the target. In the design known as the line-focus principle, the target is angled allowing a larger area for the electrons to strike while maintaining a small, effective focal spot. The effective focal spot size is the area projected onto the patient or detector. It is also the value quoted when identifying a small or large focal spot. The smaller the target angle, the smaller the focal spot size. Although the spatial resolution (the ability of the system to visualize individual microcalcifications as separate entities.) is related to the focal spot size, changes in the SID, OID, and size of the collimated field do not affect the focal spot size[3,5] (Figure 2-5).

10. **(B)** Mammography units generally have 2 focal spot sizes. The large focal spot may be 0.4 or below (generally 0.3 mm) and the small focal spot ranges from 0.15 to 0.1 (generally 0.1 mm). Routine work utilizes the large focal spot size. The small focal spot size is used for magnification.[3,5]

11. **(C)** The repeat/reject analysis is performed quarterly. The visual checklist is performed monthly, the phantom image check is often taken weekly (daily on mobile units), the CNR can be taken daily, weekly, or even monthly depending on the manufacturer.[7,8]

12. **(B)** The criteria for the number of objects on the phantom necessary to pass the ACR are a minimum of 4 largest fibers, 3 largest speck groups, and 3 largest masses (Figure 2-6). There are a few exceptions. The Hologic and

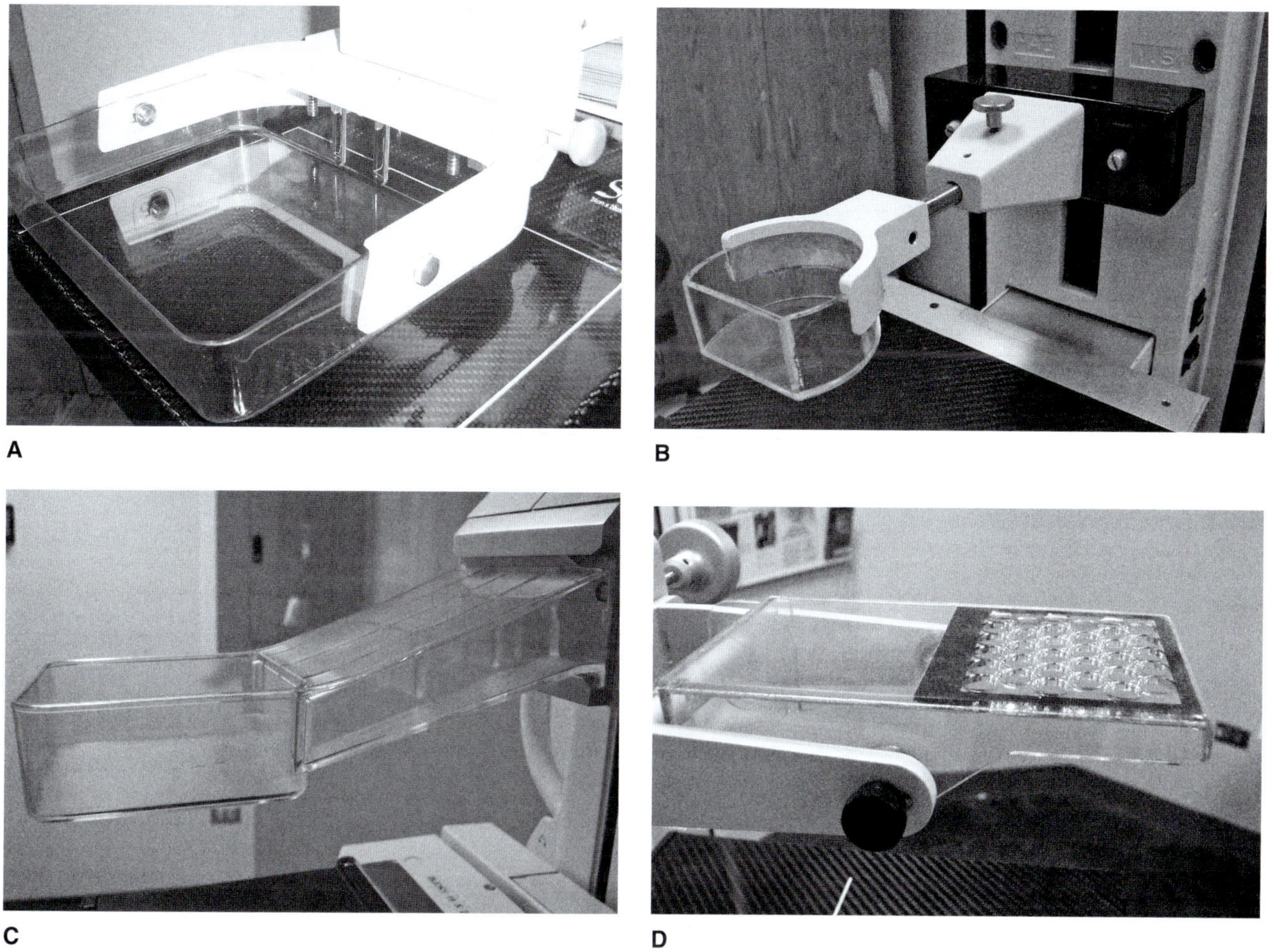

Figure 2-2. Mammography compression plates can be styled for different uses (A) routine imaging plate, (B) spot compression plate, (C) spot compression, (D) biopsy compression.

Siemens digital units require 5 fibers, 4 speck groups, and 4 masses. In addition to the above criteria, the number of test objects of each group type (fibers, specks, and masses)

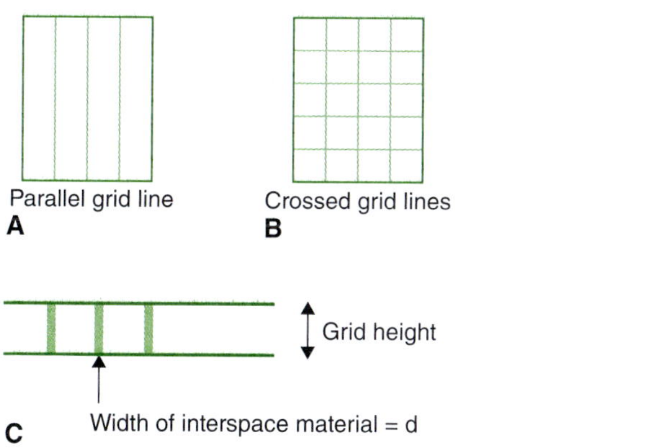

Cross-section of the grid showing the grid strips between the interspace material

Grid ratio = h/d

Grid frequency = number of grid strips per inch or per centimeter

Figure 2-3. Schematic diagram showing (A) a parallel grid typical of mammography grids, (B) the cross grid such as the HTC grid, and (C) cross-section of a grid.

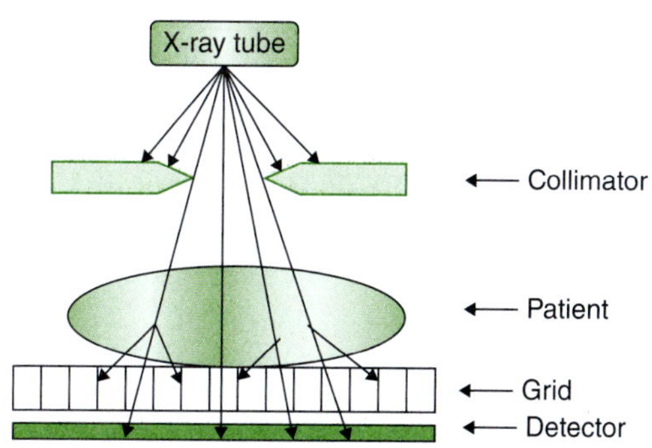

Figure 2-4. A cross-section of a typical grid. The grid strips will transmit x-rays traveling straight while absorbing any scattered rays.

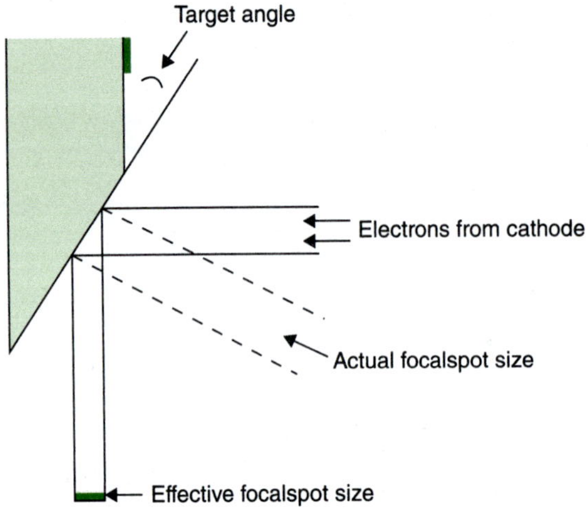

Figure 2-5. The target is angled to allow a smaller effective focal spot size to be matched with a larger actual focal spot. This allows greater anode heat capacity. (Reproduced with permission from Peart O: Mammography and Breast Imaging PREP: Program Review and Exam Prep. New York, NY: McGraw-Hill Education; 2012.)

visible in the phantom image should not decrease by more than one-half.[7,8,9]

13. **(A)** The towels protect the detector surface and prevent damage to the compression device. The amount of automatic compression applied is a function of the unit and will not be altered by the presence or absence of a towel. However, the force of the compression device hitting the scale could damage the compression device or the detector[7,8,9] (Figure 2-7).

14. **(C)** The repeat analysis is used to identify problem areas within the department. Most units can automatically generate a repeat rate based on the mammographer's input of the reason why a new projection is taken or a projection is discarded. The final percentage of repeats and rejects is calculated as a percentage of the total image taken. The percentage of repeats for each category is calculated as a percentage of the total repeat rate (Figure 2-8). However, for the analysis to be meaningful a sufficient patient volume is needed. The MQSA recommends a meaningful volume of at least 250 patients every 3 months.[7,8,9]

15. **(D)** The purpose of quality control testing is to ensure optimal conditions before clinical images are processed. Whenever a test fails, the first corrective action is to verify that the equipment is operating correctly, and then repeat the test to determine whether the change is real or not. However, the phantom test is a check of the detector on mammography unit, the monitor capabilities and the

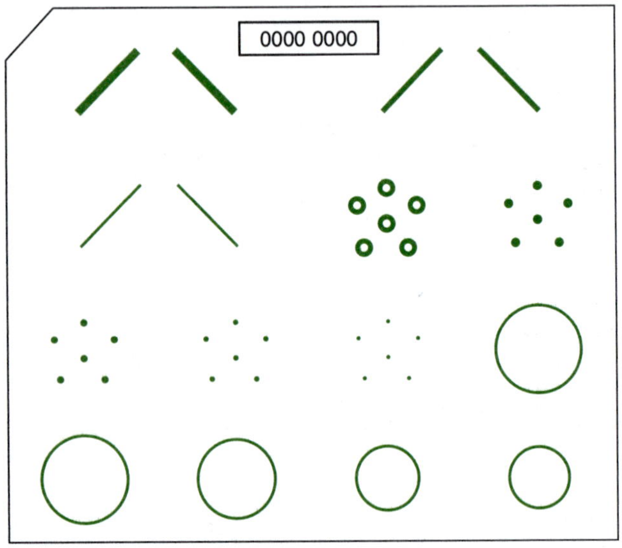

A

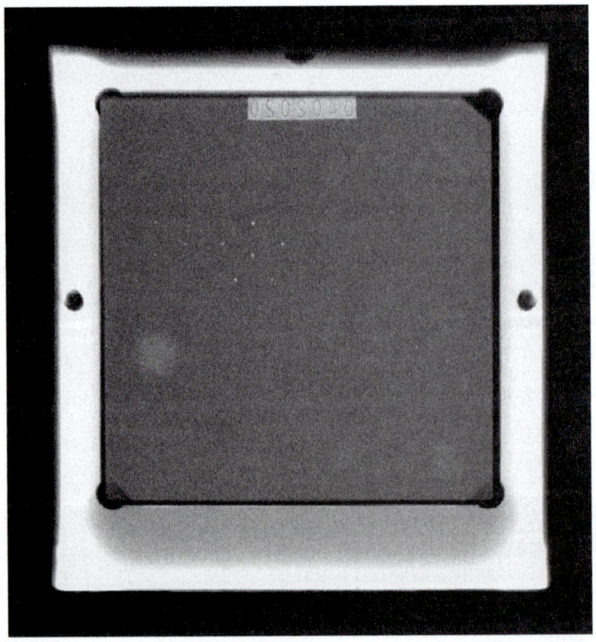

B

Figure 2-6. (A) A schematic diagram of the phantom showing the relative position of the different objects embedded within the phantom, (B) radiograph of a phantom. (Reproduced with permission from Peart O: Mammography and Breast Imaging PREP: Program Review and Exam Prep. New York, NY: McGraw-Hill Education; 2012.)

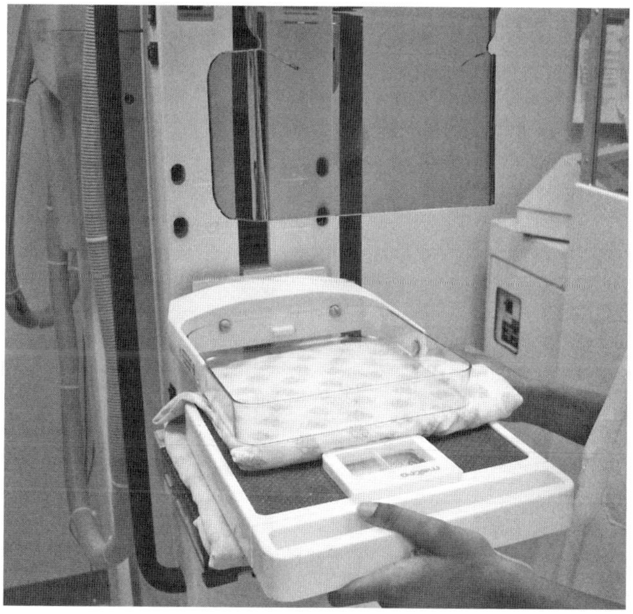

Figure 2-7. A towel, gowns, or sheet can be used to protect the surface of the detector and the compression plate from scratches during the compression test. (Reproduced with permission from Peart O: Mammography and Breast Imaging PREP: Program Review and Exam Prep. New York, NY: McGraw-Hill Education; 2012.)

printer if images are printed. Flat field test for the monitor and the QC test for printer must be performed before phantom test. This will direct attention to the correct source of the problem: the mammography unit, monitor or printer. In digital units the flat field and other test can be accessed from the quality control menu on the device. The medical physicist or the equipment service personnel should be called if problems cannot be isolated or corrected by the mammographer.[7,8,9]

16. **(C)** Repeated images are those that had to be repeated and resulted in additional exposure to the patient, e.g., images with motion. Rejected images are all discarded images, including repeated images. Rejected images can include those used for quality control purposes.[7,8,9]

17. **(D)** Repeat analysis testing is carried out every 3 months (quarterly), unless the patient volume is less than 250 in the quarter.[7,8,9]

18. **(B)** Under MQSA rules, accreditation and certification are 2 separate processes. Both are required by the FDA. Effective on May 2002, certification is permitted only by the FDA or certain states—States as Certifiers (SAC). The SAC permitted are Illinois, Iowa, and South Carolina. States can certify only facilities within their state. Accreditation is a process administered by an FDA-approved accreditation body, which can be a private, nonprofit organization or a state agency approved to accredit mammography facilities. The FDA has approved 4 accreditation bodies—the American College of Radiology (ACR) and the states of Arkansas, Iowa, and Texas. State accreditors can only accredit facilities within their state. These 4 bodies all have the authority to implement the MQSA standards through the accreditation process.[8,9]

19. **(C)** Analog units use molybdenum or rhodium targets matched with the same element as the filter. Tungsten targets are now used for many digital mammography systems. Tungsten has a higher Bremsstrahlung production efficiency and a higher tube loading than molybdenum and rhodium. However, because the unfiltered tungsten spectrum contains a large proportion of unwanted lower keV range photons (L-shell electrons), a minimum filter thickness of 0.05 mm rhodium or silver is used for fatty and dense breasts, respectively. Another filter option is aluminum. Aluminum filters has a lower atomic number. If used, a minimum of 0.7 mm aluminum is necessary to attenuate the L-electrons. In the Hologic digital tomosynthesis unit contrast is provided by tomographic image reconstruction therefore breast dose can be reduced by using aluminum filtration which allows the transmission of the higher energy x-rays. Higher kVp means that lower mAs can be used with resultant lower radiation dose to the patients. Beryllium is a low attenuating element used as the window material in x-ray tubes.[1]

20. **(A)** Examples of visual checklist items are a check of mechanical locks or display lighting. Many items are for the mammographer's convenience; some, however, are essential for patient safety and the production of quality images. If the mammographer cannot replace

Mammography Repeat-Reject Analysis Date From 9/3/01 To 12/28/01

	Projection Repeated Check One for Each Repeated Film						Number of Films	% of Repeats
Reason for Reject	Left CC	Right CC	Left MLO	Right MLO	Left Other	Right Other		
1. Positioning			✓✓	✓✓✓			5	19.2
2. Patient Motion		✓			✓		2	7.7
3. Light Films			✓	✓	✓		3	11.5
4. Dark Films	✓	✓					2	7.7
5. Black Films			✓				1	3.8
6. Static, Artifacts				✓	✓✓		3	11.5
7. Fog		✓	✓				2	7.7
8. Incorrect ID or Double Exposure							0	
9. Equipment Error			✓	✓			2	7.7
10. Technologist Error		✓✓	✓	✓			4	15.4
11. Good Film (No Apparent Reason)			✓✓				2	7.7

12. Clear Film	6
13. Wire Localization	10
14. Quality Control	7

		Number	Percentage
	Repeats (1-11)	26	1.17
	Rejects (all – 1-14)	49	2.21

Total Films Used	2216

Comments	
Action Taken	

Figure 2-8. Repeat analysis. Most mammography units will automatically generate a repeat analysis. This sample shows the calculation of the repeat or reject rates. (Reproduced with permission from Peart O: Mammography and Breast Imaging PREP: Program Review and Exam Prep. New York, NY: McGraw-Hill Education; 2012.)

or repair missing or broken items, the equipment service personnel should be called.[8,9]

21. **(A)** Any printer used for FFDM must meet FDA 510(k) clearance for digital mammography. Most digital printers offer daylight film loading features and use a photothermographic dry laser system which combines laser exposure and thermal development. After exposure to an ultraprecise laser, the photosensitive film is then uniformly heated using unique thermal element technology. The image quality produced by a FFDM printer depends on a number of factors including resolution, noise, image color, interpolation, and overall contrast and density. Any FFDM printer should be able to produce a D-max of 3.5 or greater and have a base-plus-fog level of less than 0.25. The image color should be blue/black similar to analogy mammography imaging. A printer should accept and process up to 16-bit images, as well as print those images with at least 12-bit gray levels. Disadvantages of the laser-printed film are: expense and the lower optical density and latitude. Screen-film mammography uses single emulsion films. Because of their lower spatial resolution, double emulsion films are not used in mammography. In the past, the laser printer used

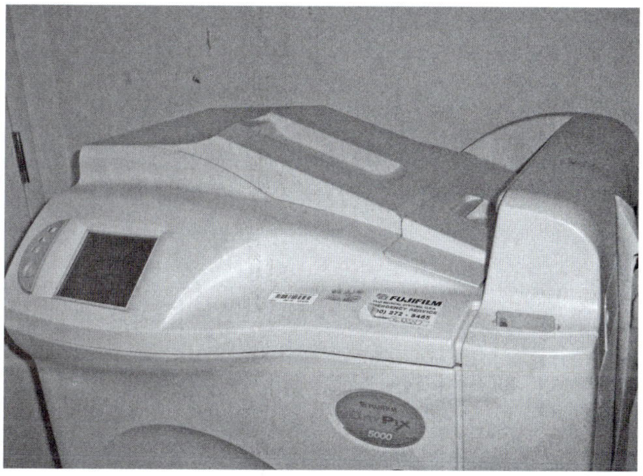

Figure 2-9. Digital printer.

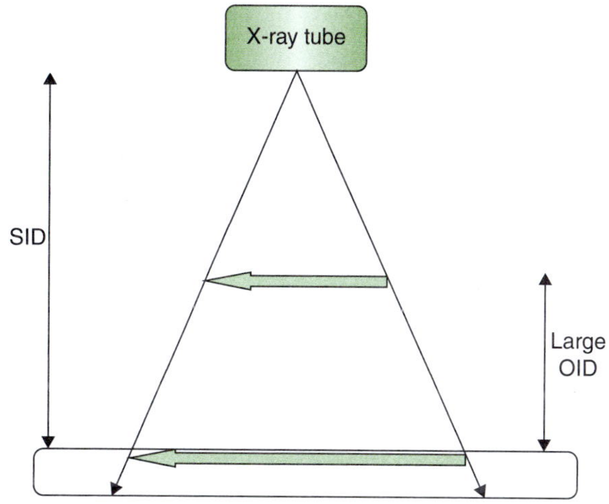

Figure 2-10. Schematic diagram demonstrating magnification mammography.

a single emulsion film that is sensitive to the red light emitted by the laser, similar to how blue- and green-sensitive films are used in conventional systems. These laser films must be handled in total darkness and were used mainly in computed tomography (CT) imaging[3] (Figure 2-9).

22. **(C)** A single binary digit of data such as "0" or "1" is a bit. The computer can use as many bits as necessary to express a decimal digit. A bunch of 8 bits is called a byte. The matrix is a box of cells with numeric values arranged in rows and columns. A digital image is a matrix of picture elements (pixels). Each cell corresponds to a specific location in the image. The size of the image matrix is determined by the number of pixels in the rows and columns. It is expressed by listing the number of pixels in each dimension (length and width).[3,4]

23. **(C)** To achieve magnification, the OID is increased. As the magnification factor increases, the focal spot must be reduced or the thickness of the part decreased to maintain sharp images. Both of these factors are used in breast magnification. The SID in mammography units is fixed and cannot be adjusted. Magnification factor = SID/SOD or image size/object size (Figure 2-10).[3,4]

24. **(C)** Magnification mammography is necessary to enhance microcalcifications or the borders of a lesion. Grids are necessary in routine mammography image to improve contrast and spatial resolution; however, with magnification a smaller effective focal spot is used to compensate for the loss of image detail and the air gap (large OID) acts like a grid in reducing the amount of scattered radiation reaching the film or electronic detector. The main disadvantage of magnification mammography is the higher skin dose (almost double the routine skin dose because the breast is closer to the radiation source). Grid use in magnification would further increase exposure times, increasing tube loading, and thus increased motion artifact owing to long exposure times. Radiation dose to the patient would also increase (see Figure 2-9).[3,4,6]

25. **(B)** The large air gap acts like a grid and reduces scatter, thus improving subject contrast. Positioning the breast away from the image receptor takes advantage of the inverse square law: the intensity of the scattered radiation is reduced because the distance between the image receptor and the object is increased. In magnification, mammography motion is controlled by vigorous breast compression. Grid use in magnification would further increase overall technical factors including the exposure times (see Figure 2-9).[5,6]

26. **(A)** Whenever the relationship between the source, object, and image are altered, as in magnification, there is an increase in focal spot blur. To keep focal spot blur at a minimum, to maintain subject contrast and image detail, and to compensate for the reduced resolution during magnification, a small focal spot must be used.[5,6]

27. **(C)** The magnification factor equals the source-to-image receptor distance divided by source-to-object distance (SID/SOD). Radiation intensity is related to the square of the distance; therefore, as the patient's breast is moved closer to the x-ray tube the SOD decreases and patient's dose increases. With a greater magnification factor, there is a greater skin dose because the SOD will be smaller. Also, as the magnification factor increases, a small focal spot must be used to maintain a sharp image. Scatter is insignificant during magnification because of the air gap[5,6] (see Figure 2-9).

28. **(D)** Magnification is ideal for imaging small areas such as the surgical site of a patient with a lumpectomy, specimen radiography, or microcalcifications. With magnification, microcalcifications that would otherwise be missed can be seen. Magnification should not be used in routine imaging of the entire breast because the entire breast may not be imaged, and patient dose is increased.[5,6]

29. **(A)** The focal spot blur (*penumbra* or *geometric unsharpness* are the old terms) is caused by a large effective focal spot. Whenever the relationship between the source, object, and image is altered, as in magnification, there is an increase in focal spot blur. To keep focal spot blur at a minimum, a small focal spot is used. The small focal spot necessitates a lower mA output and thus results in increased exposure time and risk of motion. Motion unsharpness is controlled by vigorous compression. The increase in patient dose is related to the smaller SOD used in magnification.[5,6]

30. **(B)** Unfortunately, magnification results in increased patient skin dose. Magnification factor equals SID/SOD or image size/object size. Using a magnification factor of 1.4 may actually double the radiation dose to the patient because the breast is placed closer to the radiation source. The OID must be increased to achieve magnification. Since the SID is fixed therefore the SOD will decrease. In magnification, subject contrast and motion unsharpness are controlled by using a small focal spot size with vigorous breast compression.[5,6]

31. **(A)** In a mammography unit, the back-up timer is activated if the initial test exposure—delivered to check if the exposure is adequate to penetrate the breast—fails. This could avoid a repeat due to underexposure. The density compensation circuit and the mAs should not be increased; because the primary reason for back-up time is that the beam has low-energy photons that are unable to penetrate the breast. Increasing the compensation circuit does not increase the energy of the beam. Each step on the compensation circuit generally results in a 12%-15% change in mAs. Increasing the mAs increases the overall optical density in analog units and increases the patient dose in both analog and digital imaging, but similar to the compensation circuit, this does not increase the penetrating power of the beam. In analog imaging, selecting another AEC setting may result in an underpenetrated image if the new AEC setting is placed over a less dense area of the breast[3,4,5] (Figure 2-11).

32. **(B)** The molybdenum anode will produce x-ray photons with energies in the range of 17-20 keV (kilo electron volt). The most prominent of these x-ray photons are characteristic and will account for 30% of the total x-rays in the molybdenum beam at 30 kVp. The emission spectrum shows almost no Bremsstrahlung x-rays because Bremsstrahlung x-rays are produced more easily in target atoms with high atomic numbers, such as tungsten. Coherent or classical scattering describes the interaction of very low-energy x-rays with atoms in the target. These energies are too low to impact breast imaging. Compton is the most common scattered

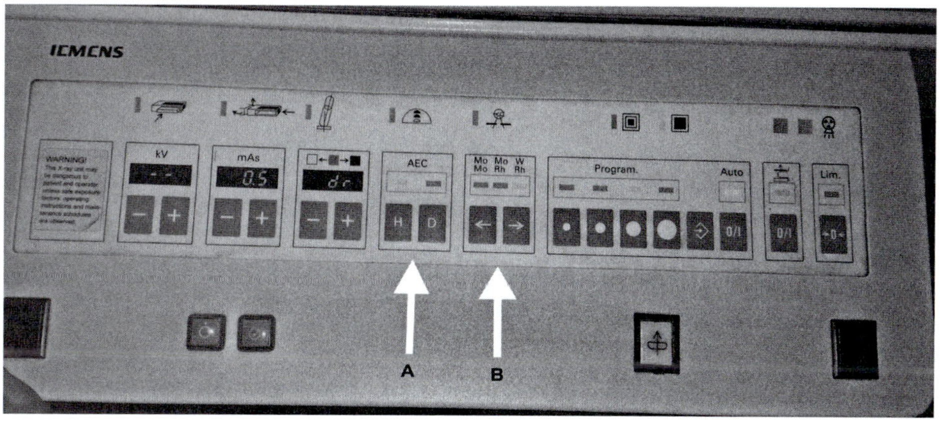

Figure 2-11. Feature on a control panel. Using the density compensation is not common since the advent of digital. Arrows indicate the controls (A) density compensator, (B) filter selection.

radiation in imaging. The Compton effect occurs when the incident x-ray interacts with an outer-shell electron and ejects it from the atom, ionizing the atom. The ejected electron is called a Compton electron or secondary electron. Compton-scattered x-rays can deflect in any direction and can retain up to two-thirds of its original energy[5,10] (Figure 2-12).

33. **(D)** Added filtration in mammography improves the energy distribution of the x-ray spectrum by removing energies below the useful range that would only contribute to skin dose and the highest energies that would reduce differential absorption in breast tissue. The elements used as filters are molybdenum (Mo), rhodium (Rh), and silver (Ag). These elements all have K-absorption edge energies between 20 and 27 keV (Figure 2-13).[1]

34. **(C)** The labeling guideline under MQSA rules is divided into 3 areas: required, strongly recommended, and recommended.

    Required labeling includes:

    - Name of patient (first and last) and additional patient identifier such as a unique medical record number.
    - Date of examination.
    - Projection and laterality (right or left) (placed near the axilla using the standardized codes approved by the FDA).
    - Facility name and location, including the city, state, and zip code.
    - Technologist/mammographer identification.
    - Mammography unit identification—if there is more than 1 unit.
    - Cassette/screen identification (on analog units).

    Strongly recommended labels include:

    - A flash card with a permanent patient identification system (analog units).

    Recommended labeling includes:

    - Technical factors (including target filter, kVp, mAs, and exposure time).
    - Compression force.
    - Compressed breast thickness.
    - Degree of obliquity.
    - Date stickers—enable easy reading of dates with overhead lights (analog units).[8,9]

35. **(C)** Sharpness is the ability to see fine detail on the mammography image, and patient motion is the most common form of unsharpness. Motion blurring is common with exposure above 2 seconds and can be prevented by proper communication. Good compression will reduce breast thickness, therefore allowing shorter exposure times. Geometric unsharpness or focal spot blur is caused by increase in focal spot size or OID or by a decrease in SID. Printer artifacts are caused when debris on the mirror in the laser printer causes fine white lines on the image. Plate

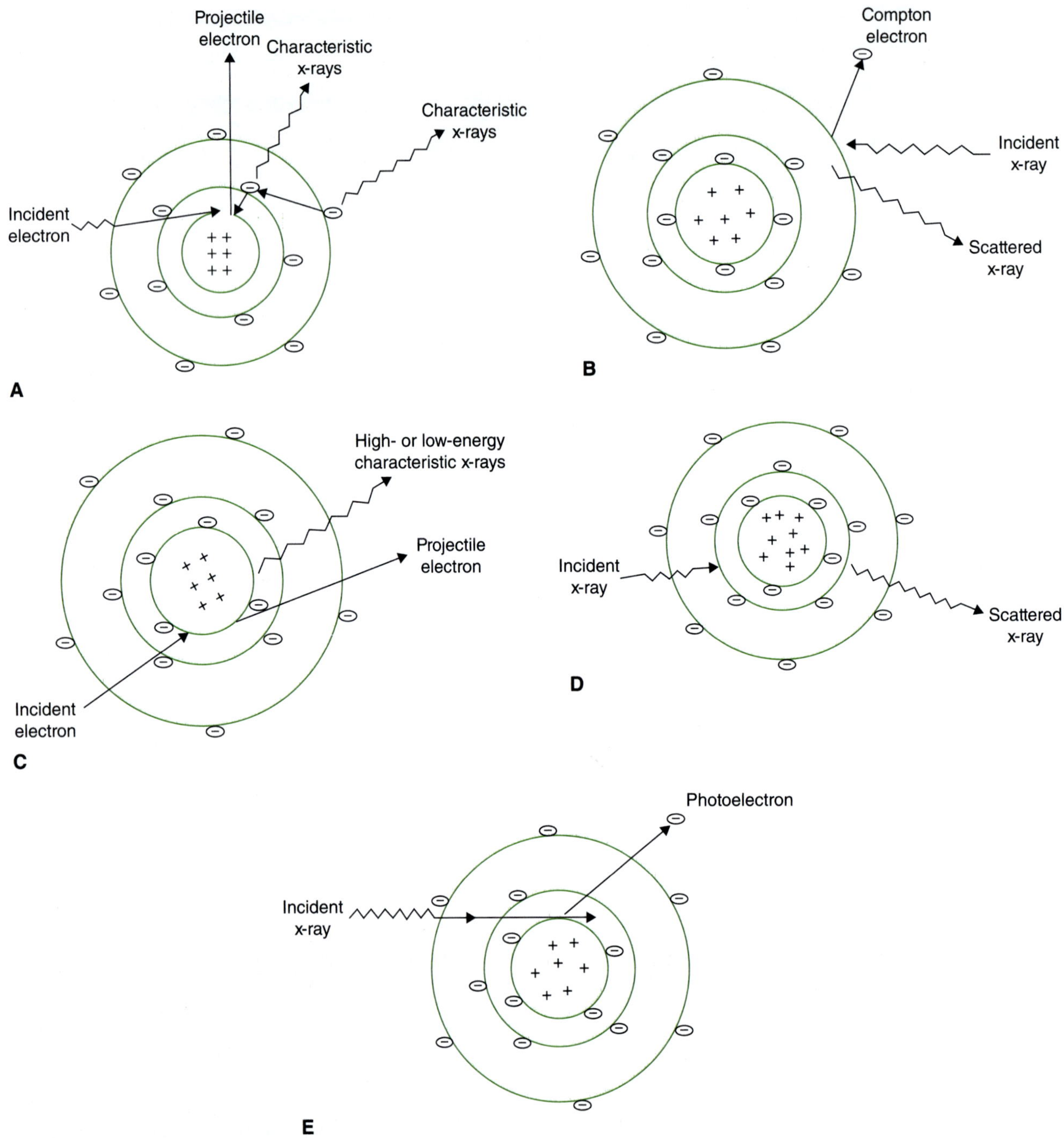

Figure 2-12. Schematic diagrams of the production of (A) characteristic radiation, (B) Compton effect, (C) Bremsstrahlung radiation, (D) Coherent scatter, (E) and photoelectric effect. (Reproduced with permission from Peart O: Mammography and Breast Imaging PREP: Program Review and Exam Prep. New York, NY: McGraw-Hill Education; 2012.)

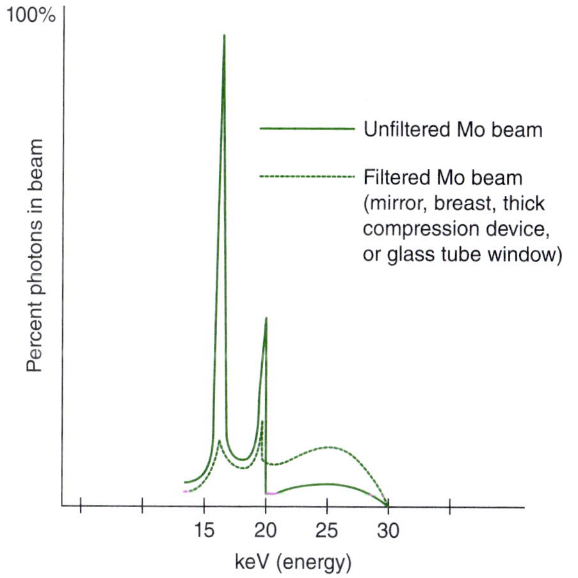

Figure 2-13. The emission spectrum of molybdenum beam filtered and unfiltered. Note that the filter beam removes the lower energies (16 keV) that would contribute only to skin dose. (Reproduced with permission from Peart O: Mammography and Breast Imaging PREP: Program Review and Exam Prep. New York, NY: McGraw-Hill Education; 2012.)

reader artifacts are the result of problems in the plate reader's electronics.[3,4,5]

36. **(C)** Facilities must have a system in place to collect and resolve serious consumer complaints such as poor image quality, missed cancers, personnel not meeting applicable training requirements, failure to send medical or lay person reports. Serious complaints must be forwarded to the FDA or State certifying agency. The facility must have a written policy for collecting and resolving patient's complaints with instructions on how to proceed with serious unresolved complaints. Records of each serious complaint must be maintained for 3 years.[8,9]

37. **(A)** The *Society of Motion Picture and Television Engineers, SMPTE* founded in 1916, is an international professional association, based in the United States, of engineers working in the motion imaging industries. SMPTE is a test pattern used to measure the resolution of a digital system. In checking the communication between the printer and the detector the pattern can be printed and values calculated (the test pattern can be displayed on a monitor to check the monitor). CNR checks consistency of image contrast and is a measure of contrast to noise ratio. Contrast is the minimum density difference between 2 tissues that can be detected in the image as different densities. Signal-to-noise ratio (SNR) is a measurement of noise and noise is the random background information—due to constant flow of current in the circuit. Noise does not contribute to image quality. On the digital, image noise looks like quantum mottle. The flat field test checks the monitor for brightness nonuniformity, high-frequency modulation (HFM), SNR nonuniformity, bad region of interest (ROI), or bad pixel verification. The flat field test should be performed before phantom tests (Figure 2-14).[3,7]

38. **(D)** Grids are not used with magnification mammography, Hologic tomosynthesis—a flat-panel detector system—and photon-counting systems. In the photon-counting system x-rays leave the x-ray tube via a slit scanning device and passes through a slot collimator before entering the breast. After leaving the breast, the beam again passes through a slot collimator before the individual rays are collected by the detector. The overall effect of the double collimation is a 97% reduction in scatter. By virtually eliminating scatter, a grid is not necessary, allowing a further reduction in patient dose. In the Hologic digital tomosynthesis system,

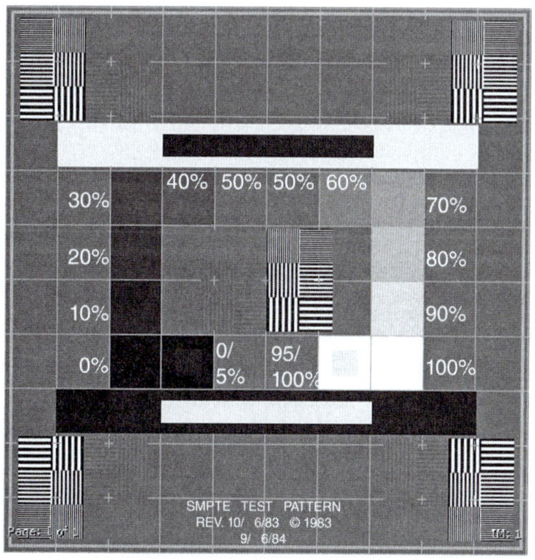

Figure 2-14. A SMPTE test pattern. (Reproduced with permission from Peart O: Mammography and Breast Imaging PREP: Program Review and Exam Prep. New York, NY: McGraw-Hill Education; 2012.)

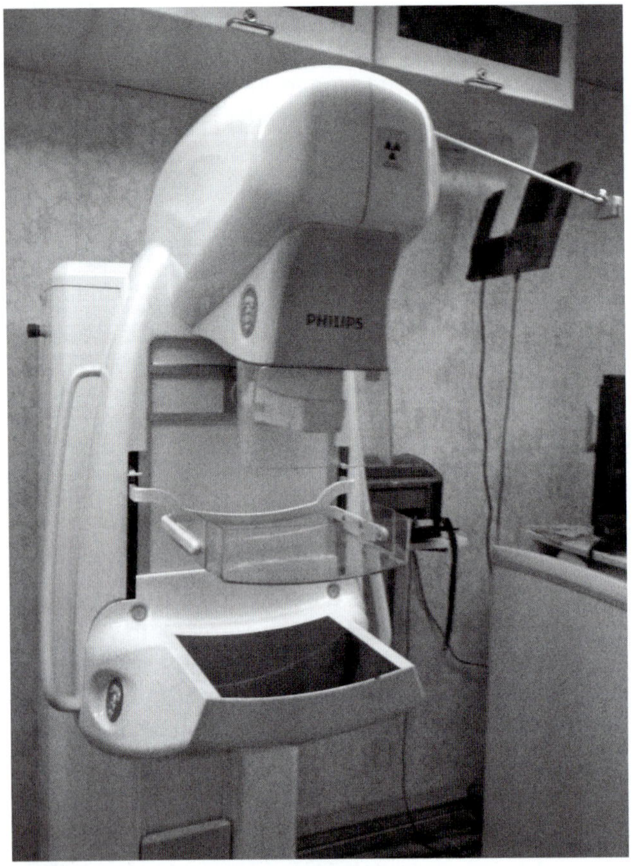

A

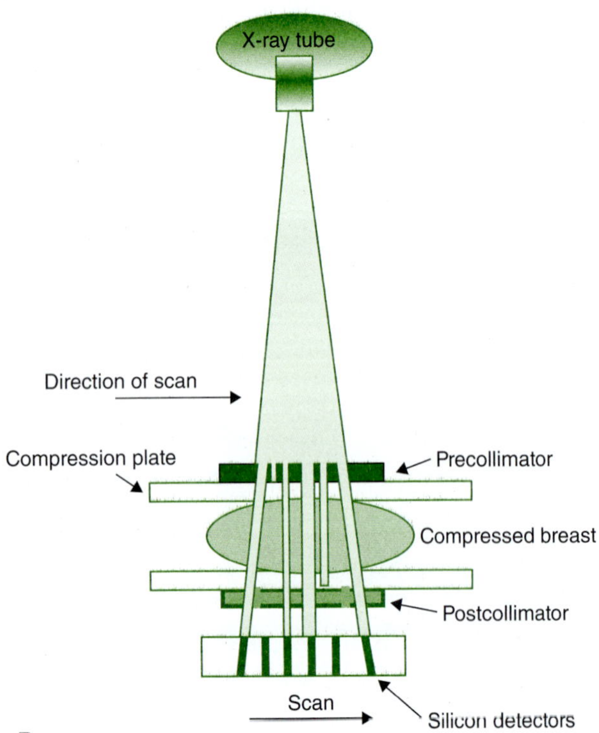

B

Figure 2-15. (A) Photon-counting unit. (B) The photon-counting systems utilize slit scanning and a precollimation and postcollimation system to reduce scatter.

the image contrast is provided by the tomographic image reconstruction processes. Magnification mammography utilizes the air gap which effectively removes scatter. Computed mammography (CM) uses a grid to control scattered radiation. The system adapts an analog imaging system to digital. It uses an imaging plate (IP) instead of a cassette. The IP contains the photostimulable phosphor (PSP). After the exposure the IP is physically removed from the unit and inserted into the computer reader for processing (Figure 2-15).[6,11,12]

39. **(A)** Aluminum (Al) is used as the filtration in Hologic digital tomosynthesis units and photon-counting imaging systems to allow higher energy x-ray and therefore reduce breast dose.

- For example, 0.70 mm Al for tomosynthesis
- For example, 0.50 mm Al for photon counting

In analog units, the filters used are often the same element as the x-ray tube target. Matching the filter to the same element as the x-ray tube target will allow the K-characteristic x-rays, produced with molybdenum and rhodium targets, to pass while blocking the higher and lower energy Bremsstrahlung x-rays.

- Molybdenum (Mo) targets
  - For example, 0.03 mm Mo (30 μm Mo) filtration or 50 μm Rh filtration
- Rhodium (Rh) targets
  - For example, 0.025 mm Rh (25 μm Rh) filtration

If the tube target is tungsten, rhodium (Rh) can be used for fatty breast and silver (Ag) for large or dense breast.

- For example, 0.05 mm Rh
- For example, 0.05 mm Ag

Some tungsten targets use molybdenum (Mo) for fatty breast and rhodium (Rh) for dense breast.[1]

40. **(C)** Detector elements (DELs or dexels) are located on the thin-film transistor and are a part of the complex circuit device of the TFT. The DEL is the sensitive component of the TFT that collects electrons emitted from either a-Se or a-Si and represent individual components of a digital image. DEL size controls the recorded detail, or spatial resolution, for the flat-panel device. Automatic exposure control (AEC) in analog imaging is used to control the length of the exposure therefore determining the density of the final image. IP is a rigid cassette device with a radiolucent front, made of a hard plastic or similar radiolucent material to allow x-rays to enter and expose the PSP. X-ray photon energy strikes the phosphor crystals in the PSP to form the latent image in CM systems.[1,3]

41. **(B)** DEL size is set by the manufacturers and is not under the technologist's control. The DELs or dexels are located within rows and columns on the TFT and are part of the complex circuit device of the TFT. DEL is the sensitive component of the TFT that collects electrons emitted from either a-Se or a-Si to represent individual components of a digital image. After the exposure, the DELs read those electrons in a sequential pattern that matches their location within the detector matrix.[1,3]

42. **(C)** Tubes are positioned with an SID of about 65 cm. Therefore in order to achieve adequate coverage on the anterior side of the field, and also to allow the central axis of the x-ray beam to run perpendicular to the plane of the detector at the chest wall, the tube must be tilted so that the effective anode angle (actual anode angle plus the physical tube tilt) is at least 22 degrees for coverage of a 24 × 30 cm field area. A tube with a 0-degree anode angle requires a tube tilt of about 22 degrees to achieve an effective anode angle of 22 degrees. A 16-degree anode angle requires a tube tilt of 6 degrees for an effective angle of 22 degrees[1,3] (Figure 2-16).

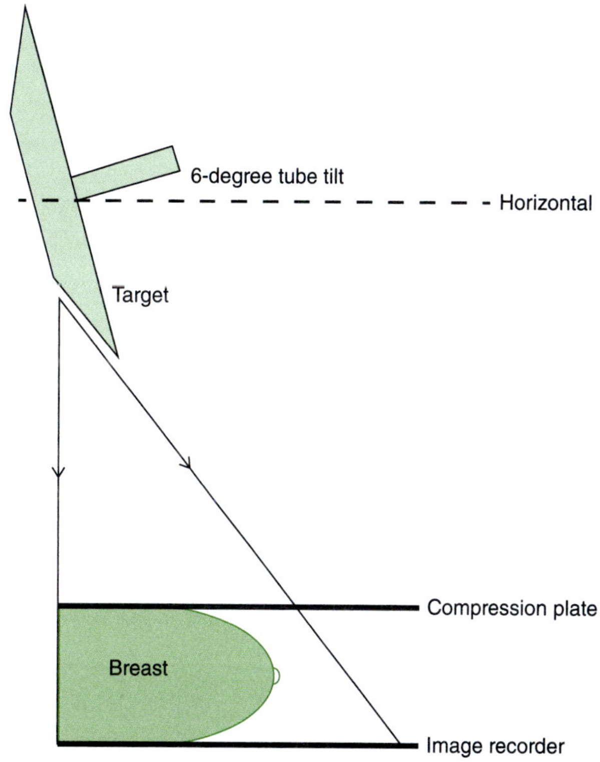

Figure 2-16. Tubes are positioned with an SID of about 65 cm; therefore, in order to achieve adequate field coverage on the anterior side of the field, and also to allow the central axis of the x-ray beam to run perpendicular to the plane of the IP at the chest wall, the tube must be tilted so that the effective anode angle (actual anode angle plus the physical tube tilt) is at least 22 degrees for coverage of a 24 x 30 cm field area. A tube with a 0-degree anode angle requires a tube tilt of about 22 degrees and a tube with 16-degree anode angle requires a tube tilt of 6 degrees.

References

1. Bushberg JT, Seibert JA, Meidholdt EM, Boone JM. Mammography. In: *The Essential Physics of Medical Imaging*. 3rd ed. Philadelphia, PA: Lippincott Williams & Wilkins; 2012:238-281.
2. Selenia Dimensions with acquisition workstation 8000. Product and Clinical Education Training manuals. Courtesy of Hologic Inc. www.hologic.com. Accessed December 2013.
3. Bushong SC. Advanced x-ray imaging. In: *Radiologic Science for Technologists—Physics, Biology and Protection*. 10th ed. St. Louis, MO: Mosby; 2004:371-384.
4. Fosbinder R, Orth D. Special imaging techniques. In: *Essentials of Radiologic Science*. Philadelphia, PA: Lippincott Williams & Wilkins; 2012:204-252.
5. Peart O. Mammography equipment. In: *Mammography and Breast Imaging: Prep*. New York, NY: McGraw-Hill; 2012:117-156.
6. Bushong SC. The radiographic image. In: *Radiologic Science for Technologists—Physics, Biology and Protection*. 10th ed. St. Louis, MO: Mosby; 2004:161-264.
7. Papp J. Mammography quality standards. In: *Quality Management in the Imaging Sciences*. 3rd ed. St. Louis, MO: Mosby; 2006:195-229.
8. Peart O. The US Mammography Quality Standard Act (MQSA). In: *Mammography and Breast Imaging: Prep*. New York, NY: McGraw-Hill; 2012:437-500.

9. Compliance Guidance: The Mammography Quality Standards Act Final Regulations: Preparing For MQSA Inspections; Final. http://www.fda.gov/MedicalDevices/DeviceRegulationandGuidance/GuidanceDocuments/ucm094420.htm. Last Updated: 07/19/2013. Accessed March 24, 2014.
10. Bushong SC. X-radiation. In: *Radiologic Science for Technologists—Physics, Biology and Protection.* 10th ed. St. Louis, MO: Mosby; 2004:83-160.
11. Weigel S, Berkemeyer S, Girnus R, et al. Digital mammography screenning with photon-counting technique: can a high diagnostic performance be realized at low mean glandular dose? In: *Radiology,* 2014; 271:345-355.
12. Schmitzberger FF, Fallenberg EM, Lawaczeck R, et al. Development of low-dose photon-counting contrast-enhanced tomosynthesis with spectral imaging. In: *Radiology* 2011; 259:259-564.

CHAPTER 3

Anatomy, Physiology, and Pathology of the Breast

Summary of Important Points

MAMMARY GLANDS

- Mammary glands are accessory glands of the female reproductive system. They are a specific type of sudoriferous or apocrine sweat glands specialized in manufacturing colostrums and milk, which is needed for the newborn. Mammary glands are also sometimes referred to as modified sebaceous glands.
- In humans the mammary glands are also regarded as a sexual asset therefore the loss or scarring of these glands can have devastating psychological implication for women.

Shape and Size of the Breast

- Spherical in shape with size varying with age, menstrual cycle, and lactation.
- Hormonal stimulation causes the breasts to grow, and will also affect breast shape and size.

Muscles Associated with the Breast

- The pectoralis major muscle lies immediately below the breast.
- Serratus anterior lies to the lateral aspect of each breast.
- The pectoralis minor muscle, a thin flat triangular muscle, lies deep to the pectoralis major muscle and covers the serratus anterior and the external oblique muscles.
- The latissimus dorsi muscle runs from the lateral aspect of the breast across the midaxillary line to the lower back.

Retromammary Space

- The retromammary space is a layer of adipose or fatty tissue that separates the breast from the pectoral muscle.
- The retromammary space is seen on the mediolateral projection in mammography imaging but only on 20% of the craniocaudal projections.

Exact Location of the Breast

- The breast extends vertically from the clavicle at the second or third rib, to meet the abdominal wall at the level of the sixth or seventh rib.
- Medially the breast extends from the midsternum to the midaxillary line and to the latissimus dorsi muscle, laterally.

Surface Anatomy of the Breast

- **The skin** of the breast, like the skin of the body, is filled with sweat glands, sebaceous glands (oil glands), and hair follicles that produce hair on the skin surface. The skin of the breast is thickest at the base, thinning as it approaches the nipple.
- **The nipple** lies at the center point of the breast. The nipple itself contains multiple crevices, within which are 15-20 orifices, or ducts that transfer milk from the lactiferous ducts to the exterior. Normally the nipple can be either flattened or inverted, both unilaterally and bilaterally. However, a nipple that suddenly becomes inverted or flattened can indicate malignancy.
- **The areola is** the smooth, circular darkened area surrounding the nipple and contains many small protrusions on its surface called

Morgagni tubercles. These tubercles are formed by opening of the ducts of the Montgomery glands, specialized sebaceous-type glands found on the areola. *Montgomery glands* usually become more prominent during pregnancy and lactation. The glands secrete a fatty lubricant, which protects the nipple during nursing.

- The pigmentation of the areola is partly dependent on estrogen levels. In younger women it is more prominent, but tends to fade at menopause. However, estrogen use at any age will increase pigmentation of the areola.

Location Terminology

- The breast is generally described in terms of the face of a clock or 4 quadrants. The breast can also be divided into 4 regions.

Four-Quadrant Method

- The 4 quadrants are: the upper-outer quadrant (UOQ), upper-inner quadrant (UIQ), lower-outer quadrant (LOQ), and lower-inner quadrant (LIQ). The exact locations within the quadrant are represented by viewing each breast separately as a clock face. The UOQ, which extends toward the axilla, is known as the axillary tail, tail of the breast or tail of Spence.

Clock Face

- Viewed as a clock, there are 4 main clock positions (12 o'clock, 3 o'clock, 6 o'clock, and 9 o' clock).

Region Method

- The breast can also be divided into 4 regions. The posterior region is closest to the chest wall. The middle region refers to the middle of the breast and the anterior region is located behind the nipple. There is also the subareola region immediately behind the areola.

Deep Anatomy of the Breast

- The breast is made up of a varying mixture of adipose or fatty tissue, glandular or secretory components, lymphatic vessels, and blood vessels.
- The fibrous and glandular tissues within the breast are generally described as fibroglandular densities.
- In general, the amount of fat and glandular tissue varies with age. Glandular tissue predominates in younger women, whereas fatty tissue predominates in older patients.
- Fatty tissue is more radiolucent and therefore shows as higher optical density areas on mammograms, while fibrous and glandular tissue are less radiolucent and will show as lower optical density on the mammograms.
- The pattern and distribution of the glandular tissue is usually the same bilaterally with most glandular breast tissue found centrally, extending laterally toward the axilla in the UOQ.
- *Cooper ligaments* are fibrous bands that predominate in the upper parts of the breast where they are also called suspensory ligaments.

Arterial Supply

- The breast receives its arterial supply from the axillary artery via the lateral thoracic artery and acromiothoracic branches. Perforating branches of the internal thoracic artery and the intercostal artery also supply the breast. Arteries appear as low-density structures on the radiograph. However, they can be sharply outlined when calcified.

Veins Drainage

- Veins form a venous network under the nipple called the circulus venous. This network then drains into the axillary and internal mammary veins. Mammographically, they appear as low-density radiopaque vessels. Like arteries, veins can be outlined by calcifications. Veins are larger and more superficially located than arteries.

Lymphatic Drainage

- There are both superficial and a deep plexus of lymphatic vessels draining the breast. The main direction of drainage from the central and lateral half of the breast tends to be into the pectoral group of axillary lymph nodes and from the medial half into the internal mammary lymph nodes. From the internal mammary nodes drainage tends toward the mediastinal nodes and others may cross the costal margin therefore communicating with the opposite breast.

The Lymph Node

- A typical lymph node is less than 2 cm in size and has a kidney-shaped appearance.

Nervous Supply

- The breast is supplied with sensory and sympathetic functions by the anterior and lateral cutaneous branches of the fourth, fifth, and sixth intercostal nerves.

Ductal System

- The ductal system begins with the lobules deep in the breast. Milk produced in the lobules travel through the segmental or mammary ducts to the nipple. The ducts gradually increase in size as they approach the nipple. Immediately behind the nipple is the pouch-like orifice called the ampulla or lactiferous sinus. Between the nipple orifice and the ampulla is a connecting duct called the lactiferous duct.

Terminal Ductal Lobular Unit

Milk production begins in the lobule or terminal ductal lobular unit (TDLU). They have the most rapidly dividing cells.

Lobes

- The average female breast will eventually develop 15-20 lobes containing numerous glandular lobules held together by connective tissue, blood vessels, and mammary ducts.

Each of the 15-20 lobes in the breast contains a tree-like pattern of ductal structures radiating out from the nipple. Each lobe can have 10-100 terminal ductules.

Factors Affecting Breast Tissue

Increased or decreased glandularity of the breast can be related to *menarche or hormonal fluctuations* whether normal or synthetic, pregnancy, lactation, or menopause. Increase in glandularity is also dependent on a woman's genetic predisposition.

Age

- The female breasts are inactive during childhood because there are no lobules. The breast will consist of small ducts within fibrous tissue. As the female ages, the ovaries begin to produce estrogen and progesterone and breast development begins.

Hormones

- At puberty the secondary sex characteristics including the breast will manifest and a woman begins to menstruate. This first menses is called menarche.
- The 2 most prominent hormones, active in breast development are *estrogen*, which is responsible for ductal proliferation, and *progesterone*, which is responsible for lobular proliferation and growth. Estrogen and progesterone are produced by the ovaries. The production of both hormones will also affect menstrual cycle and pregnancy.
- Once a woman starts producing estrogen the changes in the breast can be spotty causing lumps or increased interstitial fluids (cysts), but will generally result in an overall increased glandular tissue.
- During each menstrual cycle there is fluctuation in the hormone levels in the body, which causes structural changes in the breast tissue. The breast can increase in size, density, and nodularity, as well as sensitivity, during the 3-4 day prior to the start of menstruation. Within 5-10 days after the start of the menstrual period this condition will diminish.

Lactation

- Changes in the breast will begin within the first few weeks of conception. The corpus luteum and the placenta both produce estrogen and progesterone and will influence the proliferation and development of the mammary tissues. Lactation is made possible by the production of the hormones prolactin and secretions from the adrenal cortex. The lobules become bigger and increase in size, the alveoli are dilated and the lactiferous ducts are distended with milk. The overall effect is a denser and larger breast.

Parity

- Parity is the terminology used if a woman carries a pregnancy to a point of viability (24-26 weeks of gestation) regardless of the outcome.

Weight Gain or Loss

- Both conditions can change the tissue composition by increasing or decreasing the fat content of the breast tissue, thereby affecting the overall glandularity of the breast.

Involution

- The young breast will have fibroglandular tissue with very little fat. Gradually the percentage of ovulation cycles will decrease and the level of estrogen and progesterone in the body begins to fluctuate. This period for women is called perimenopause and can last several years. During this time the breast undergoes involution where the glandular, supportive, and connective tissue is replaced by fatty tissue producing a smaller breast or a larger more pendulous one. Involution will occur normally with age. Atrophy of the glandular tissue generally begins first in the medial posterior aspect of the breast then moves forward to the nipple.

- Although this composition change takes place as a woman ages, it is still possible to find older women with extremely dense, glandular breast.

Menopause

- At menopause generally there is atrophy of mammary structures. The ovarian hormones are no longer stimulated and the secretory cells and alveoli will degenerate.
- Menopause does not officially begin until a woman is period free without spotting, being pregnant, breast-feeding, taking medications, or surgery for at least a year. Menopause can occur anytime between ages 45 and 54.

Hormone Replacement Therapy

- Hormone replacement therapy (HRT) will increase the amount of glandular tissue in the breast of menopausal women, making the breast appear denser on mammograms. It also appears that HRT inhibits the involution process. HRT also causes increase in the size of fibroadenomas and the development or increase in the size of cysts in the breast.

Positive Effects of HRT

- With menopause comes a drop in estrogen and progesterone with resultant symptoms that can last for years and can vary tremendously from woman to woman. The most common symptoms are hot flashes or flushes, sweats, and sleep disturbances. Women can also experience mood swings, irritability, fatigue, osteoporosis, vaginal dryness, memory loss, and insomnia. But the drop in estrogen also can contribute to other symptoms, such as changes in the vaginal and urinary tracts, which often causes painful intercourse, urinary infections, and the need to urinate more often. HRT relieves most of the symptoms of menopause.

Negative Effects of HRT

- The use of estrogen alone is known to promote the enlargement of cysts and fibroadenomas and a combination of estrogen and progesterone are often associated with diffuse increasing densities in the breast that can mimic carcinoma.
- New studies continue to find negative effects from long-term use of HRT. Results of the Women's Health Initiative Memory Study (WHIMS) published in May 2003 in the Journal of the American Medical Association (JAMA) showed that women who use HRT appear to be at increased risk for developing breast and uterine cancer and also asthma. Although the risk of asthma is still low the study also found women older than 65 years were at an increased risk for dementia. Recent studies have also linked HRT with an increased risk for heart attacks and strokes.

Visualization of Breast Tissue on the Mammogram

- Mammographically, the breast will be visualized as less dense areas of fat (which appear black on the radiograph) and denser glandular areas (which appear white or gray on the radiograph). Often blood vessels can be seen, especially if they are calcified, and occasionally lymph nodes are visualized within the breast as kidney-shaped oval densities with lucent centers.

Breast Augmentation

- The process of increasing the size of the breast is termed augmentation. Common methods include using saline or silicone implants.
- Implants can be placed in front of the pectoral muscle (subglandular or retromammary implants) or behind the pectoral muscle (subpectoral or retropectoral implants).

Breast Reduction

- Reduction is a technique used to reduce total breast size for cosmetic or medical reasons such as macromastia (large breast) or postsurgery to maintain equal breast size. Most techniques involve elevation of the nipple and removal of some of the glandular tissue.

Classifying Lesions

- A lesion can only be classified by a histological or cytological analysis.

Halo Sign

- The halo is a curved radiopaque line seen around lesions containing fat. Lesions with a "halo" sign usually indicate the presence of a benign lesion, e.g., a cyst. The absence of a halo does not necessarily prove malignancy.

Skin Lesions

- Occasionally a skin lesion can mimic a breast lesion because the mammographic images are 2-dimensional. The lesion will appear to lie within the breast tissue. Skin lesions can include moles, keratosis, skin tags, and epidermoid cysts.

Characteristics of Benign Lesions

- Circumscribed—circular or oval in size/shape. The most common circular oval lesions are cysts and the fibroadenomas. They can be poorly outlined/obscured, lobulated, solitary, or multiple. These are often aligned with the trabecular structures of the breast. They are often symptomatic and are detected by the patient as a palpable mass.
- Low density or radiolucent. In these lesions the surrounding parenchymal structures can be seen through the lesion, e.g., lipoma, galactocele, fibroadenoma, cyst.
- Radiolucent and radiopaque combined. It may be more difficult to visualize the parenchymal structures through these lesions, e.g., lymph node, fibroadenolipoma, galactocele, and hematoma.
- *Halo sign*: A lesion with a halo can suggest a cyst although the content must be assessed. Malignant exceptions are: intracystic carcinoma, papillary carcinoma, carcinoma within a fibroadenoma.

Characteristics of Malignant Lesions

- A spiculated border is a strong indication for malignancy. However, these are indicators only, and will not necessarily determine the presence or absence of carcinomas.
- Irregular or obscured borders. If the borders are obscured more testing may be needed.
- Multiple lobulated and randomly orientated (not aligned along the trabecular structure of the breast), e.g., sarcomas.
- Radiopaque and high-density radiopaque. High-density lesions where the trabeculae cannot be seen through the lesion are often malignant, although some structures such as veins are high density and benign. Malignant examples are invasive ductal carcinoma or sarcoma. Other benign exceptions are: abscess, calcified hematoma, calcified galactocele, and epidermoid cyst.

Characteristics of Spiculated or Stellate Lesions

- These lesions can have a solid central tumor with radiating structures and ill-defined borders.
- Breast cancer can present mammographically as a spiculated lesion, although a very small spiculated lesion can be difficult to perceive.
- With malignant spiculated lesions, if the spicules reach the skin, muscle, or areola region, it can cause retraction and disruption of the lymphatics, leading to localized skin thickening.
- Benign lesions such as postsurgical fibrosis, fat necrosis, abscess, and hematomas can mimic spiculated lesions.

Changing Lesion Size

- Generally, benign lesions will not change much in size or shape over time or will grow evenly, whereas a malignant lesion can grow significantly over a 1-year period.

Architectural Distortion

- Asymmetric breast tissue is usually identified when comparing one breast with the other. The breasts usually present a mirror image although 3%-5% of normal breast can show asymmetric densities in the outer quadrant or axillary tail.
- Areas of architectural distortion can represent a malignancy or a benign process such as surgical scars, sclerosing lesions, or posttraumatic fat necrosis.
- In-drawing or tenting of the breast parenchyma can be a sign of malignancy.

Calcification Morphology

- Calcifications within the breast may or may not be associated with a tumor, but should be evaluated separately from any associated tumor. Magnification mammography technique is extremely useful in evaluating calcification. Morphology as it relates to calcifications describes the form and structure of the calcifications, e.g., coarse, linear, round, casting, amorphous, or pleomorphic.
  - **Density**—Low- or high-density radiopaque and any combination in between.
  - **Distribution**—Placement of the calcifications within the breast.
  - **Change over time**—Variation in density, distribution, number, morphology, or size over time.
  - **Number**—Single or in clusters where a cluster of microcalcifications are described as 3-5 calcifications within an area no larger than 0.5-1 cm.
  - **Size**—Varying from microcalcifications in the millimeter range to macrocalcifications in the centimeter range. Malignant-type calcifications are often microcalcifications.
  - **Coarse**—Calcifications larger than 0.5 mm in diameter.
  - **Linear or rod-like**—Calcifications over 1 mm in diameter and often associated with ducts.
  - **Round or punctuate**—if the calcifications are smaller than 0.5 mm in diameter.
  - **Casting type**—Fine, linear, or branching calcifications that can be fragmented with irregular contours and are often malignant.
  - **Amorphous or indistinct**—Calcifications forming multiple flake-like irregular clusters that can be micro or macro and typically of intermediate concern.
  - **Pleomorphic or granular**—Calcification of different shapes, irregular in form, size, and density and are typically malignant.

Benign Breast Calcifications

Appearance

- Smooth contours, high uniform density, e.g., plasma cell mastitis.
- Evenly scattered, homogenous, e.g., calcified arteries.
- Sharply outlined, spherical or oval, e.g., oil cysts.
- Pear-like densities resemble teacups or pearl drops on the lateral projection, e.g., milk of calcium.
- Bilateral and evenly scattered following the course of the ducts throughout much of the parenchyma, e.g., plasma cell mastitis.
- Ring-like, hollow, e.g., sebaceous gland calcifications.
- Eggshell-like, e.g., oil cyst, papilloma.
- Large bizarre size, e.g., hemangiomas.

- **Milk of calcium** is often due to cystic changes and can be associated with a micro cyst containing granules of calcified debris (milk of calcium). The calcifications are located within the lobules and because they are mobile, they will take the shape of the cavity where they are located. On the 90-degree lateral they will settle in the dependent portion of the lobules and are viewed as a crescent shape, resembling a teacup.
- **Dermal calcifications** are calcifications in the skin.
- **Sutural calcifications** are often seen in the breast after surgery and radiation therapy. Effects from radiation therapy may cause delays in the reabsorption of sutures. Calcium deposits on the sutures over time. These calcifications have a tubular appearance and are rarely seen if the patient does not have a history of radiation therapy.
- **Vascular calcifications** are calcified arteries or veins. Vascular calcifications are very distinctive and are seen mammographically as 2 parallel lines or broken tubular patterns.
- **Oil cysts** show mammographically as high-density tumors with lucent centers and eggshell-like calcifications. They usually form as a result of fat necrosis or are calcifying hematomas.
- **Sclerosing adenosis or ductal hyperplasia** is usually a result of increased cellular activity in the ducts and surrounding tissues. The condition can produce calcifications that tend to be linear and segmental but are sometimes malignant appearing.
- **Ductal ectasia or plasma cell mastitis** produces large calcifications that are the result of secretions within dilated ducts, whether periductal or intraductal. Periductal calcifications will have radiolucent centers representing the noncalcified centers of the duct. Because the

calcifications are within the ducts they are linear and fragmental, forming along the long axis and pointing toward the nipple with only occasionally branching. Often these calcifications are bilateral and symmetrical in distribution.

Skin Thickening Syndrome

- Skin thickening can be the result of benign or malignant causes. Some causes include:
  - Late malignancy either from direct invasion by the tumor or obstruction of the lymphatic or venous return.
  - Inflammatory carcinoma will often result in diffuse unilateral skin thickening because there is direct tumor invasion of the dermal lymphatics.
  - Infection and axillary lymphatic obstruction. These conditions can be secondary to breast carcinoma, metastases, or lymphomas.
  - Radiation to the axilla.
  - Cardiac failure or vena cava obstruction.
  - Chronic renal failure.

Peau d'orange is used to describe generalized skin thickening. The skin will appear obviously thickened, most often in the lower dependent portion of the breast and takes on the appearance of an orange skin with prominent pores, hence the term—*Peau d'orange.* Mammographically, because the overall density of the breast is increased due to the high fluid content, there is a coarse reticular pattern on the mammogram.

MALIGNANT DISEASES

Location of the Breast Cancers

- The majority of breast diseases occur in the TDLUs; however, cancer can also grow in fibrous tissue, connective tissue, and larger ducts.

Common Breast Cancers

- The 2 main classifications of breast cancer are ductal and lobular carcinoma. Ductal carcinoma is the most common, accounting for about 90% of all breast cancers. Lobular carcinoma accounts for 5%-10% of all breast cancers.
  - Ductal carcinoma in situ: The cancer is confined to the duct and does not invade the duct walls. There is a lot of controversy on the cancerous nature of this condition. This is commonly referred to as stage 0 carcinoma.
  - Invasive or infiltrating ductal carcinoma: The cancer has spread from the ducts into the surrounding stromal tissue and may or may not extend into the pectoral fascia and muscle.
  - Lobular carcinoma in situ is often not seen mammographically. The abnormal cells grow within the lobules but do not penetrate through the lobule walls. Lobular carcinoma in situ is sometimes referred to as lobular neoplasia and it is often considered to be a premalignant lesion that identifies women at an increased risk for subsequent development of invasive breast cancer.
  - Invasive lobular carcinoma is often difficult to perceive on a mammogram and is better visualized using other modalities.

Other Breast Cancers

- Inflammatory, infiltrating medullary, mucinous or colloid, comedo, tubular, mucinous, papillary, and other breast cancers account for less than 10% of the total breast cancer cases and, apart from inflammatory carcinoma, they all have a better prognosis than infiltrating ductal or infiltrating lobular cancers.

Mammography Terminology

- **Adenosis** is enlargement and/or development of new lobular units.
- **Apocrine metaplasia** is a change occurring in the epithelial cells which exhibit characteristics of apocrine sweat glands.
- **Biopsy** is the pathologic examination of body tissue that has been removed from the body.
- **Carcinoma** is a malignant neoplasm or growth that can be visualized on a mammogram.
- **Cysts** occur in the TDLU when the extralobular terminal duct becomes blocked. The normal ductal secretions are not reabsorbed quickly enough and fluid begins to accumulate. Accumulating fluid causes pressure and the TDLU loses its shape as the cyst is formed.
- **Duct ectasia** is a benign process consisting of widened ducts containing thickened material. The cause is unknown.
- **Epithelial hyperplasia** describes an increase in the number of epithelial cells lining the duct. Certain stages can be considered premalignant.

- **Fibroadenoma** is a radiographically dense, encapsulated, round, and movable benign tumor seen frequently in women younger than 30 years. It develops from epithelial and fibroblastic tissue brought on by higher than normal estrogen levels.
- **Fibrosis** is the formation of fibrous tissue stemming from the connective and supportive stroma. Upon autopsy, up to 50% of all women have been found to have fibrocystic breasts.
- **Fibrocystic changes** represent development of benign cystic spaces within the ducts due to monthly hormone fluctuations that cause cysts to form throughout the breast tissue. Fibrocystic changes can mask or hide other malignant tumors.
- **Fine-needle aspiration** is a biopsy technique using a fine needle to aspirate or remove cells from a localized breast lesion for pathologic evaluation.
- **Gynecomastia** is the most common disorder that results in excessive development of the male breast from physiologic, hormonal, or pharmacologic causes.
- **Hormone replacement therapy** (HRT) is the prescribing of hormones for postmenopausal women to maintain their hormone levels to decrease symptoms and complications that could arise from declining estrogen levels.
- **Intraductal papilloma** is a benign, lobulated neoplasm, composed of benign epithelial tissue and located in the walls of ducts of the breast. It has a "berry-like" shape.
- **Involution** is the process of lobular regression. As a woman ages, the lobules will reduce in number and size with a decrease in the number of acini per lobule. The acini are the milk producing elements in the lobules. There is also replacement of the intralobular stroma with the dense collagen of breast connective tissue and over time there is progressive fatty replacement of the glandular elements.
- **Lactation** describes milk secretion from the breast.
- **Lumpectomy** is the removal of a tumor with excision of surrounding tissue. Lymph nodes are sometimes removed during the procedure.
- **Mammography Quality Standards (MQSA)** is the legislation passed by the United States Congress on October 1994, to ensure quality mammograms for all patients and to improve and standardize breast imaging.
- **Mastectomy** is the removal of the breast.
- **Mastitis** is inflammation of breast tissue.
- **Mastorrhagia** is the copious discharge of blood from the breast.
- **Microcalcifications** are minute calcium deposits in the breast that could possible indicate the presence of malignancy, although they can be benign.
- **Multiparity** is the condition of having carried more than 1 pregnancy past the point of viability (24-26 weeks of gestation) regardless of the outcome.
- **Nulliparity** describes a woman who has never given birth to a viable offspring. The nulliparous breast involutes more slowly than that of multiparous women and multiparity is generally associated with breasts that involute earlier.
- **Parity** is a condition of being pregnant and carrying a pregnancy past the point of viability or delivering a child.
- **Postsurgical scarring** can mimic a radial scar. It follows a surgical intervention and can appear as an area of architectural distortion or an irregular shaped lesion with spiculated margins. It may or may not be associated with calcifications. Typically, the surgical scar will resolve over time.
- **Radial scar** has a central fibrous core with radiating arms made up of benign epithelial growth and sclerosis .They are not truly scars and are often unrelated to prior surgery or trauma. Some possible causes of the radial scar are localized inflammatory reaction or chronic ischemia with a slow infection. The radial scar can be a benign condition, but can be associated with premalignant—atypical ductal hyperplasia—and malignant conditions.
- **Sclerosing adenosis** is adenosis with sclerosing of the intralobular stroma. This can present as calcifications or masses and is considered benign, and not a premalignant condition.
- **Symmetry** of the breast refers to breasts that are similar in size, shape, and composition of anatomy, so that one breast is a "mirror image" of the other.

Questions

1. A lesion located in the upper-outer quadrant of the right breast is located in the
   (A) 5 o'clock position
   (B) 2 o'clock position
   (C) 10 o'clock position
   (D) 7 o'clock position

2. Morgagni tubercles are usually found
   (A) on the nipple
   (B) on the lateral border of the breast
   (C) in the terminal duct lobular unit (TDLU)
   (D) on the areola

3. An inverted nipple
   (A) always indicates breast cancer
   (B) sometimes indicates breast cancer
   (C) never indicates breast cancer
   (D) usually indicates breast cancer

4. The most mobile margins of the breast are
   (A) medial and lateral aspects
   (B) inferior and superior aspects
   (C) medial and superior aspects
   (D) inferior and lateral aspects

5. The normal breast may have
   (A) 0-5 lobes
   (B) 15-20 lobes
   (C) 30-40 lobes
   (D) 340-350 lobes

6. The structure that supports the breast and contributes to breast shape is called
   (A) Montgomery ligament
   (B) Cooper ligament
   (C) fibroglandular tissue
   (D) fatty tissue

7. The breast extends vertically from the
   (A) first through the ninth rib
   (B) second through the tenth rib
   (C) second through the sixth rib
   (D) third through the tenth rib

8. The thickest skin portion of the breast is at the
   (A) areola
   (B) nipple
   (C) tail of Spence
   (D) inframammary crease

9. Cooper ligaments attach anteriorly to the
   (A) deep fascia of the lobes
   (B) fascia of the skin
   (C) posterior surface of the breast
   (D) connective and supporting stroma

10. Fatty tissue is generally _______ and on the mammogram is seen as areas of _______ optical density.
    (A) radiolucent/lower
    (B) radiopaque/higher
    (C) radiolucent/higher
    (D) radiopaque/lower

11. Typically, a patient with dense fibrous and glandular tissue throughout the entire breast on a baseline mammogram is
    (A) age 20 or younger
    (B) between ages 50 and 60
    (C) above 70
    (D) below 45

12. Glandular tissue is usually found in the _______ of the breast.
    (A) medial and lower-inner quadrant
    (B) central and upper-outer quadrant
    (C) medial and lower-outer quadrant
    (D) central and upper-inner quadrant

13. Lymph drainage from the medial half of the breast is generally directed to the
    (A) internal mammary lymph nodes
    (B) external mammary lymph nodes
    (C) axillary lymph nodes
    (D) mediastinal nodes

14. Immediately behind the nipple, there is a widened area of the collecting duct called the
    (A) lactiferous sinus
    (B) ampulla acinus
    (C) TDLU
    (D) segmental duct

15. The portion of the breast that holds the milk-producing element is the
    (A) ampulla
    (B) segmental duct
    (C) lobule
    (D) lactiferous sinus

16. Veins are normally located
    (A) in the periphery of the breast
    (B) in the central areas of the breast
    (C) in the axilla area of the breast
    (D) in the medial areas of the breast

17. The TDLU consists of the
    (A) mammary ducts and the extralobular terminal ducts (ETDs)
    (B) intralobular terminal duct (ITD) and the segmental ducts
    (C) the ETDs and the lactiferous ducts
    (D) both the ETDs and the ITDs

18. A patient began taking synthetic hormones 6 months prior to her current mammogram. The mammogram is most likely to
    (A) be unchanged from the previous year
    (B) show increased glandular tissue when compared to her previous mammogram
    (C) show decreased glandular tissue compared to her previous mammogram
    (D) show increased fatty tissue compared to her previous mammogram

19. A baseline mammogram shows that the patient's breast consists primarily of adipose tissue. This patient is most likely to be
    (A) on hormone therapy
    (B) above 60
    (C) below 20
    (D) between 35 and 40

20. A patient is to have a routine baseline mammogram, but it is determined that the woman is lactating. What should be done and why?
    (A) Lactating breasts are extremely sensitive to compression; the mammogram should be postponed.
    (B) The mammogram should be done; radiation has no effect on lactation.
    (C) Although lactating breasts are extremely dense, the mammogram should not be rescheduled.
    (D) Lactation results in increased glandularity; the mammogram should be postponed.

21. The craniocaudal mammograms of the same woman prior to menopause and 1 year after the onset of menopause are compared. The woman has never taken synthetic hormones. What is the most likely difference?

    (A) The mammogram taken prior to menopause shows signs of atrophy.
    (B) The mammogram taken after the onset of menopause shows signs of atrophy.
    (C) There will be little or no change in the glandularity of the breast.
    (D) The mammogram taken after menopause will show increased glandularity.

22. Which of the following will affect the ratio of glandular tissue to total breast tissue?

    1. the woman's genetic predisposition
    2. ratio of total body adipose tissue to total body weight
    3. drastic weight gain or weight loss

    (A) 1 only
    (B) 1 and 2 only
    (C) 2 and 3 only
    (D) 1, 2, and 3

23. Hormone replacement therapy could be recommended to?

    1. relieve insomnia symptoms
    2. vprevent osteoporosis
    3. reduce weight gain

    (A) 1 only
    (B) 1 and 2 only
    (C) 2 and 3 only
    (D) 1, 2, and 3

24. A woman is referred to as nullipara. This means

    (A) she has never given birth to a viable offspring
    (B) the woman has had only 1 child
    (C) the woman has given birth to more than 1 viable offspring
    (D) she carried a pregnancy past the point of viability regardless of the outcome

25. An asymptomatic patient presents with an oval, lobulated tumor with unsharp margins. There is no evidence of a halo sign.

    (A) If the lesion is also radiolucent it is likely to be benign
    (B) The lesion could be malignant
    (C) All oval lesions are benign
    (D) The absence of a halo indicates malignancy

26. The tumor seen in Figure 3-1 is characteristic of

    (A) ductal carcinoma in situ
    (B) a mammographically malignant tumor
    (C) a mammographically benign tumor
    (D) a low-density tumor typical of benign lesions

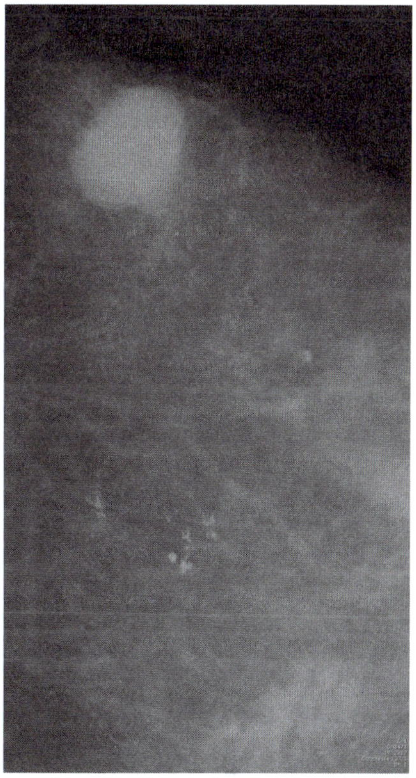

Figure 3-1.

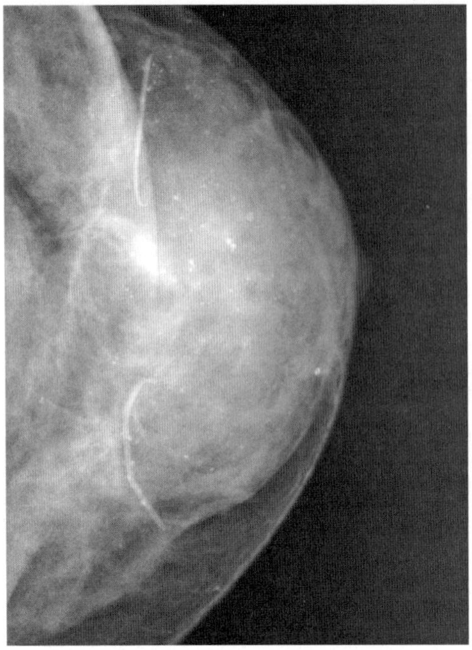

Figure 3-2.

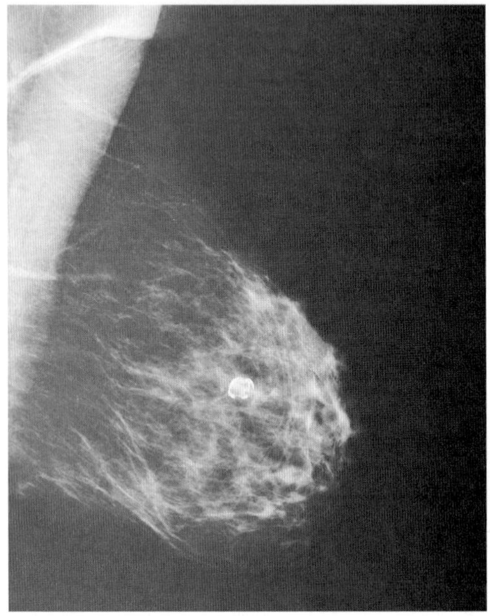

Figure 3-3. (Reproduced with permission from Peart O: Lange Q&A: Mammography Examination, 2nd ed. New York, NY: McGraw-Hill Education; 2008.)

27. The calcifications seen in Figure 3-2 have the typical appearance of

    (A) mammographically malignant-type calcifications
    (B) mammographically benign-type calcifications
    (C) calcifications typical of an oil cyst
    (D) calcified microhematomas

28. Characteristics of a malignant stellate tumor include which of the following?

    1. The spicules are generally bunched together.
    2. The presence of a central tumor mass.
    3. The larger the tumor, the longer the spicules.

    (A) 1 only
    (B) 1 and 2 only
    (C) 2 and 3 only
    (D) 1 and 3 only

29. The calcifications seen in Figure 3-3 have the typical appearance of

    (A) an oil cyst
    (B) plasma cell mastitis calcification
    (C) a small calcified hematoma
    (D) a calcified sebaceous gland

30. Postsurgical scaring

    1. can sometimes be mistaken for carcinoma
    2. has a solid dense central tumor
    3. is usually not associated with skin thickening or dimpling over the lesion

    (A) 1 only
    (B) 1 and 2 only
    (C) 2 and 3 only
    (D) 1 and 3 only

31. A mammogram shows a low-density radiopaque tumor. It is oval, lobulated, and a halo is seen along 1 border only. The next step should be

    (A) pneumocystogram
    (B) ultrasound
    (C) biopsy
    (D) no further testing; the tumor is benign

32. A galactocele

(A) is always radiolucent
(B) is usually associated with trauma
(C) is associated with nursing
(D) usually has irregular borders

33. A lipoma

(A) is generally seen as a high-density radiopaque lesion on the mammogram
(B) can be a huge encapsulated lesion occupying the entire breast
(B) may have irregular borders typical of malignant lesions
(B) is usually difficult to image mammographically

34. A rare form of cancer that presents with swelling, warmth, or erythema and mammographically with skin thickening describes

(A) inflammatory carcinoma
(B) invasive ductal carcinoma
(C) invasive lobular carcinoma
(D) papillary carcinoma

35. Sometimes described as an oil cyst, this lesion represents an encapsulated area on the mammogram and can be caused by surgery, biopsy, trauma, or radiation therapy.

(A) stellate lesion
(B) galactocele
(C) fat necrosis
(D) lipoma

36. A benign self-limiting breast tumor that is the result of new disorganized cell growth is

(A) sarcoma
(B) radial scar
(C) invasive lobular carcinoma
(D) hamartoma

37. An infusa-port can be used to

(A) provide radiation therapy treatment
(B) allow repeated access to the venous system
(C) infuse radioactive tracers directly into the breast lesion
(D) infuse radioactive isotopes directly into the arterial system

38. The low-density radiopaque lesions seen in Figure 3-4 is characteristic of a

(A) benign fibroadenoma
(B) skin mole
(C) galactocele
(D) keratosis

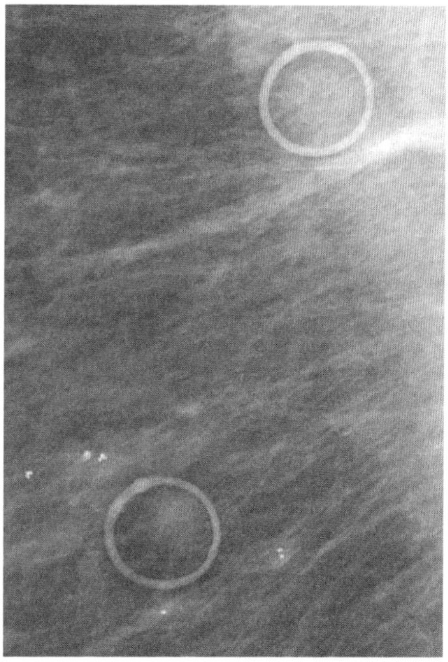

Figure 3-4.

39. The calcifications in Figure 3-5 are characteristic of

(A) a definite malignant
(B) benign skin calcifications
(C) benign calcifications but further tests are needed
(D) benign calcifications

40. The circular mixed-density lesions seen in Figure 3-6 are characteristics of

(A) calcified microhematomas
(B) galactocele, calcified
(C) malignant calcification
(D) epidermoid cyst

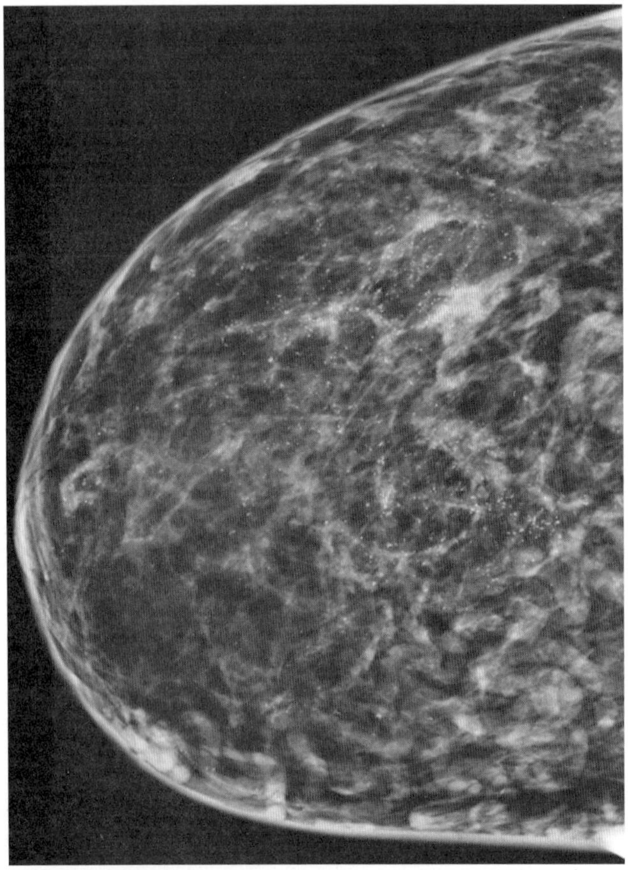

Figure 3-5.

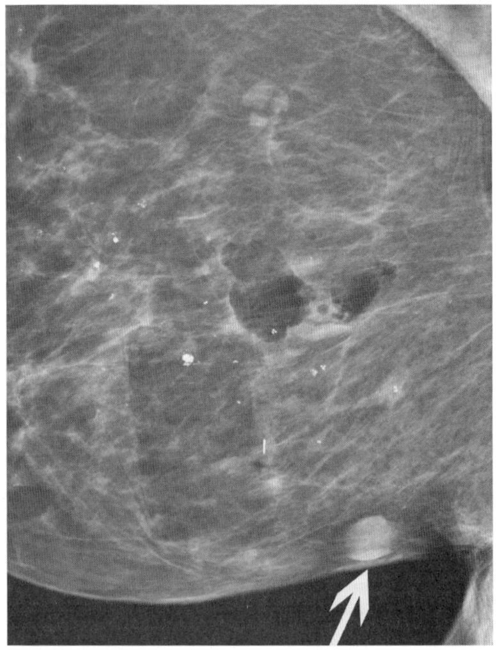

Figure 3-6. (Reproduced with permission from Peart O: Lange Q&A: Mammography Examination, 2nd ed. New York, NY: McGraw-Hill Education; 2008.)

Answers and Explanation

1. **(C)** Each breast can be divided into 4 quadrants: the upper-outer quadrant (UOQ), upper-inner quadrant (UIQ), lower-outer quadrant (LOQ), and lower-inner quadrant (LIQ). The exact locations within the quadrant are represented by viewing each breast (separately) as a clock face (Figure 3-7). Lesions can also be described in relation to the nipple (e.g., subareolar or below the nipple).[1]

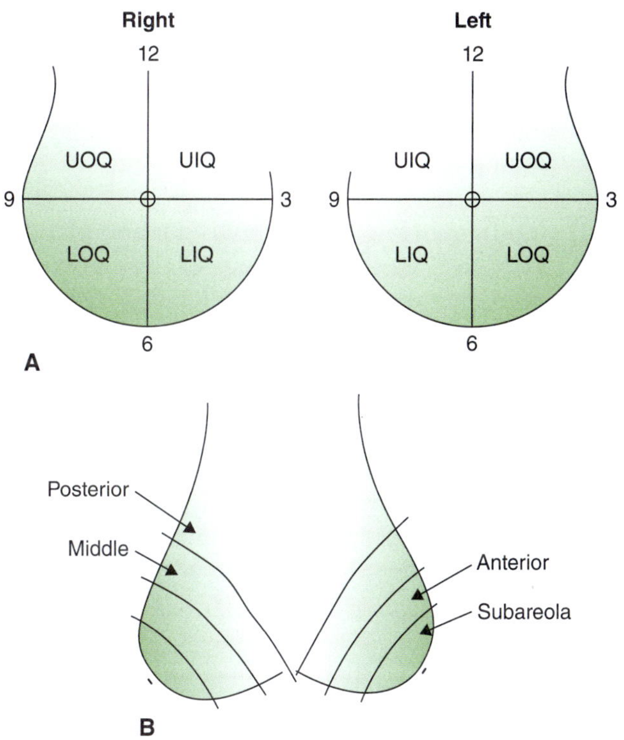

Figure 3-7. (A) Breast localization pictures. The breast can be viewed in different ways: (1) As a clock with clock-time descriptions within the breast. (2) Using the 4-quadrant method: the upper-outer quadrant (UOQ), the upper-inner quadrant (UIQ), the lower-outer quadrant (LOQ), and the lower-inner quadrant (LIQ). Note that the 4-o'clock position on the right breast represents the lower-inner quadrant but on the left breast would indicate the lower-outer quadrant. (B) Lesions can also be localized using the region method. (Reproduced with permission from Peart O: Mammography and Breast Imaging PREP: Program Review and Exam Prep. New York, NY: McGraw-Hill Education; 2012.)

2. **(D)** Morgagni tubercles are elevations formed by the opening of the ducts of the Montgomery glands, which are specialized sebaceous-type glands found on the areola, not the nipple. The terminal ductal lobular unit (TDLU), also called the lobule, is located at the very beginning of the ductal system.[1,2]

3. **(B)** The normal nipple can be either flattened or inverted, both unilaterally and bilaterally. However, a nipple that suddenly becomes inverted or flattened can indicate malignancy.[1,2]

4. **(D)** The breast is most secured at the superior and medial aspects. The lateral borders of the breast and the inferior aspect (inframammary crease) are the most mobile portions. To maximize compression of breast tissue, the most movable parts of the breast are pulled onto the detector before applying compression.[1,2]

5. **(B)** On an average, a breast has 15 lobes. The number can, however, be as low as 10 or as high as 20.[1,2]

6. **(B)** Cooper ligaments are a network of fibrous and elastic membranes. They incompletely sheath the lobes of the breast. The ligaments start at the most posterior portion (base) of the breast and extend outward to attach to the anterior superficial fascia of the skin. Fibroglandular and fatty tissues make up the breast parenchyma. Montgomery is a gland, not a ligament. It is located on the areola (Figure 3-8).[1,2]

7. **(C)** The breast extends vertically from the clavicle (the second or third rib) to meet the abdominal wall at the level of the sixth or

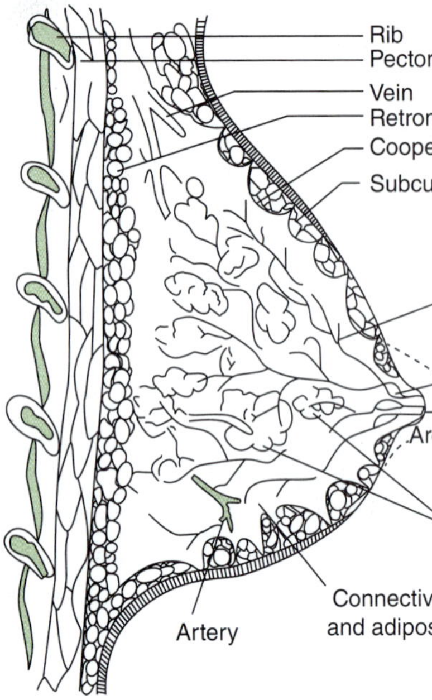

Figure 3-8. A schematic diagram showing the anatomy of the breast. (Reproduced with permission from Peart O: Lange Q&A: Mammography Examination, 2nd ed. New York, NY: McGraw-Hill Education; 2008.)

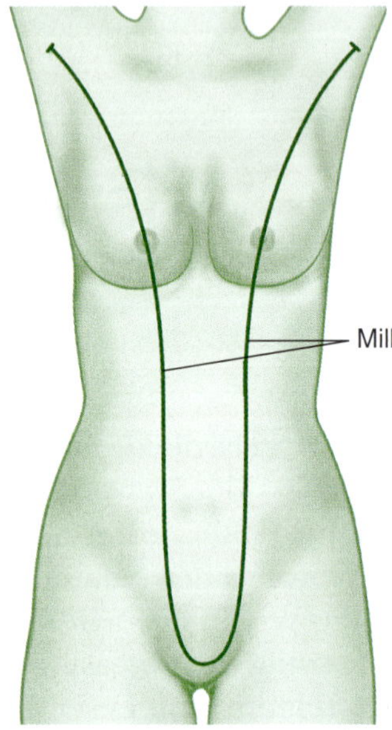

Figure 3-9. Diagram showing the milk line also called milk ridge or mammary line. This line extends from the armpits in the axilla to the groin region of the body. (Reproduced with permission from Peart O: Mammography and Breast Imaging PREP: Program Review and Exam Prep. New York, NY: McGraw-Hill Education; 2012.)

seventh rib and horizontally from the midsternum to the midaxillary line (the latissimus dorsi muscle). However, breast tissue can form anywhere along the milk ridge or line, also called the mammary line. This line extends from the armpits in the axilla to the groin region of the body (Figure 3-9).[1,2]

8. **(C)** The UOQ, which extends toward the axilla, is known as the axillary tail or the tail of Spence. It is the thickest portion of the breast. The nipple is the center point of the breast and it is surrounded by the areola. The inframammary fold or crease (IMF) is the lowest extent of the breast where it attaches to the chest wall. (See Figure 3-8.)[1,2]

9. **(B)** Cooper ligaments are strands of connective tissue that run between the skin and deep fascia to support the lobes of the breast. They start at the most posterior portion (base) of the breast, extend outward, and attach to the anterior fascia of the skin.[1,2]

10. **(C)** Fatty tissue is radiolucent and will therefore show as higher optical density areas on mammograms (black). Fibrous and glandular tissues are less radiolucent and will show as lower optical density on the mammograms (white or gray) (Figure 3-10).[1,2]

11. **(D)** In general, the amount of fat and glandular tissue varies with age. Glandular tissue predominates in younger women, whereas fatty tissue predominates in older patients. A patient below 20 is unlikely to have regular mammograms.[1,2]

12. **(B)** The majority of glandular tissue is distributed in the breast bilaterally and is located centrally and laterally toward the UOQ, extending toward the axilla. Most breast cancer arises from the glandular tissue.[1,2]

13. **(A)** The main direction of drainage from the lateral half of the breast tends to be into the pectoral group of axillary lymph nodes and from the medial half of the breast into the internal mammary lymph nodes. The axillary lymph nodes receive about three quarter of the lymphatic drainage from the breast via the pectoral lymph nodes. There are generally 20-30 axillary lymph nodes arranged in 5 groups. The anterior or pectoral group lies below the pectoralis major muscle and along the lower border of the pectoralis minor, the

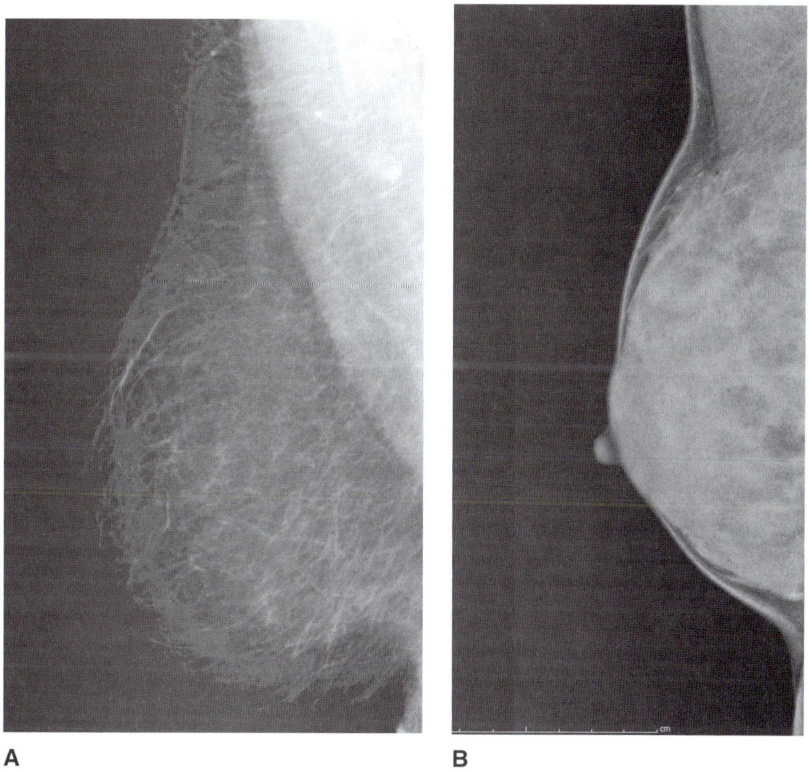

Figure 3-10. Different density beast tissue. (A) All fatty. (B) Extremely dense.

posterior or subscapular group lies along the subscapular vessels, the lateral group lies along the axillary vein, the central group lies in the axillary tissues and are easily palpable and the apical group which lies above the pectoralis minor and behind the clavicle. Lymph also travels along the tributaries of the internal thoracic vessels and the lateral perforating branches of the intercostal vessels to drain to the internal mammary nodes. There can also be cross-mediastinal drainage from the medial portion of one breast to the opposite breast (Figure 3-11).[1,2]

14. **(A)** Starting at the TDLU, the collecting ductal system gradually widens in tree-like branches forming segmental ducts. Immediately behind the nipple it further distends to form an ampulla, also called the lactiferous sinus. This is a pouch-like structure immediately behind the nipple. The ducts again narrow to end at the nipple (Figure 3-12).[1,2]

15. **(C)** Starting at the TDLU, the collecting ductal system gradually widens in tree-like branches forming segmental ducts. Immediately behind the nipple it further distends to form an ampulla, also called the lactiferous sinus. This is a pouch-like structure immediately behind the nipple. The TDLU is lined with a single layer of epithelial cells and a peripheral layer of myoepithelial cells and can be further divided into extralobular terminal ducts (ETD), which is a small duct leading into the terminal ductules, and the intralobular

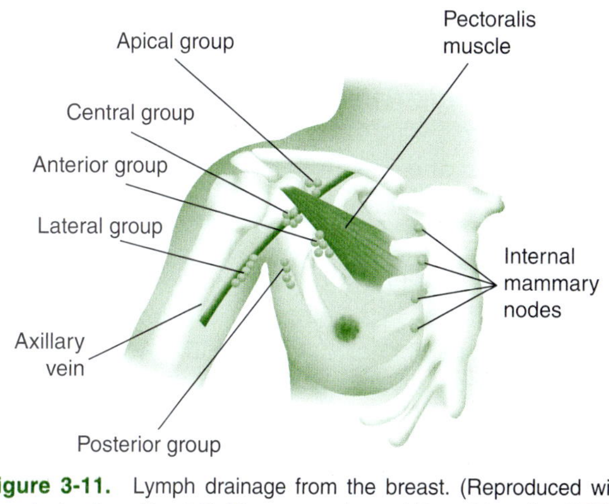

Figure 3-11. Lymph drainage from the breast. (Reproduced with permission from Peart O: Mammography and Breast Imaging PREP: Program Review and Exam Prep. New York, NY: McGraw-Hill Education; 2012.)

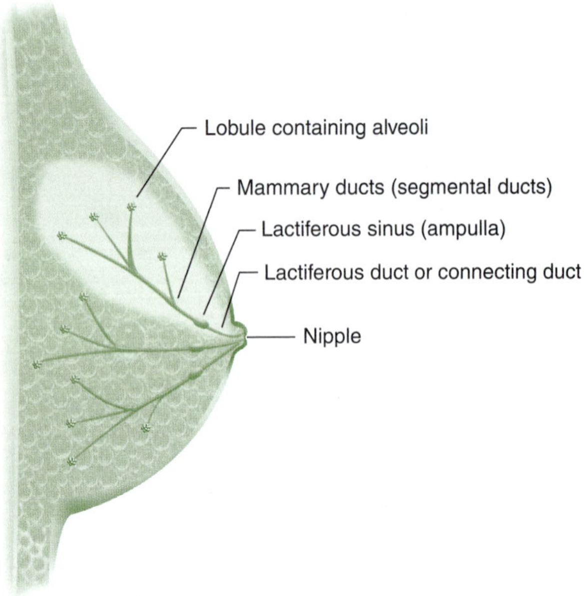

Figure 3-12. A schematic diagram of the breast showing the branching distribution system of a collecting duct within one lobe (Clear area). The nomenclature of the duct system is varied. (Reproduced with permission from Peart O: Mammography and Breast Imaging PREP: Program Review and Exam Prep. New York, NY: McGraw-Hill Education; 2012.)

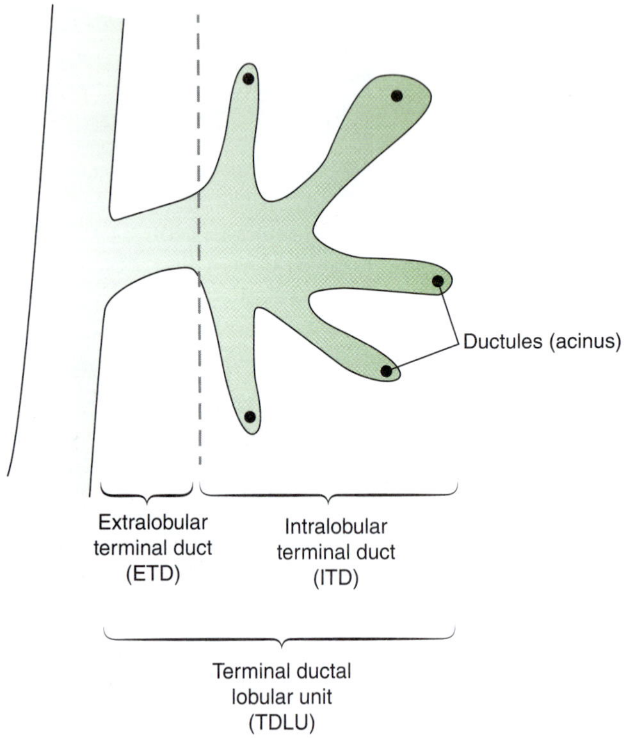

Figure 3-13. The TDLU showing the ETD and ITD divisions. (Reproduced with permission from Peart O: Mammography and Breast Imaging PREP: Program Review and Exam Prep. New York, NY: McGraw-Hill Education; 2012.)

terminal ducts (ITD), located at the end of the terminal ductules. The ITDs hold the acinus within the alveolar glands, which are the milk-producing elements of the breast (Figure 3-13).[1,2]

16. **(A)** Veins are larger than arteries. Unlike arteries, they are normally located peripherally and easily seen. Mammographically they appear as low-density, radiopaque vessels. Both arteries and veins can be outlined by calcifications (Figure 3-14).[1,2]

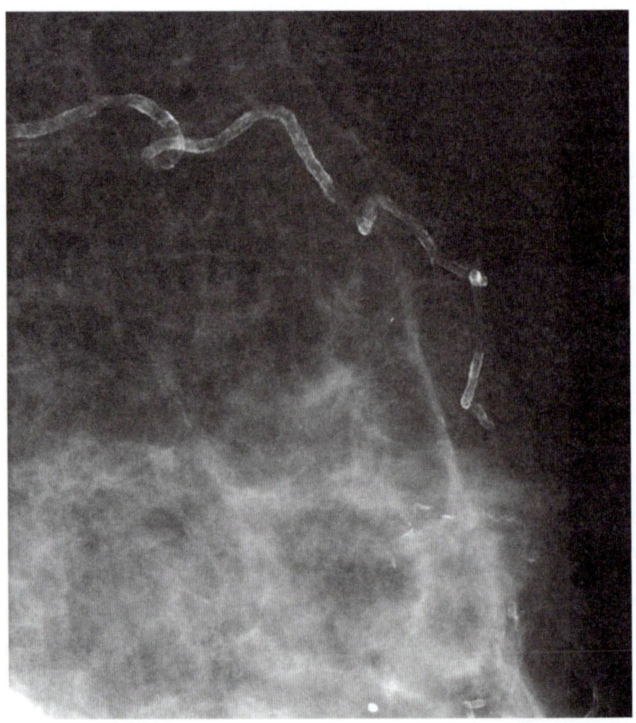

Figure 3-14. Calcified arteries and veins. Arteries are smaller and more centrally located than veins.

17. **(D)** The TDLUs are responsible for milk production and it is here that most cancers originate. The ductal system begins at the TDLU. The TDLU increase and decrease in size and number, depending on menstrual cycle, pregnancy, lactation, and hormone use. The TDLU is further divided into the extralobular terminal duct or ETD, which is a small duct leading into the terminal ductules, and the intralobular terminal duct or ITD, located at the end of the terminal ductules. The ETD is surrounded by elastic tissue and lined by columnar cells. The ITD has no surrounding

elastic tissue and contains cuboidal cells. The ITD holds the milk-producing elements of the breast, called the ductules or acinus (plural, acini). Each lobule can have 10-100 terminal ductules. (See Figure 3-13.)[1,2]

18. **(B)** Increased or decreased glandularity of the breast is a part of the normal physiological changes that take place. Glandularity can be related to menarche, hormonal fluctuation whether normal or synthetic, pregnancy, lactation, or menopause; however, increasing glandularity is usually related to an increase in any of the 2 most prominent hormones active in the breast. These are estrogen (responsible for ductal proliferation) and progesterone (responsible for lobular proliferation and growth).[1,2]

19. **(B)** As a person ages, there is a decline in hormones (perimenopause) eventually leading to menopause after which the glandular breast tissue will atrophy. The breast then loses its supportive and connective tissue to fat. Patients above 60 will most likely have fatty breast; glandular tissues predominate in young women and adipose tissue (fat) predominate in older women. Patients below 20 usually have dense breasts, but are also less likely to have a mammogram. Hormone therapy is likely to increase the glandular nature of the breast.[1,2]

20. **(D)** Ideally, a mammogram should not be scheduled during lactation unless the patient is symptomatic, has a personal history of breast cancer, or is very high risk. In such cases, the total time of lactation may exceed the recommended time interval for screening. If a mammogram must be done during lactation, the patient should nurse just prior to the mammogram to remove as much milk as possible from the breast which will improve visualization of the breast tissue. Because this is a routine baseline mammogram on an asymptomatic patient, the mammogram could be postponed. During lactation, the increased blood supply, milk production, and overall physiologic changes cause increased glandularity that reduces the accuracy of the mammogram, making it less effective as a diagnostic tool. Also, the increased density results in increased radiation exposure to the patient.[1,2]

21. **(B)** Generally, atrophy of mammary structures begins at menopause and ends 3-5 years later. After menopause, the breast loses its supportive tissue to fat, producing a smaller breast, or a larger, more pendulous one. This process is called involution.[1,2]

22. **(D)** The total amount of glandular tissue increases and decreases with hormonal fluctuations, use of synthetic hormones, and menopause. The amount of glandular tissue versus fatty tissue will also depend on a woman's genetic predisposition and total body fat. It is therefore possible to find young women with fatty breasts and older women with extremely dense, glandular breasts. Weight gain and loss also increase or decrease the fat content of the breast tissue, thereby affecting the overall glandularity of the breast.[1,2]

23. **(B)** Hormone replacement therapy (HRT) will relieve symptoms of menopause which can include hot flashes, sleep disturbance, fatigue, osteoporosis, and insomnia. HRT can cause increase in glandular tissue, increase in fibroadenomas, and an increase in the development of breast cyst, but it can inhibit the involution process. The negative effects of HRT can be severe and include breast and uterine cancer, asthma, dementia, heart attacks, strokes, and blood clots. Most women are now advised to consult their doctors regularly if taking HRT or consider on long-term solutions not involving HRT.[1,3]

24. **(A)** Nulliparous is the condition of not having given birth to a viable offspring. Nullipara would then refer to a woman who has never produced a viable offspring. Parity is the terminology used if a woman carries a pregnancy to a point of viability (24-26 weeks of gestation) regardless of the outcome. Other terminology is multiparity, regarded as having carried 1 or more fetuses to viability regardless of the outcome, and primipara, a woman who has delivered a child of 500 g (or greater

than or equal to 20 weeks' gestation) regardless of its viability.[1,3]

25. **(B)** Although a halo is typically present in benign lesions, absence of a halo does not necessarily prove malignancy. The borders or shape of breast masses may be round, oval, lobulated, irregular, or spiculated. A spiculated border is a strong indication for malignancy, whereas a smooth border is a strong indication for a benign abnormality. These, however, are indicators and will not necessarily determine the presence or absence of carcinoma. Typically, any circumscribed radiopaque tumor with unsharp borders and no demonstrable halo sign would be considered suspicious for malignancy, regardless of density (Figure 3-15).[3,4]

26. **(B)** The mammogram shows a stellate tumor. Although the mammogram can suggest carcinoma and may be highly suspicious for carcinoma, only a microscopic analysis (histological or cytological analysis) will reveal the exact type. The presence of a central tumor mass with associated spicules is typical of malignant stellate tumors. The spicules are dense and sharp, radiate from the tumor surface, and usually are not bunched together. When they extend to the skin or areolar region, they cause retraction and local thickening. In general, the larger the tumor, the longer the spicules. (See Figure 3-1.)[3,5]

27. **(A)** These calcifications are typical of mammographically malignant-type casting or granular microcalcifications. Casting calcifications are produced when carcinoma in situ fills the ducts and their branches. The shape of the cast is determined by the uneven production of calcifications and the irregular necrosis of the cellular content. (The cells are reproducing or growing at such a fast rate that they outstrip their blood supply and die—the results are seen as calcifications.) The contours of the cast are always irregular in density, size, and length and the casts are always fragmented. A calcification is seen as branching when it extends into adjacent ducts. Also, the width of the ducts determines the width of the castings. Granular-type calcifications are seen as mammographically similar in appearance to granulated sugar or crushed stones. These are also malignant-type calcifications. Oil cysts are generally seen mammographically as eggshell-like calcifications and a microhematoma or calcified microhematoma can be high-density or a mixed-density oval or circular calcification (see Figure 3-2).[4,6]

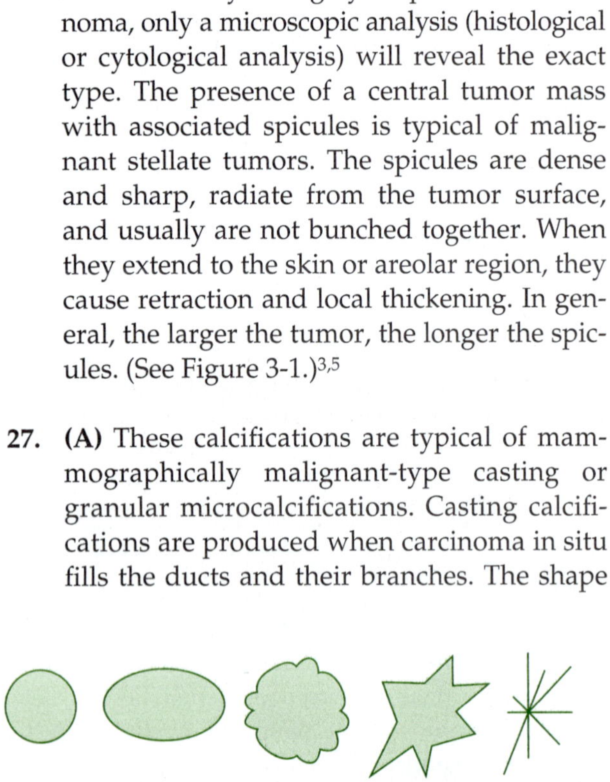

Figure 3-15. The borders of lesions in the breast can be round, oval, lobulated, irregular, or spiculated. (Reproduced with permission from Peart O: Lange Q&A: Mammography Examination, 2nd ed. New York, NY: McGraw-Hill Education; 2008.)

28. **(C)** A typical malignant stellate tumor has a central tumor with dense spicules radiating in all directions. The spicules are separate and increase in length with increased tumor size. If the spicules reach the skin, there can be localized dimpling or skin thickening.[4,5]

29. **(A)** This calcification has the typical appearance of an oil cyst. Oil cysts are generally seen mammographically as eggshell-like calcifications. Plasma cell mastitis calcifications follow the course of the ducts. Some may be elongated and branching, some needle-like, and some ring-like or oval, but all are sharply outlined, high density, and have smooth borders. If they are periductal, they have central lucencies. Calcified sebaceous glands are typically ring-like oval calcifications with lucent centers; there are 2 types, depending on where the calcifications started. Calcifications within a sebaceous gland are hollow or ring-like calcifications; calcifications within the cavity are punctuate calcifications. A microhematoma or calcified microhematoma can be high-density or a mixed-density oval or circular calcification (Figure 3-16).[4,6]

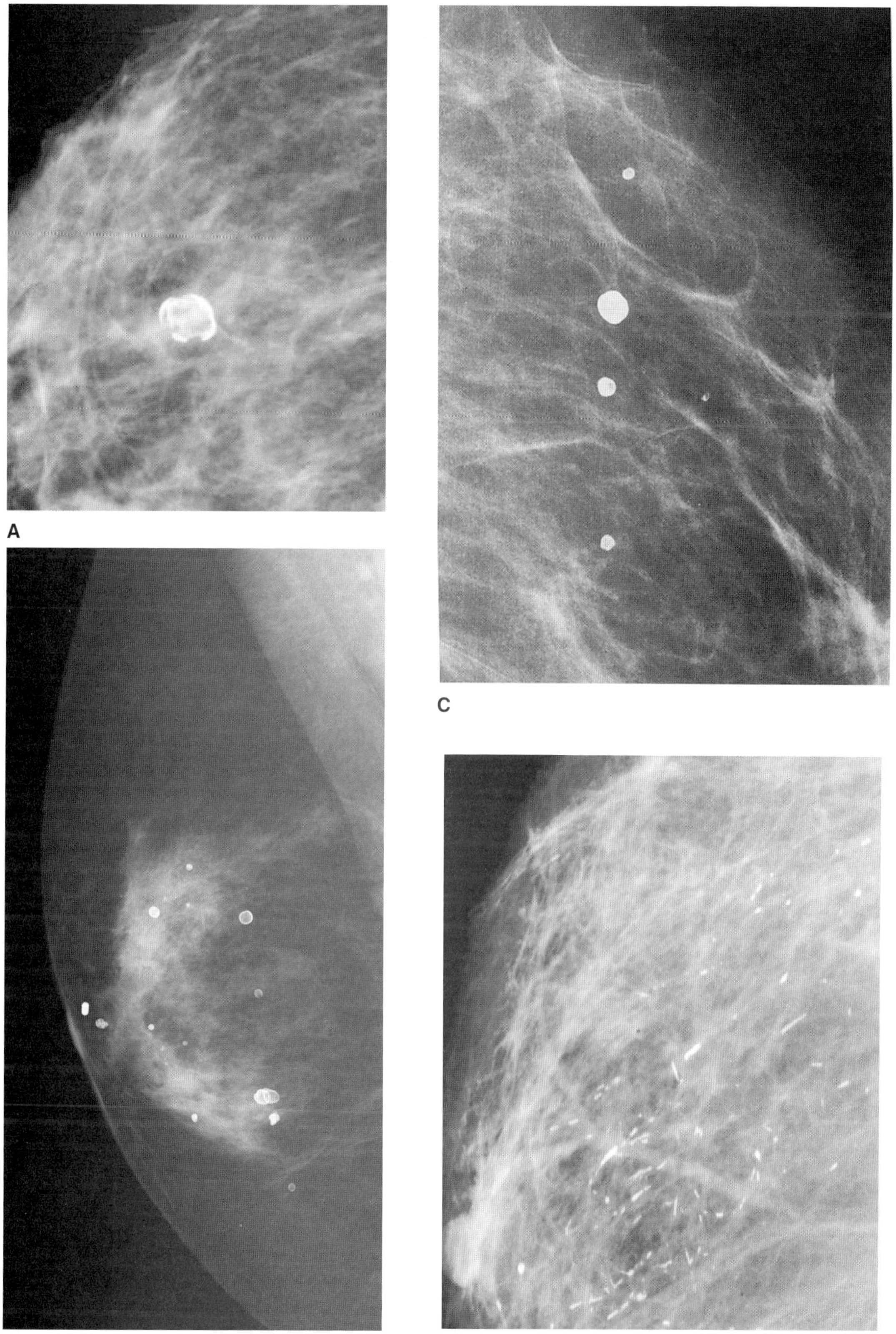

A B C D

Figure 3-16. Pictogram of breast calcifications benign and malignant (A) benign oil cyst, (B) developing oil cyst and hematoma, (C) microhematoma, (D) plasma cell mastitis (benign), (E) sebaceous glands calcified, (F) galactocele, (G) deodorant calcification, (H) dermal calcifications, (I) malignant calcifications, IDC, (J) malignant calcifications, (K) malignant calcifications. (Figure 3-16 B, F, I: Reproduced with permission from Peart O: Lange Q&A: Mammography Examination, 2nd ed. New York, NY: McGraw-Hill Education; 2008.)

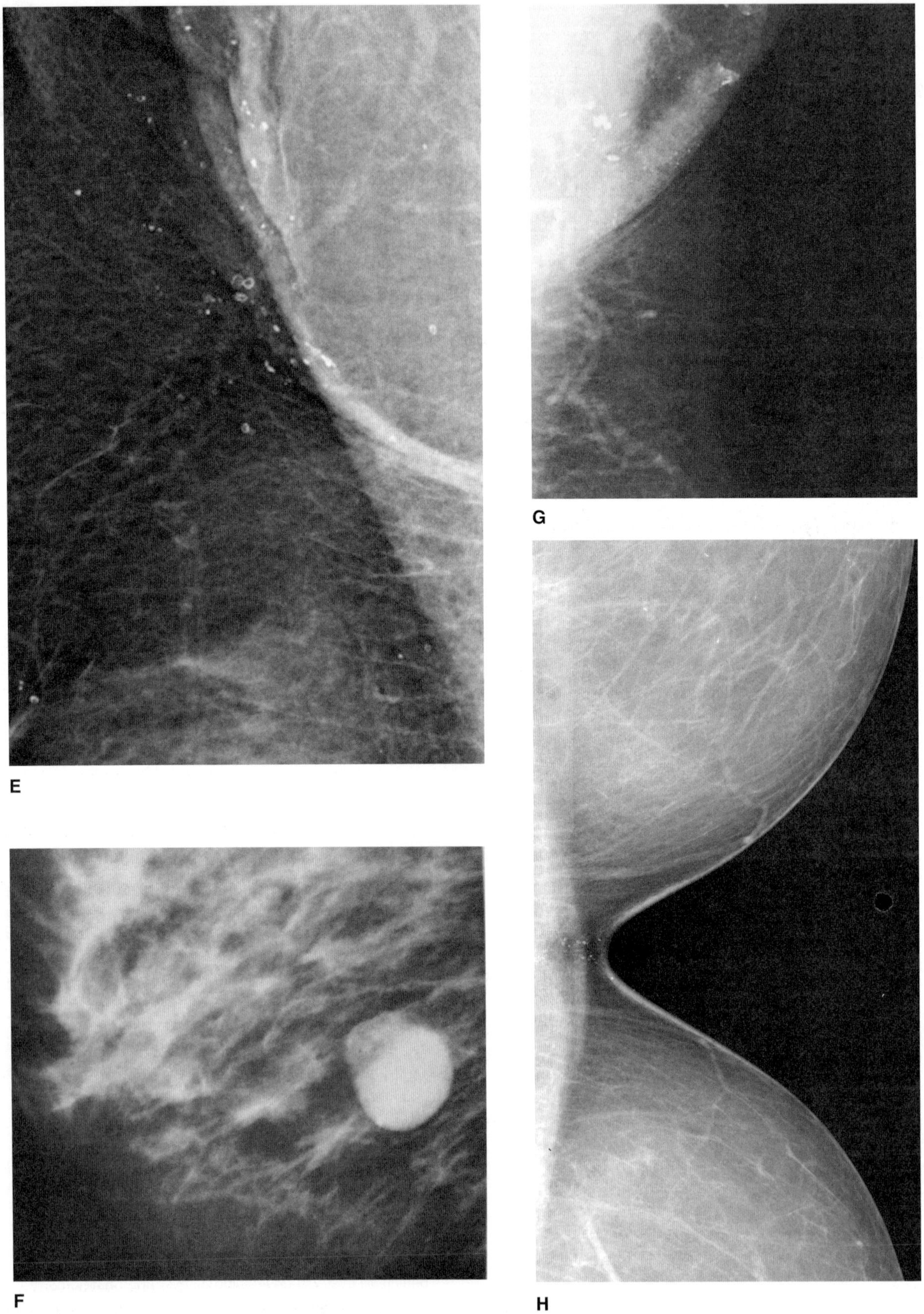

Figure 3-16. *(continued)*

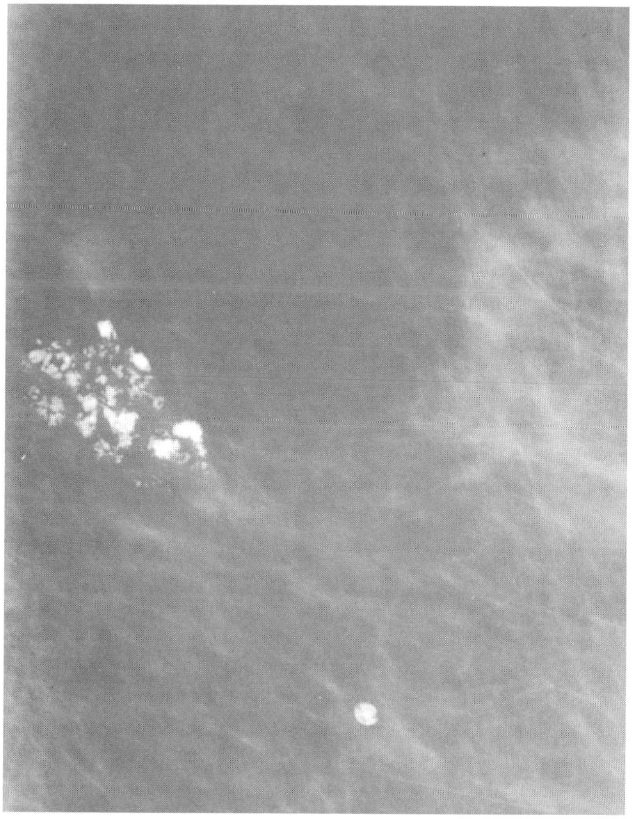

I

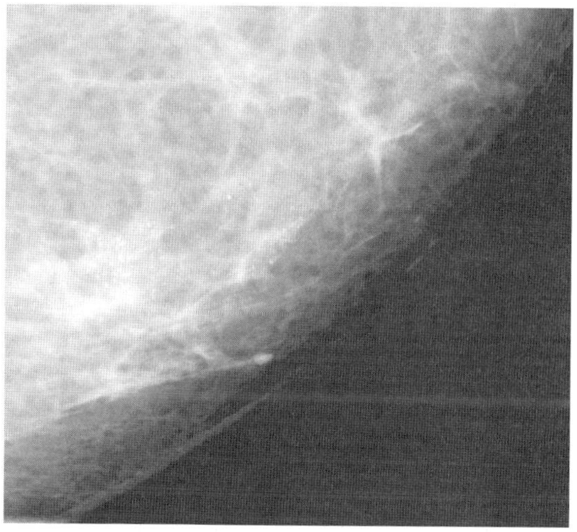

J

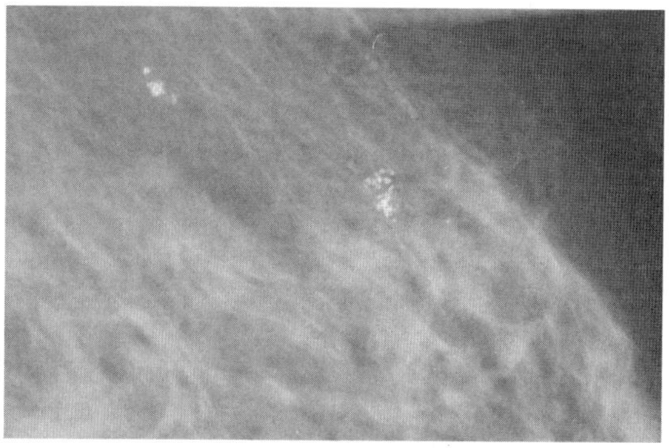

K

Figure 3-16. (continued)

30. **(D)** Postsurgical scarring can mimic a malignancy or radial scar but it is a benign lesion that often resolves over time. Like the radial scar it is rarely palpable. It has no central tumor and regardless of the lesion's size there is no associated skin thickening or dimpling (Figure 3-17).[4,5]

31. **(B)** Most highly suspicious lesions will be recommended for biopsy, but if the lesion is suspected to be benign further testing is done to prove the benign nature of the lesion. A partial halo around a lesion suggests a mammographically benign tumor. An ultrasound would be the best next step to differentiate that a lesion is solid versus a cyst. After the ultrasound, a pneumocystogram could be used to assess the inside margins of the tumor (Figure 3-18).[4,5]

32. **(C)** A galactocele is a benign, milk-filled cyst with high fat content. These lesions are generally associated with lactation. They are usually circular, with sharply defined borders and have densities that are a combination of radiolucent and radiopaque. They are often left alone, but if painful they can be drained using needle puncture. Often they yield a yellow fluid. The galactocele can calcify to a high-density circular or oval radiopaque lesion (Figure 3-19).[3,4]

33. **(B)** A lipoma is a fatty tumor. It is radiolucent with smooth borders and can be huge, growing to occupy the entire breast. It is easily seen mammographically and is not metastatic.[3,4]

34. **(A)** Inflammatory carcinoma is a rare form of invasive carcinoma accounting for 1%-4% of all breast cancers. It generally presents with swelling, warmth, erythema, and skin thickening. The symptoms result from vascular or lymphatic invasion of the carcinoma but are

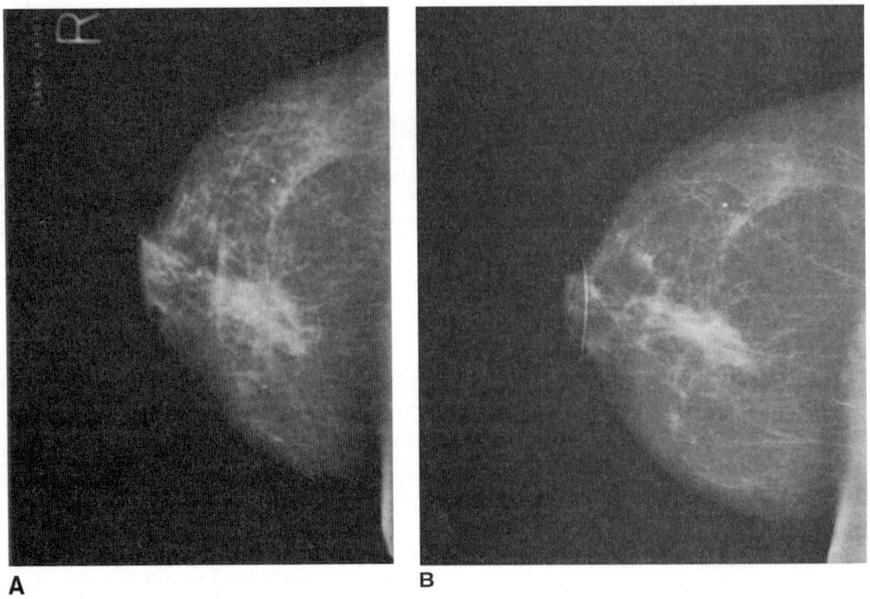

Figure 3-17. (A) Postsurgical scaring. (B) Resolving postsurgical scar.

unfortunately very similar to symptoms of a severe infection (Figure 3-20). Invasive ductal carcinoma accounts for more than 90% of all breast cancers. It usually presents as a central tumor with radiating spicules and often the associated malignant microcalcifications. Invasive ductal carcinoma is the most common of all breast cancers. This form of cancer is often associated with a tumor and malignant appearing calcifications. Invasive lobular carcinoma is often difficult to perceive on a mammogram and is better visualized using other modalities. On the mammogram it may show as a spider web appearance or cause skin retraction. Papillary carcinoma is frequently seen as a circumscribed mass on older women. It is often indistinguishable from a cyst mammographically, but on ultrasound is identified as a complex or solid mass. It is a slow-growing tumor with good prognosis.[4]

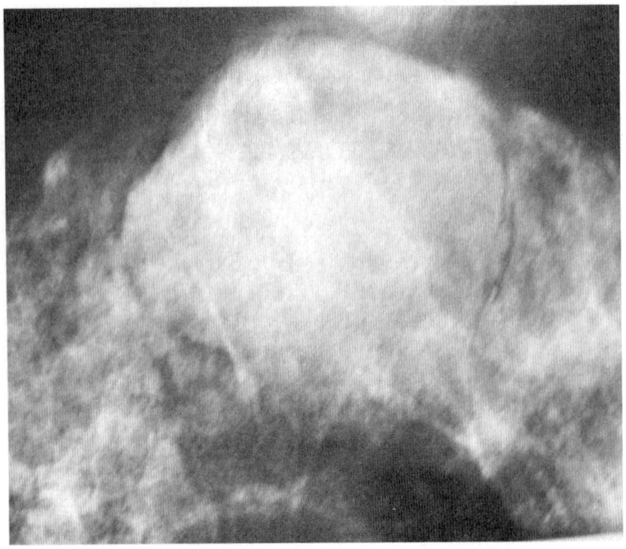

Figure 3-18. The halo on a partially obscured lesion.

35. **(C)** Fat necrosis can be caused by surgery, biopsy, trauma, or radiation therapy. At the site of the injury there may be hemorrhage, then as the tissue dies, liquefied fat necrotic material and blood remains. The area becomes encapsulated by a thin layer of calcification, which appears on the mammogram as eggshell-like calcification described as an oil cyst. Stellate lesions such as invasive ductal carcinoma have a distinct central mass and sharp, dense fine lines of variable length radiating in all directions—the larger the central tumor mass, the longer the spicules. A galactocele is a benign, milk-filled cyst with high fat content. These lesions are generally associated with lactation and can calcify to a high-density radiopaque circular or oval lesion. A lipoma is a fatty tumor. It is

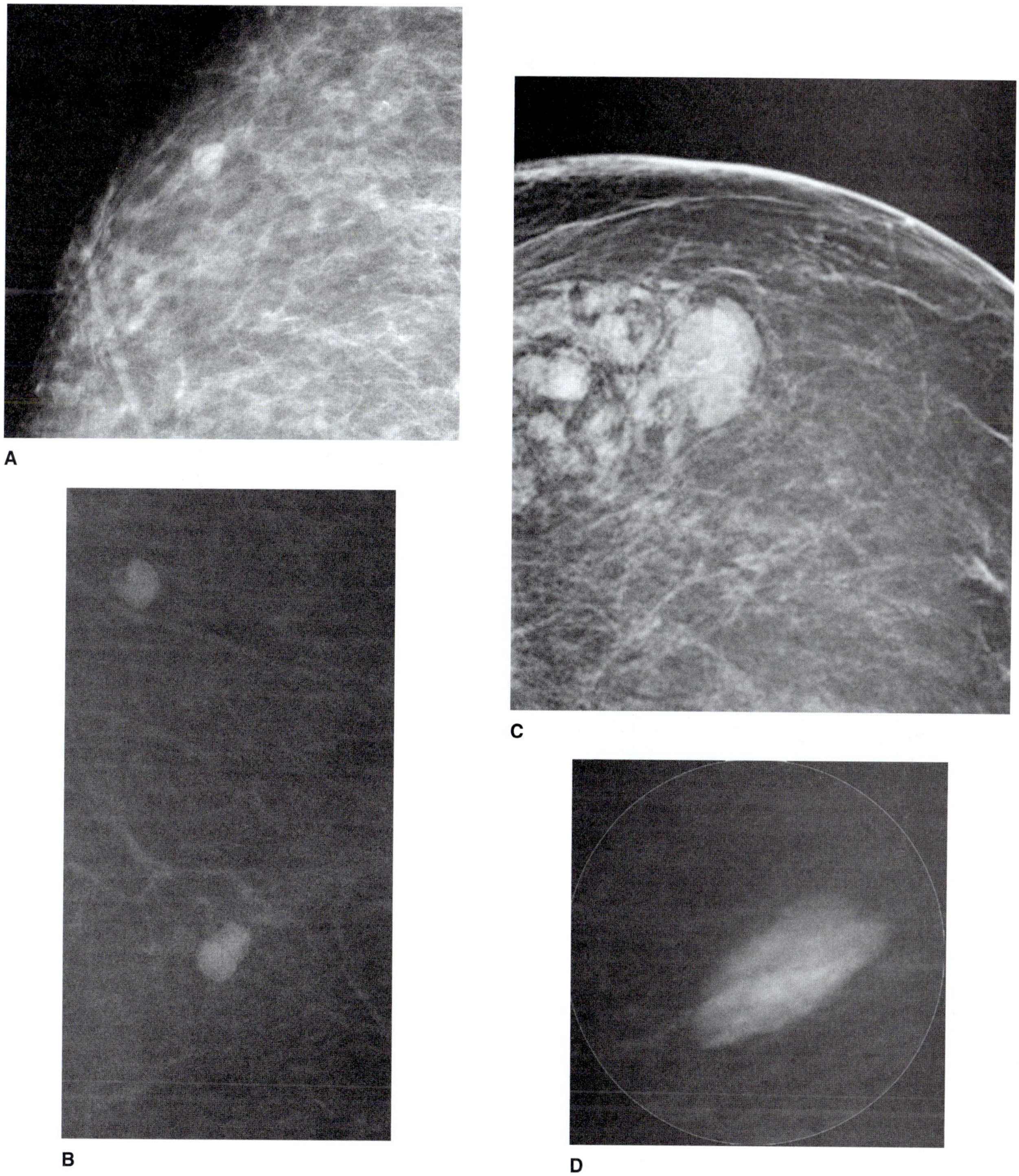

Figure 3-19. Pictogram of breast lesions (A) fibroadenoma, (B) lymph nodes, (C) hamartoma, (D) rhemangeoma, (E) spot compression of a lesion, (F) air in breast after biopsy, (G) fat necrosis, (H) cyst, (I) malignant oval lesion, (J) stellate lesion, (K) stellate lesion with nipple retraction. (Figure 3-19C: Reproduced with permission from Peart O: Mammography and Breast Imaging PREP: Program Review and Exam Prep. New York, NY: McGraw-Hill Education; 2012; Figure 3-19 H, J: Reproduced with permission from Peart O: Lange Q&A: Mammography Examination, 2nd ed. New York, NY: McGraw-Hill Education; 2008.)

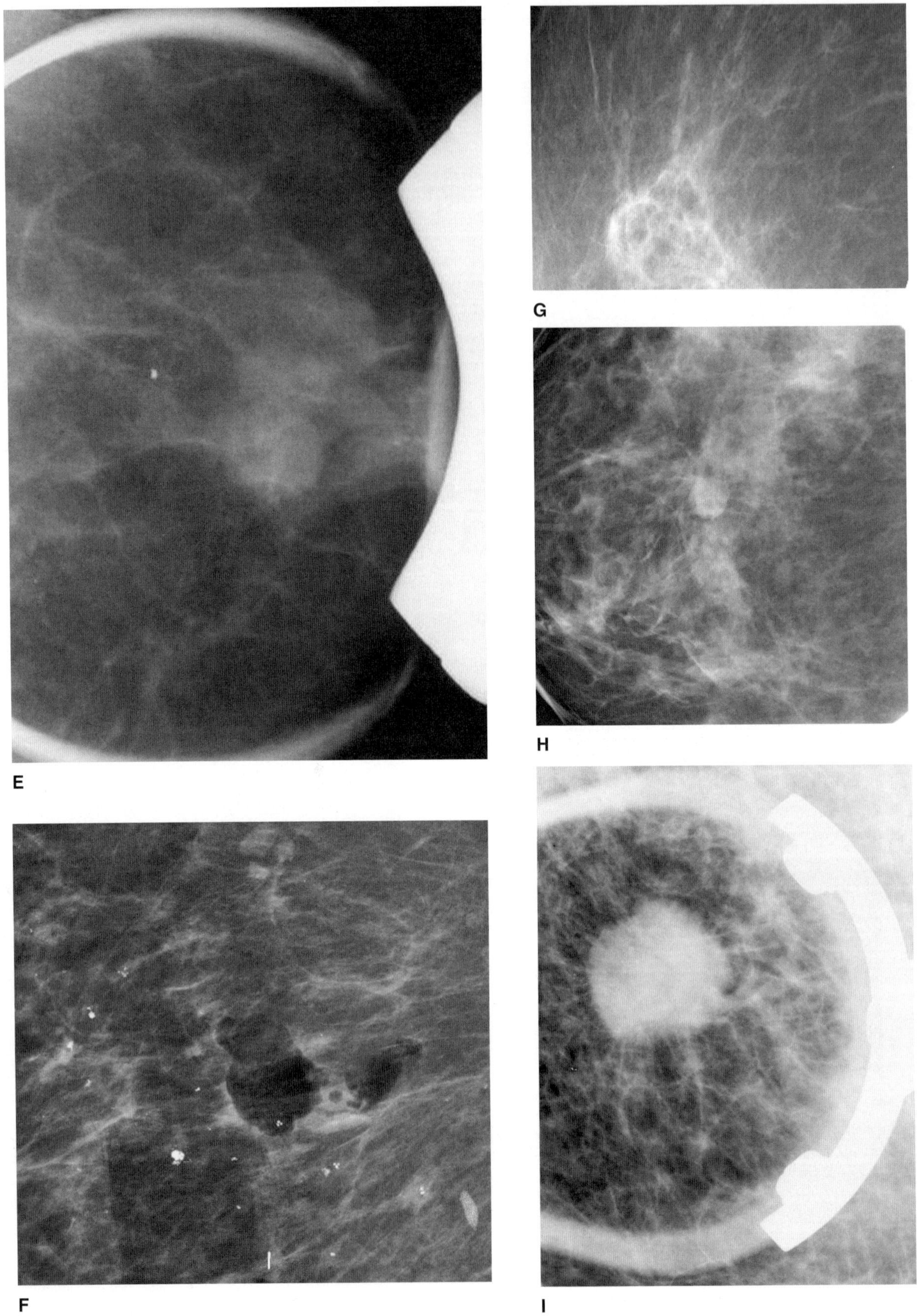

Figure 3-19. *(continued)*

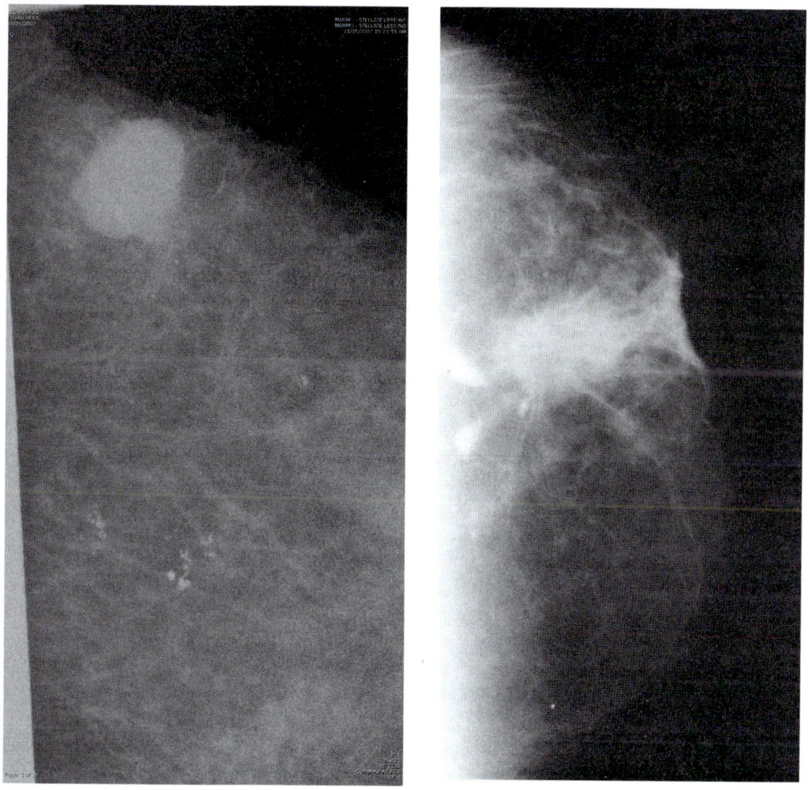

J K

Figure 3-19. (*continued*)

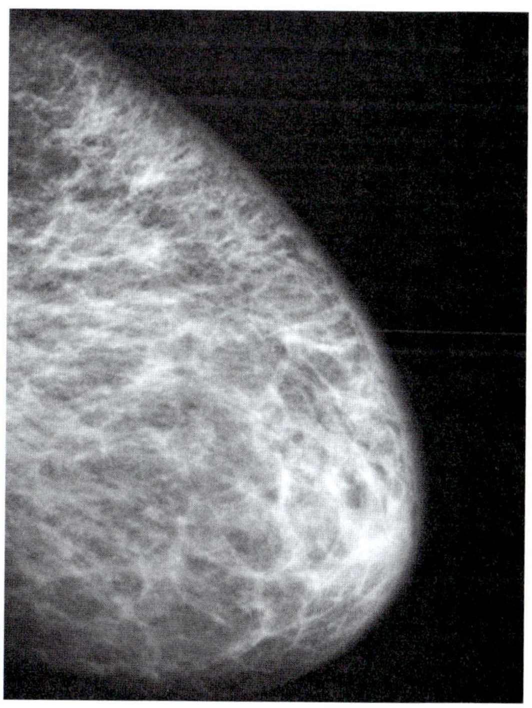

Figure 3-20. Skin thickening as seen on a mammogram.

radiolucent and may be huge, occupying the entire breast. It is easily seen mammographically and is not metastatic (Figure 3-21).[4,5]

36. **(D)** Hamartomas or fibroadenolipomas result from an abnormal formation of normal tissue. The cells of the tumor grow in a disorganized mass and are composed of tissue elements normally found at the site. Unlike a cancerous tumor, the hamartoma rarely invade or compress surrounding structures. The cells grow spontaneously, reach maturity, and then do not reproduce. This growth is self-limiting and benign. Radial scars are complex sclerosing lesions. They are not truly scars and are often unrelated to prior surgery or trauma. Some possible causes of the radial scar are localized inflammatory reaction or chronic ischemia with a slow infection. The radial scar can be a benign condition, but can be associated with premalignant—atypical ductal hyperplasia—and

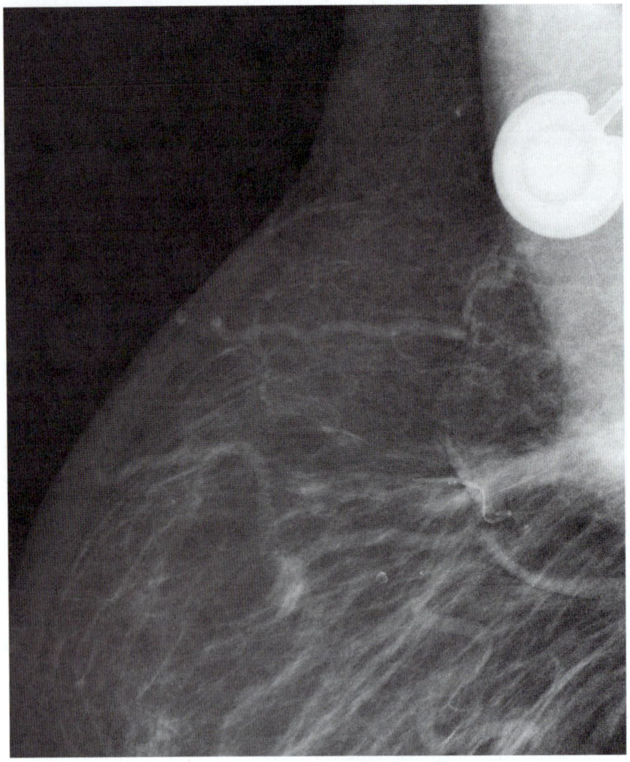

Figure 3-21. A mammogram showing a port-a-cath or infusa-port.

malignant conditions. A benign radial scar has no central tumor, although there may be long spicules radiating from the center of the lesion. Regardless of the size of the spicules in the benign radial scar, there is no associated skin thickening, dimpling, or nipple reaction. Because of the possible association with malignancy it is recommended that all stellate lesions, including radial scars, should be excised. A sarcoma is a cancerous tumor from mesenchymal tissue such as muscle or bone. Lobular carcinomas are often difficult to diagnose. Invasive lobular carcinoma is a malignant condition where the cancer has spread from the lobular into the surrounding tissue. On the mammogram this can show as a spiderweb appearance or cause skin retraction (see Figure 3-19).[4,5]

37. **(B)** Infusa-ports are designed to permit repeated access to the venous system for the parenteral delivery of medications, fluids, and nutritional solutions and for the sampling of venous blood. In the treatment of breast cancer the infusa-port or port-a-cath are often used to deliver chemotherapy treatment and are sometime referred to as central venous access devices (CVAD). They are surgically implanted completely under the skin. Patients with infusa-ports can leave the hospital and continue their treatment at home. The infusa-port must be inspected daily for signs of infection. When imaging a patient with an infusa-port the location of the port can make imaging difficult. Radiation treatment exposes a specific body area to various high-energy radiations to destroy cancer cells. Radioactive tracers or radioactive isotopes are injected directly into the breast tissue in a technique known as lymphoscintigraphy or sentinel node mapping, the idea being to track the path of metastatic cancer (Figure 3-21).[3,7]

38. **(B)** The skin markers suggest that these are visible skin lesions. Epidermoid cysts, keratosis, moles, calcified sebaceous glands, and skin tags are the most common. These are skin moles. The epidermoid cyst can appear as firm, round, mobile lumps just below the skin surface. These cysts are sometimes incorrectly referred to as sebaceous cysts but they are not of sebaceous origin. Mammographically, they are seen as mixed-density circular or oval lesions and can be mistaken for an internal lesion if not marked. The keratosis often presents as a raised lesion on the skin surface. Unlike warts, which they resemble, they are not caused by the human papilloma virus. They tend to have a very rough surface with bumps and crevices. Mammographically, they appear as oval mixed-density lesions, often radiolucent but the crevices will appear as higher density areas on the mammogram. Moles, known medically as nevi, can come in a range of colors, but are usually dark brown spots. In rare cases, a mole can become cancerous, but usually they are harmless clusters of pigmented cells. Mammographically, the mole can appear as a radiolucent circumscribed lesion and can be mistaken for an internal lesion if not identified. Calcified sebaceous glands are typically ring-like oval calcifications with lucent centers. A skin tag is a benign skin growth that looks like a small piece of hanging skin. Mammographically, it is seen as a

low-density circumscribed lesion and can be mistaken for an internal lesion if not identified. The fibroadenoma is a benign radiolucent and radiopaque combined lesion within the breast. The galactocele is often circular or oval with mixed density and is also located within breast tissue. It is associated with lactation (Figure 3-22).[3,4]

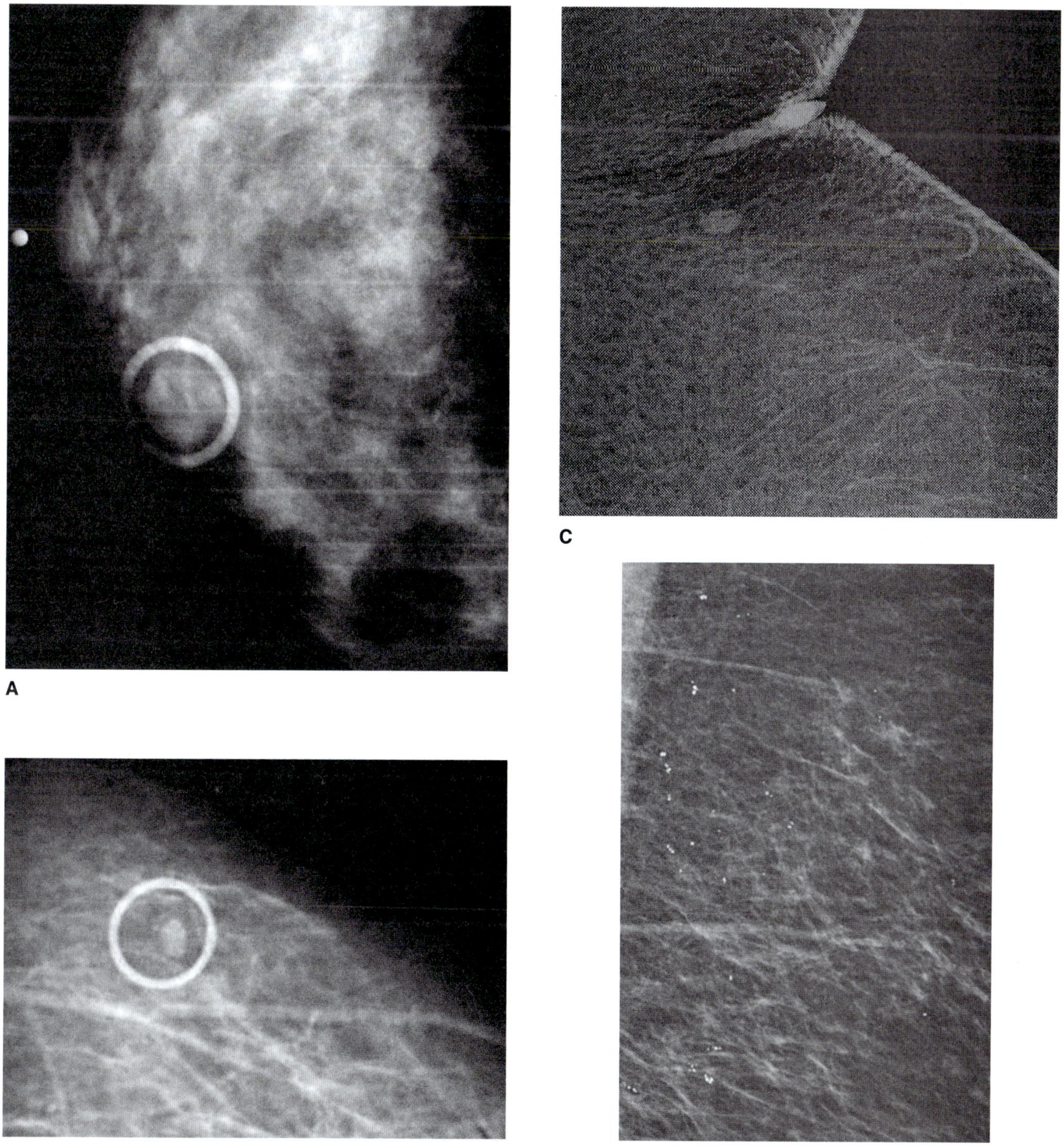

A B C D

Figure 3-22. Pictogram of breast skin lesions (A) keratosis, (B) skin mole, (C) skin tags, (D) calcified sebaceous glands, (E) epidermoid cyst. (Reproduced with permission from Peart O: Mammography and Breast Imaging PREP: Program Review and Exam Prep. New York, NY: McGraw-Hill Education; 2012.)

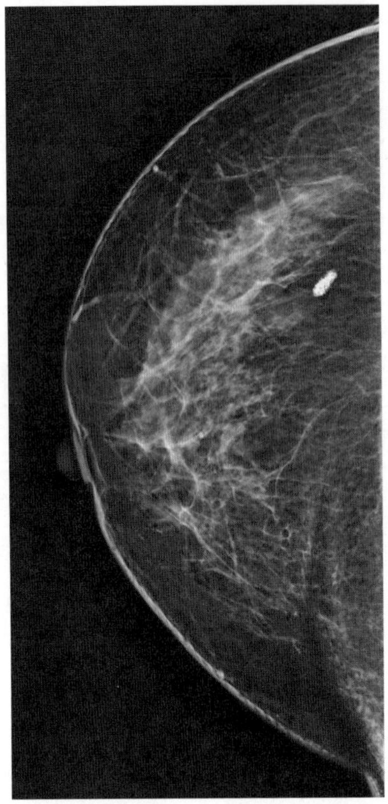

E

Figure 3-22. (continued)

39. **(C)** These calcifications are due to fibrocystic changes. Calcifications can sometime be hard to define and in the absence of previous studies or a clear clinical history further testing (spots, magnification, or even a biopsy) is often necessary. Malignant type calcifications can be: casting type, fine, linear, or branching calcifications that are fragmented with irregular contours; amorphous or indistinct calcifications forming multiple flakes; pleomorphic or granular calcification of different shapes, irregular in form, size, and density. Typically benign calcifications are: smooth contours, high uniform density, e.g., plasma cell mastitis; evenly scattered, homogenous, e.g., calcified arteries; sharply outlined, spherical, or oval, e.g., oil cysts; pear-like densities resembling teacups or pearl drops on the lateral projection, e.g., milk of calcium; bilateral and evenly scattered following the course of the ducts throughout much of the parenchyma, e.g., plasma cell mastitis; ring-like, hollow, e.g., sebaceous gland calcifications; eggshell-like, e.g., oil cyst, papilloma; or large bizarre size, e.g., hemangiomas. (See Figure 3-19.)[8]

40. **(D)** Epidermoid cysts are often incorrectly referred to as sebaceous cysts, but they are not of sebaceous origin. The epidermoid cysts appear as firm, round, mobile lumps just below the skin surface. Mammographically, they are seen as mixed-density circular or oval lesions and can be mistaken for an internal lesion if not marked. A microhematoma or calcified microhematoma can be mixed-density or a high-density oval or circular calcification. A galactocele is a benign, milk-filled cyst with high fat content. These lesions are generally associated with lactation. They are usually circular, with sharply defined borders and have densities that are a combination of radiolucent and radiopaque. The calcified galactocele is usually seen mammographically as a circular or oval high-density radiopaque lesion. Malignant-type calcifications are often seen in clusters and are typically

casting or granular in appearance. Casting calcifications are produced when carcinoma in situ fills the ducts and their branches. The shape of the cast is determined by the uneven production of calcifications and the irregular necrosis of the cellular content. The contours of the cast are always irregular in density, size, and length and the casts are always fragmented. A calcification is seen as branching when it extends into adjacent ducts. Also, the width of the ducts determines the width of the castings. Granular-type calcifications are seen as mammographically similar in appearance to granulated sugar or crushed stones. (See Figures 3-16 and 3-22.)[3,4]

References

1. Peart O. Breast anatomy, physiology and pathology of the breast. In: *Mammography and Breast Imaging: Prep*. New York, NY: McGraw-Hill; 2012:263-332.
2. Tortora GJ, Derrickson B. The reproductive systems. In: *Principles of Anatomy and Physiology*. 12th ed. New York, NY: John Wiley & Sons; 2009:1110-1112.
3. Venes D, Biderman A, Adler E. *Taber's Cyclopedic Medical Dictionary*. 21st ed. Philadelphia, PA: F.A. Davis; 2005:1-2518.
4. Peart O. Breast benign and malignant diseases of the breast. In: *Mammography and Breast Imaging: Prep*. New York, NY: McGraw-Hill; 2012:263-332.
5. Tabár L, Dean PB. Stellate/spiculated lesions and architectural distortion. In: *Teaching Atlas of Mammography*. 4th ed. New York, NY: Thieme; 2011:93-148.
6. Tabár L, Dean PB. Calcifications in the mammogram In: *Teaching Atlas of Mammography*. 4th ed. New York, NY: Thieme; 2011:149-238.
7. Peart O. Treatment options. In: *Mammography and Breast Imaging: Prep*. New York, NY: McGraw-Hill; 2012:397-432.
8. Peart O. Breast imaging mammography. In: *Mammography and Breast Imaging: Prep*. New York, NY: McGraw-Hill; 2012:213-262.

CHAPTER 4

Mammographic Technique and Image Evaluation

Summary of Important Points

ROUTINE BREAST IMAGING

Breast Compression

Breast compression is under the discretion of the mammographer and will depend on the patient's breast sensitivity and size. In general, the breast should be compressed until taut to fingertip pressure to ensure adequate compression. Often, after the automatic compression stops, manual compression must be applied to adequately immobilize and compress the breast. Although too little compression will compromise image quality, the compression should not be applied to cause the patient severe pain.

Main Reason for Breast Compression

- Compression allows a uniform density by flattening the posterior breast to the same degree as the more anterior regions, permitting optimal imaging of the entire breast on 1 exposure.

Added Advantages of Breast Compression

- The tissue thickness of the compressed breast is less than that of the uncompressed breast which means that lower radiation is needed to penetrate the compressed breast allowing reduced radiation dose to the patient.
- Compression brings lesions closer to the detector for more accuracy when evaluating fine detail.
- Compression reduces the possibility of motion by immobilizing the breast during the exposure.
- Compression allows the use of lower peak kilovoltage (kVp) which allows increased contrast.
- Compression separates superimposed areas of glandular tissue by spreading apart overlapping tissue, allowing visualization of the borders of circumscribed lesions.
- Compression assists in capturing the breast tissue to include the posterior chest wall anatomy.

Routine Breast Imaging Projections

Typically, the routine 4-projection series in mammography involves imaging in the craniocaudal (CC) and the mediolateral oblique (MLO) of both breasts. The CC and MLO projections are complementary. The idea behind the 4-projection routine in mammography is to image both breasts with minimal radiation dose to the patient and to include the maximum amount of breast tissue possible.

Areas Best Demonstrated on the CC Projection

The CC projection breast demonstrates the anterior, central, medial, and posteromedial portions of the breast, but is poor at visualizing the lateral breast tissue. It is critical to include the medial breast on the CC projection. The medial breast may be inadvertently eliminated on the MLO because the breast is less mobile and cannot be stretched at its medial aspect (the sternum side).

Key Points of the CC Projection

- Position the detector at the level of the raised inframammary crease. The breast must be elevated before positioning the detector.
- Turn the patient's head away from the side being examined.

- Position the patient's feet apart with weight equally distributed.
- The ipsilateral arm is positioned by patient's side.
- The contralateral arm is raised and the patient can hold the machine for support.
- Optimal compression is achieved if the patient is relaxed. To aid relaxation of the shoulder, place your hand on the ipsilateral shoulder and gently push down.
- Expose on suspended respiration but try to avoid telling the patient to take a deep breath before the exposure.

CC Evaluation

- The nipple should be in profile.
- The nipple should be centered on the radiograph; however, do not eliminate breast tissue to center the nipple.
- The medial and lateral aspects of the breast must be included in the collimated area.
- If possible, include the cleavage and a small amount of contralateral breast at the medial margin.
- The pectoralis major muscle is seen in approximately 30%-40% of the cases. If the pectoral muscle is seen on all cases imaging may be losing medial breast tissue.
- Appropriate markers and labeling must be used as required by Mammography Quality Standard Act (MQSA).
- The CC should include, within 1 cm, the posterior nipple line (PNL) measurement of the MLO.
- Dense areas of the breast should be adequately penetrated.

Areas Best Demonstrated on the MLO Projection

- The MLO projection demonstrates the extreme posterior and upper-outer quadrant but there is distortion of the anterior, central, and medial breast tissue.
- In imaging in the MLO projection, the detector must be parallel to the pectoralis muscle, which can vary from 30 to 60 degrees.
- The more parallel the detector is to the pectoralis muscle the more tissue will be included in the image.

Key points of the MLO Projection

- The degree of tube angulation will vary between 30 and 60 degrees, depending on the patient's body habitus. Thin patients require steeper angulation than heavier patients.
- The correct detector or compression paddle size is needed to avoid stretching the pectoralis major muscle.
- Too much pectoral muscle under the compression plate, especially when imaging the male breast, will reduce compression to the anterior portions of the breast.
- The ipsilateral arm should be draped over the top of the detector.
- The detector should rest in the armpit, posterior to the midaxilla and anterior to the latissimus dorsi muscle.
- Compression must adequately support the anterior breast tissue to preventing sagging and distortion of the ductal architecture.
- Appropriate markers and labeling must be used, as required by MQSA.
- Expose on suspended respiration, but try to avoid telling the patient to take a deep breath before the exposure.

MLO Evaluation

- The pectoral muscle should be wide superiorly with a convex anterior border and should extend to or below the level of the PNL.
- The inframammary fold should be open.
- Dense areas of the breast should be adequately penetrated.
- There should be no drooping of the anterior breast and distortion of the architectural structures.
- Abdominal tissue should not overlap the breast tissue.

Supplementary Projection

- Supplementary projections become useful when the standard projections are inadequate.
- Supplementary projections can be used to image a patient when medical or surgical history or body build makes the standard projections difficult to obtain.
- Supplementary projections can be used to provide more details of a suspicious lesion or microcalcifications.

Supplementary Projections, Recognized by the ACR and ARRT

- 90-degree mediolateral (ML)
- 90-degree lateromedial (LM)
- Lateromedial oblique (LMO)
- Tangential projection (TAN)
- Exaggerated craniocaudal lateral or medial (XCCL or XCCM)
- Caudocranial or from below (FB)
- Cleavage or "valley view" (CV)
- Axillary tail (AT)
- Superoinferior oblique (SIO)

Other Modified Positions

- Rolled medial (RM) or rolled lateral (RL)
- Rolled inferior (RI) or rolled superior (RS)
- Magnification (M)
- Spot compression

The ACR also accepts that ruling out an abnormality could involve imaging the breast using *any* manipulation or technique that is not a part of the routine or supplementary series.

Mediolateral

This is a 90-degree lateral projection of the breast with the x-ray beam passing medial to lateral.

- Used to improve detail of a lesion located in the lateral aspect of the breast.
- Used to verify a finding or to localize a lesion in another dimension, e.g., during localization.
- Used to image breast tissue missed on the MLO, e.g., at the inframammary fold area.
- To triangulate a lesion seen on the MLO but not seen on the CC projection. When comparing the MLO and ML projections:
  - Medial lesions move up on the lateral from their position on the MLO.
  - Lateral lesions move down on the lateral from their position on the MLO.
  - Central lesions will not change significantly from the MLO to the ML.
- Used to prove benign breast calcifications, e.g., milk of calcium.

Lateromedial

This is a 90-degree lateral projection of the breast with the x-ray beam passing lateral to medial.

- Used to improve details of a lesion located in the medial aspect of the breast.
- Used to verify a finding or to localize a lesion in another dimension. (e.g., during localization).
- Used during preoperative localization, giving a true representation of inferior and/or lateral lesions.
- Used to replace the MLO when imaging patients with difficult body habitus although the study may be limited because it does not image as much posterior breast as the routine MLO projection.

Lateromedial Oblique

This is a true reverse of the MLO projection with the x-ray beam directed inferolateral to superomedial.

- Used to evaluate the medial aspect of the breast.
- Used when the standard MLO projection is difficult to obtain because of patient body build such as prominent sternum.
- Used when the patient has a pacemaker or chest surgery to avoid pulling at the scar tissue and causing discomfort.

Tangential

This provides a profile projection of the area of interest, avoiding superimposition on other breast tissue. The x-ray beam skims the skin surface of interest.

- Used to confirm or locate skin calcification or skin lesions. A BB or lead spot marker can be placed over the area of interest during the exposure.

Exaggerated Craniocaudal Lateral or Medial

This is a CC projection of the posterior or medial breast tissue. The x-ray is directed superior to inferior with the patient positioned first for the CC then turned laterally or medially.

- Used to locate lesions in the lateral or medical aspect of breast not seen on the CC projection.

Caudocranial or From Below

This is a reverse of the CC projection, with the x-ray beam traveling inferior to superior. The tube is rotated 180 degrees with detector to the top.

- Used to better visualize lesions in the superior or upper quadrants of the breast.
- Used to image small breasts or the male breast.
- Used to image the kyphotic patient or patients with pacemakers.

The Cleavage or Valley View

This projection visualizes the deep medial breast tissue with the x-ray beam directed superior to inferior.

- Used to show lesions deep in the medial aspect of the breast, the area closest to the chest wall.

The Axillary Tail

This is an oblique projection of the tail of the breast that is customized, with the angle depending on the patient's body habitus and/or radiologist request. The beam passes superomedial to inferolateral, perpendicular to the angle of the axillary tail.

- Used to visualize the tail of the breast.

The Superoinferior Oblique Projection

This is an oblique projection with the x-ray beam directed superolateral to inferomedial.

- Used to demonstrate the upper-inner quadrant and the lower-outer quadrant of the breast, free of superimposition.
- The 45-degree SIO is useful in providing a projection perpendicular to the MLO to help distinguish pseudomass from malignant lesions.
- The 45-degree SIO is useful when imaging the most posterior and inferior portion of the lower-outer quadrant of the breast.
- The 60-degree SIO can be used to visualize the breast free of implants using the Eklund technique.

Rolled Lateral or Rolled Medial

In these positions the breast is rolled laterally or medially after the patient is positioned for the CC projection. The idea is useful in removing superimposed tissue when imaging dense breast. The lesion is "rolled" off or away from the dense tissue.

- **RL**—after positioning the patient for the CC, the superior portion of the breast is rolled laterally and the inferior (lower) portion is rolled medially.
- **RM**—after positioning the patient for the CC, the superior portion of the breast is rolled medially and the inferior (lower) portion is rolled laterally.

Rolled Superior or Rolled Inferior

These are lateral positions used to remove superimposed tissue. The breast surface away from the detector is then rolled superiorly or inferiorly.

- **RS**—after positioning the patient for the ML, the medial portion of the breast is rolled superiorly and the lateral portion of the breast is rolled inferiorly.
- **RI**—after positioning the patient for the ML lateral, the medial portion of the breast is rolled inferiorly and the lateral portion of the breast is rolled superiorly.

Spot Compression

With spot compression more compression is applied to a localized area of interest using a small compression paddle. Spot compression can be performed in any projection or with or without magnification. It is not recommended for imaging of lesions directly behind the nipple; the small compression paddle will push or displace the lesion posteriorly.

- Used for localization of suspected abnormalities.
- Useful in applying additional compression when evaluating a suspicious area.

Magnification Mammography

Magnification images the breast with an increased OID which results in magnification of the part. A small focal spot must be used with magnification to improve the resolution and sharpness to compensate for the large OID. However, the large OID acts as an air gap in reducing the amount of scattered radiation reaching the detector. A grid is therefore not necessary.

- Used to improve visualization of fine details especially when analyzing calcifications.
- Used to evaluate the margins of lesions or the density of masses.
- Used to image specimens or surgical sites.

IMAGING IMPLANTS

The standard series of projections for a patient with an implant is the routine CC and MLO projections with limited compression, plus the Eklund projections which are often called *implant-displaced* (ID) projections. Most implants can be displaced by using the ID projections. The result is an 8-projection series.

- The "implant in place" imaging refers to the standard projection taken to demonstrate the posterior breast tissue surrounding the margins of the implant. Compression is used for immobilization only. Vigorous compression should not be applied to the implant.

- The implant-displaced technique requires pulling the natural breast tissue forward while simultaneously, pushing the implant back toward the chest wall. Maximum compression is therefore applied only to the breast tissue anterior to the implant.
- ID technique will work on all implants regardless of whether the implant is placed in front of the pectoral muscle (subglandular or retromammary implants) or behind the pectoral muscle (subpectoral implants), as long as the implant is not encapsulated.

Technique

- Before beginning positioning the mammographer must locate the extent of the implant by feeling for the edges (how far it extends).
- Next have the patient stand in the position for a routine CC or MLO.
- The patient then steps back, slightly away from the detector.
- The mammographer locates the anterior edge of the implant and places the detector anterior to the edge of the implant.
- The mammographer can use thumb and fingers to grasp the breast anterior to the implant and pull breast tissue forward.
- Compression begins while holding and pulling the breast tissue forward.
- The edge of the detector and the compression plate will help keep the implant posterior to the breast tissue and displaced from the field of view.
- The breast free of implant is compressed normally.
- If there is sufficient breast tissue to cover the detector, automatic exposure control can be use. However, if enough breast tissue does not cover the detector, manual technique must be used.

SPECIAL IMAGING SITUATIONS

Small Breast

- Manual technique is needed if the breast does not cover enough of the detector.
- The MLO is generally easier to perform and beginning the exam with the MLO will generally allow for using the AEC. Using the information provided from the MLO exposure will assist in choosing a manual technique for the CC images.
- Use a spatula if necessary.
- Roll or tilt the patient to the affected side.
- The FB can replace the CC.

Male Breast

- Imaging is similar to that of a small female breast.
- The FB is an option if the patient is mobile and especially when there is chest hair.
- Chest hair and too much pectoral muscle can present problems.

Large or Wide Breast

- Sectional imaging may be necessary.
- In any sectional imaging there must be at least 2.5 cm (1 inch) of breast tissue overlap.
- All images must be clearly labeled for proper evaluation, e.g., MLO upper or MLO lower.

Kyphotic Patients

- The FB can replace the CC or the XCCL and XCCM can be used.
- The LMO can replace the MLO.
- The LM, documented as a limited study, can replace the MLO.

Pectus Excavatum (Depressed Sternum)

- The XCCL and XCCM can replace the CC projection to image medial and lateral portions of the breast.
- The CV can be used to image medial breast.
- The LMO can replace the MLO.
- The LM, documented as a limited study, can replace the MLO.

Pectus Carinatum (Pigeon Chest—Prominent Sternum) and Barrel Chest (Prominent Ribs and Sternum)

- The XCCL and XCCM can replace the CC projection to image medial and lateral portions of the breast.
- The routine MLO plus AT can be used.

Postsurgical Breast

- Postlumpectomy imaging can include CC and ML or MLO imaging of the surgical site.
- Magnification can be used to evaluate calcifications.
- Other imaging may include a spot compression of the area of concern, and/or an AT projection.

Irradiated Breast

- Mammograms can be performed 6-12 months after completion of radiation treatment.
- Infection control is critical.

Stretcher/Cart Patients

- The CC imaging can be performed with the patient supine and the tube rotated 90 degrees.
- The FB can replace the CC with the patient supine and the tube rotated 90 degrees.
- The ML or LM, documented as a limited study, can replace the MLO with the patient lateral and the tube positioned at 0 degrees.

Wheelchair Patients

- The ML or LM, documented as a limited study, can replace the MLO.
- A bolster behind the patient can help straighten the spine and allow better positioning.
- If the chair arm is removed, the patient must be carefully monitored or supported.

Elderly Patient

- A chair examination may be necessary.
- The patient should be allowed to keep all walking aids, such as walkers or canes.
- All limitations should be documented.

Nipple Not in Profile

- Always image the entire breast first, then if necessary, image the nipple separately using nipple in profile projections.
- Using nipple markers can eliminate the need for added projections.

Skin Folds or Wrinkling of the Breast

- Skin folds or wrinkling may be impossible to avoid in the elderly.
- Smooth folds or wrinkles using the index finger during compression.
- Avoid pushing breast tissue outside of the compression field to eliminate a fold or wrinkle.
- Added projections will be needed if any breast tissue is eliminated when removing wrinkling or folds.

Breast Thickness

- When imaging for the MLO projection, the detector must be parallel to the pectoral muscle.
- Two images, the MLO and AT or the MLO and ML, for each routine projection may be necessary to image the posterior and anterior breast. Imaging the anterior portion of the breast to improve compression may be designated as "anterior compression" projections.
- Flex paddles can be used to avoid overcompression of posterior breast tissue to achieve adequate compression of anterior breast.

Protruding Abdomen

- CC and MLO imaging should start with the patient standing away from the unit and leaning forward.
- MLO imaging may need reduced tube angulation for better control of the anterior breast.

Frozen Shoulder

- The LMO or the LM can replace the MLO.
- Imaging for the MLO can be performed with the patient's ipsilateral arm down.
- Any limitations should be documented.

Specimen Imaging

The specimen is the breast tissue sample removed during a biopsy. A radiograph of the specimen is necessary to ensure the area under suspicion is totally removed and the margins are clean. In imaging the specimen:

- Speed and efficiency are important because the patient may be under anesthesia.
- Always use compression when imaging larger specimens.
- Magnification may help to visualize microcalcifications.

MQSA IMAGING REQUIREMENT

MQSA requirements for image identification include:

- Name of patient and additional patient identifier, such as hospital number or medical records number.
- Date of examination.
- Projection indicator and right or left marker, placed near the axilla using standardized codes approved by the FDA.
- Facility name and location to include city, state, and zip code.
- Mammographer's identification.
- Mammography unit identification if there is more than 1 unit at the facility.
- Cassette/screen identification for analog units.

Questions

1. Which of the following statements is true?
   (A) Compression increases image sharpness by reducing the focal spot size.
   (B) Compression decreases subject contrast by reducing the thickness of the penetrated tissue.
   (C) Compression increases the uniformity of the breast, making diagnosis easier.
   (D) The compressed breast requires increase kVp to penetrate the thicker tissue.

2. The maximum compression force applied to the breast should not exceed _______.
   (A) 111 N (25 lb)
   (B) 178 N (40 lb)
   (C) 200 N (45 lb)
   (D) none of the above

3. In assessing the degree of compression for any one patient, the mammographer should take into consideration
   1. the maximum to which the patient's breast can actually be compressed
   2. the amount of compression the patient can tolerate
   3. compression that should be just sufficient to immobilize the breast

   (A) 1 only
   (B) 1 and 2 only
   (C) 1 and 3 only
   (D) 2 and 3 only

4. Manual compression in mammography
   (A) has a fixed upper and lower limit
   (B) depends solely on breast size
   (C) depends on breast size and the patient's pain tolerance
   (D) generally depends on the patient's pain tolerance

5. Some considerations that could be given to women with painful breasts include
   1. having the patient take ibuprofen prior to the mammogram
   2. scheduling the mammogram during the menstrual cycle
   3. explaining, before the examination, the importance of compression

   (A) 1 only
   (B) 1 and 2
   (C) 2 and 3
   (D) 1 and 3

6. When imaging using the FB, the area of the breast that will likely be missed is the
   (A) medial
   (B) lateral
   (C) inferior
   (D) posterior

7. Compression allows reduced radiation to the breast by
   (A) providing a uniform breast thickness
   (B) decreasing breast thickness
   (C) decreasing motion unsharpness
   (D) separating superimposed areas of glandular tissue

8. What principle does compression use to visualize the borders of circumscribed lesions?
   1. It brings the lesion closer to the detector.
   2. It spreads apart overlapping tissue.
   3. It separates superimposed areas of glandular tissue.

   (A) 1 only
   (B) 1 and 2 only
   (C) 2 and 3 only
   (D) 1, 2, and 3

9. Ideally, breast compression is maximized when
   1. accompanied by a thorough explanation to increase patient cooperation
   2. the exposure is made on arrested inspiration to reduce motion
   3. the patient recognizes the advantage of compression in reducing radiation dose

   (A) 1 and 2 only
   (B) 2 and 3 only
   (C) 1 and 3 only
   (D) 1, 2, and 3

10. Magnification can be used to assess the

    (A) margins of a lesion
    (B) size of a lesion
    (C) location of a lesion
    (D) density of a lesion

11. With calcifications, magnification can be used to assess
    1. the number
    2. morphology
    3. distribution

    (A) 1 only
    (B) 1 and 2 only
    (C) 2 and 3 only
    (D) 1, 2, and 3

12. The last degree of compression should be applied

    (A) using manual compression
    (B) after the breast is released from compression
    (C) with the automatic compression device
    (D) with the mammographer's hand between the breast and the compression paddle

13. Which projection is used to determine if a lesion is medial or lateral to the nipple?

    (A) CC
    (B) MLO
    (C) TAN
    (D) ML

14. If any breast tissue is poorly imaged on the MLO projection, it is likely to be

    (A) medial breast tissue
    (B) lateral breast tissue
    (C) inferior breast tissue
    (D) superior breast tissue

15. The length of the posterior nipple line (PNL), visualized on the CC, should be within how many centimeters of the PNL on the MLO?

    (A) 0.25
    (B) 0.50
    (C) 1.00
    (D) 1.50

16. Which of the following conditions must be met when imaging the breast in the MLO?
    1. The pectoral muscle should extend to or below the PNL.
    2. Visualized fat should be posterior to all the fibroglandular tissues.
    3. The inframammary fold (IMF) should be open.

    (A) 1 and 2 only
    (B) 2 and 3 only
    (C) 1 and 3 only
    (D) 1, 2, and 3

17. In positioning for the CC projection, if the C-arm of the mammography unit is raised too high the IMF is overelevated, resulting in loss of

1 superior breast tissue
2. inferior breast tissue
3. posterior breast tissue

(A) 1 and 2 only
(B) 2 and 3 only
(C) 1 and 3 only
(D) 1, 2, and 3

18. The single projection that will best visualize the maximum amount of breast tissue is the

(A) CC
(B) MLO
(C) ML
(D) XCCL

19. In general, when imaging tall, thin patients the angulation is adjusted to

(A) below 30 degrees
(B) between 30 and 40 degrees
(C) close to 60 degrees
(D) over 70 degrees

20. The position used to determine whether an abnormality is superior or inferior to the nipple is the

(A) CC
(B) MLO
(C) XCCL
(D) TAN

21. The principle of mobile versus fixed tissue is used in mammography positioning to image the maximum

(A) medial breast on the MLO projection
(B) inferior breast on the CC projection
(C) superior breast on the MLO projection
(D) medial tissue on the CC projection

22. In the CC projection of the breast, the detector is positioned

(A) at the level of the raised inframammary crease
(B) below the level of the raised inframammary crease
(C) at the level of the inframammary crease
(D) just below the level of the inframammary crease

23. In positioning for the MLO, the tube is always angled

(A) 90 degrees
(B) 60 degrees
(C) 50 degrees
(D) none of the above

24. What position is shown in Figure 4-1?

(A) CC
(B) MLO
(C) CV
(D) XCCL

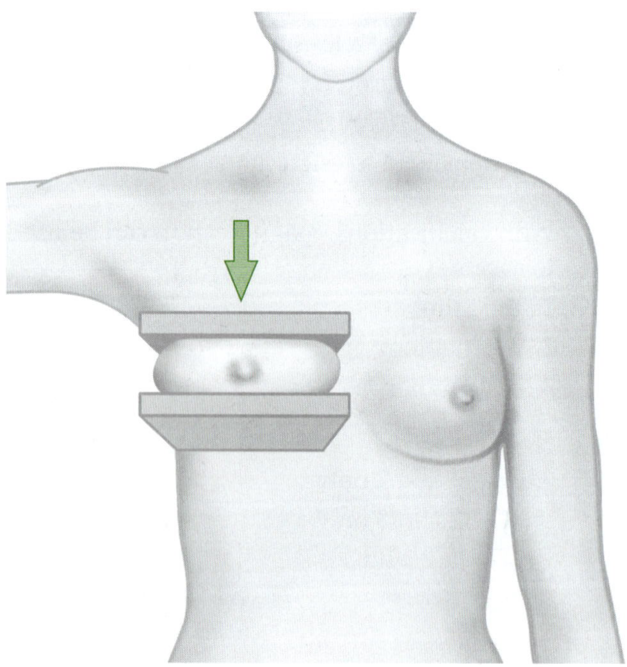

Figure 4-1.

25. When positioning for the right CC, where is the patient's left arm placed?
    - (A) Brought back. This action rotates the shoulder to remove it from the imaging area.
    - (B) Brought forward. The patient can hold the handle bar of the unit.
    - (C) Brought forward. The patient can hold the detector.
    - (D) Remains at the patient's side.

26. Your patient has had recent chest surgery and has a scarred and painful area running along the sternum. With the medial aspect of the breast immobile, which of the following is an alternative to the RMLO?
    - (A) RLMO
    - (B) LMLO
    - (C) LLM
    - (D) RML

27. Which projection is best used to visualize the tail of the breast?
    - (A) LMO
    - (B) TAN
    - (C) LM
    - (D) AT

28. Calcifications seen on the mammogram are suspected to be in the skin. The best projection necessary to prove this theory is the
    - (A) LMO
    - (B) TAN
    - (C) LM
    - (D) AT

29. The projection best used to demonstrate details of the medial breast structures of the breast is the
    - (A) LM
    - (B) AT
    - (C) ML
    - (D) TAN

30. A lesion on the lateral aspect of the breast is not seen on the CC. An additional projection used to image the lesion could be the
    - (A) CV
    - (B) XCCL
    - (C) FB
    - (D) TAN

31. Which projection can be used instead of the CC to image patients with severe kyphosis?
    - (A) ML
    - (B) TAN
    - (C) FB
    - (D) CV

32. A lesion moved up on the ML projection from its original position on the MLO. The location of the lesion within the breast is
    - (A) lateral
    - (B) medial
    - (C) inferior
    - (D) superior

33. Which projection can be used to prove breast calcifications are benign (teacup shaped)?
    - (A) CC
    - (B) XCCL
    - (C) FB
    - (D) ML

34. Which projection can be used to give a profile image of the area in question without superimposition of breast tissue?
    - (A) CV
    - (B) TAN
    - (C) LMO
    - (D) AT

35. Identify the projection shown in Figure 4-2.
    - (A) FB
    - (B) XCCL
    - (C) ML
    - (D) AT

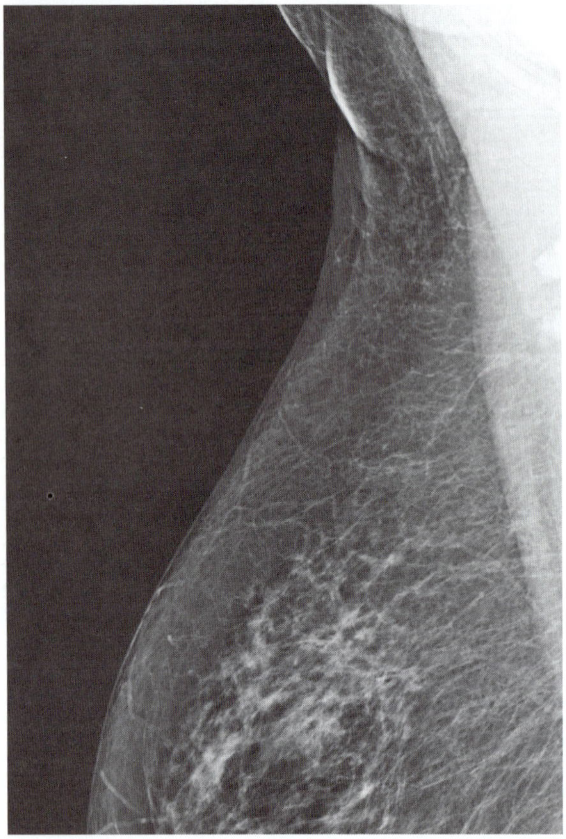

Figure 4-2.

36. A barrel-chested patient whose chest wall protrudes outward may have breast tissue extending laterally under the arm. What projection, used to image the breast with the beam directed superiorly to inferiorly, should be taken in addition to the CC?

    (A) AT
    (B) XCCL
    (C) CV
    (D) MLO

37. The FB projection can be useful in imaging
    1. patients with extreme kyphosis
    2. abnormalities high on the chest wall or superior aspect of breast
    3. inferior lesions or lesions near the IMF

    (A) 1 and 2 only
    (B) 2 and 3 only
    (C) 1 and 3 only
    (D) 1, 2, and 3

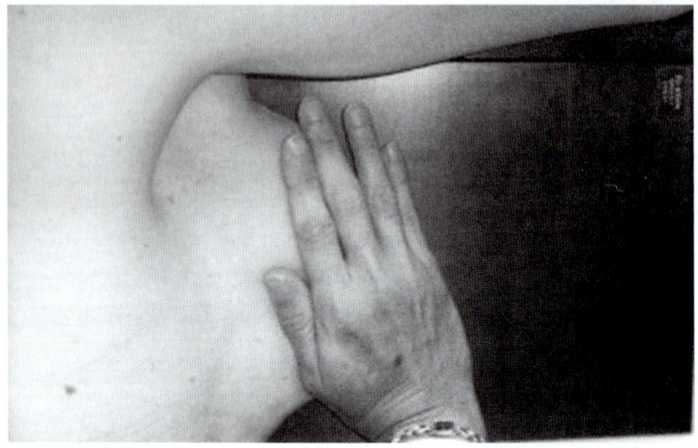

Figure 4-3.

38. Identify the position shown in Figure 4-3.

    (A) MLO
    (B) CV
    (C) LM
    (D) ML

39. Why is the MLO preferred to the ML as a routine projection?

    (A) The MLO visualizes the medial breast.
    (B) The ML does not visualize the medial breast.
    (C) The ML poorly visualizes the posterior and lateral breast.
    (D) The MLO does not distort the anterior structure of the breast.

40. Which projection best shows the extreme medial aspect of the breast?

    (A) CC
    (B) MLO
    (C) ML
    (D) CV

41. In which modified projection is the superior aspect of the breast rolled medially?

    (A) RM
    (B) RL
    (C) M
    (D) LM

42. In the LMO projection, the beam is directed from the
    - (A) upper-inner aspect to the lower-outer aspect of the breast
    - (B) inner-outer aspect to the upper-outer aspect of the breast
    - (C) lower-outer aspect to the upper-inner aspect of the breast
    - (D) superolateral aspect to the inferomedial aspect of the breast

43. Identify the projection shown in Figure 4-4.
    - (A) MLO
    - (B) CV
    - (C) LM
    - (D) ML

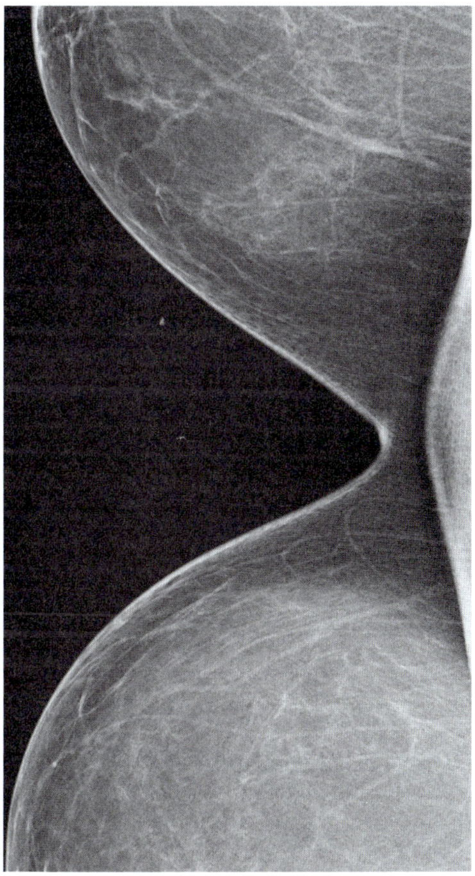

Figure 4-4.

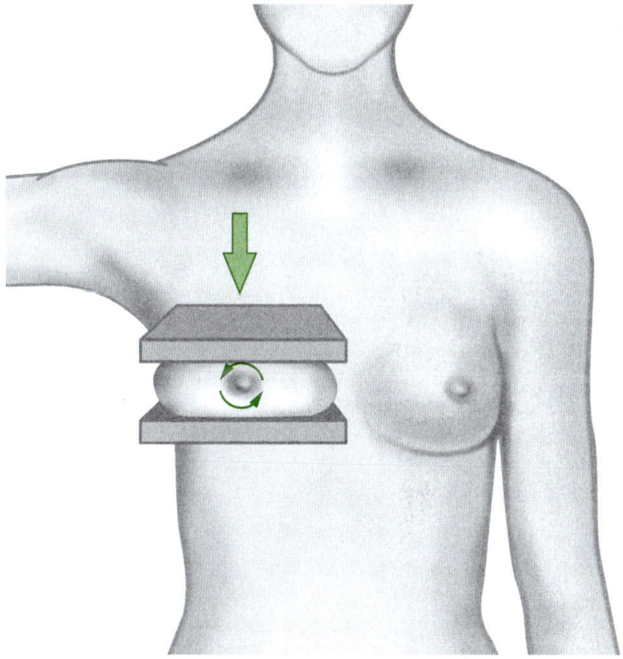

Figure 4-5. (Reproduced with permission from Peart O: Mammography and Breast Imaging PREP: Program Review and Exam Prep. New York, NY: McGraw-Hill Education; 2012.)

44. Identify the position shown in Figure 4-5.
    - (A) RM
    - (B) CV
    - (C) RL
    - (D) MLO

45. Which projection is especially useful when analyzing calcifications?
    - (A) RM
    - (B) M
    - (C) LM
    - (D) ML

46. Identify the position shown in Figure 4-6.
    - (A) RM
    - (B) CV
    - (C) RL
    - (D) MLO

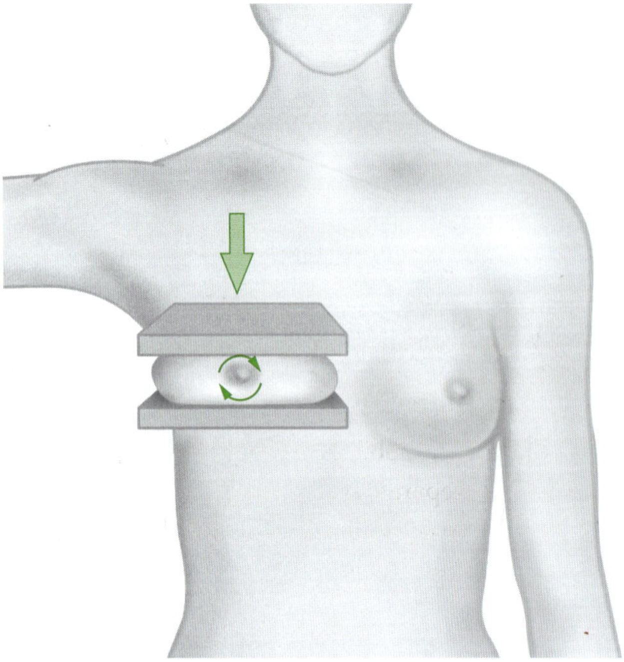

Figure 4-6. (Reproduced with permission from Peart O: Mammography and Breast Imaging PREP: Program Review and Exam Prep. New York, NY: McGraw-Hill Education; 2012.)

47. All of the following statements about magnification are true *except*
    (A) With magnification, patient dose increases.
    (B) Magnification can be used to image specimen radiographs.
    (C) Magnification can be used to assess suspicious lesions.
    (D) Magnification images the entire breast with 1 exposure.

48. In the RS position, the surface _________ the detector is rolled _______.
    (A) furthest from/inferiorly
    (B) closest to/superiorly
    (C) furthest from/superiorly
    (D) closest to/inferiorly

49. Which technique accurately describes how the breast is rolled for the RM?
    (A) The superior surface is rolled medially and the inferior surface does not move.
    (B) The superior surface is rolled laterally and the inferior surface is rolled medially.
    (C) The inferior surface is rolled medially and the superior surface does not move.
    (D) The inferior surface is rolled laterally and the superior surface is rolled medially.

50. A patient with pectus excavatum may present a positioning problem because the patient has
    (A) extensive pectoral muscle
    (B) barrel chest
    (C) kyphosis
    (D) depressed sternum

51. In imaging the augmented breast in the CC position, using the implant-displaced technique, the breast tissue is pulled/pushed
    (A) anteriorly
    (B) posteriorly
    (C) inferiorly
    (D) superiorly

52. A routine series on patients with encapsulated implants could include an additional projection such as the
    (A) TAN
    (B) CC
    (C) MLO
    (D) ML

53. Which of the following is used to spread out the tissue and improve resolution on a localized area of interest?
    (A) CV
    (B) AT
    (C) TAN
    (D) spot compression

54. How many projections are routinely required to image a patient with implant augmented breasts?

(A) 5
(B) 6
(C) 7
(D) 8

55. When is imaging of the irradiated breast recommended?

(A) immediately after treatment
(B) 1-2 months after treatment
(C) 6-12 months after treatment
(D) 1-2 years after treatment

56. Which of the following projections or positions can be performed with any patient orientation, with or without magnification?

(A) spot compression
(B) XCCL
(C) AT
(D) CV

57. In addition to the routine series, many post-lumpectomy patients can also be imaged using the

(A) CC
(B) MLO
(C) ML
(D) CV

58. The "implant in place" projections taken on patients with breast implants requires compression

(A) for immobilization only
(B) to separate the breast tissue
(C) to provide a uniform tissue thickness
(D) for improved spatial resolution

Answers and Explanations

1. **(C)** Compression makes the breast tissue more uniform and reduces the thickness through which the x-ray beam must pass. This produces uniform densities that are easier to interpret and allows the use of lower exposure factors. Compression will increase image sharpness but has no impact on the focal spot size.[1,2]

2. **(D)** The actual compression applied to the breast will depend on the size and sensitivity of the patient's breasts. However, too little compression will compromise the image; too much can damage breast tissue. The compression standards, set by the MQSA are used for testing purposes to ensure the unit's compression device is working properly. As per the MQSAs guidelines, the compression force for the initial power drive must be between 111 and 200 N (25 and 45 lb). Manual compression is always at the discretion of the mammographer and typically has limits set by the unit manufacturers. Some upper limits on the manual compression can be 267-289 N (60-65 lb).[2,3]

3. **(B)** Ideally, compression should be applied until the breast tissue is taut. However, the patient should not be in pain at maximum compression, as this will be a disincentive to return for annual mammograms. The patient will generally be able to tolerate more compression if they are prepared for it, and if it is applied slowly. Although compression immobilizes the breast and reduces motion, compression just adequate to immobilize the breast is usually insufficient to separate breast tissue.[1]

4. **(C)** In general, the amount of compression applied will depend on the patient's breast size and patient's tolerance for compression. After the initial automatic compression most patients will require more manual compression to adequately compress the breast. However, too little compression will compromise the image; too much can damage breast tissue. The compression standards, set by the MQSA are used for testing purposes to ensure the unit's compression device is working properly. As per the MQSAs guidelines, the compression force for the initial power drive must be between 111 and 200 N (25 and 45 lb). Manual compression is always at the discretion of the mammographer and typically has upper limits set by the unit manufacturers. Some upper limits on the manual compression can be 267-289 N (60-65 lb).[2,3]

5. **(D)** Often the patient will be able to tolerate more compression if the need for compression is explained to the patient. Patients with particularly sensitive breasts could benefit from pain medication prior to the mammogram. The patient must consult their physician before taking any medication. There are over the counter oral pain medications that could be taken 30 minutes before the mammogram and there are also prescription pain gels that can be applied to the breast just before compression. Also, the breast is often more sensitive to pain just before or during the menstrual period and is least sensitive 5-10 days after the start of the period.[1,4]

6. **(D)** The breast is least mobile at the medial and superior aspects and most mobile at the lateral and inferior aspects. To image the maximum amount of breast tissue, the most mobile parts of the breast must be placed adjacent to the detector while applying compression from the least mobile aspect of the breast. Since the beam is directed from below, the fixed posterior area of the superior aspect of the breast is least likely to be included on the image.[5]

7. **(B)** Although the primary goal of compression is to provide a uniform breast thickness, compression will also decrease motion unsharpness by immobilizing the breast and it will separate superimposed areas of glandular tissue. Compression also reduces radiation dose to the breast by decreasing the thickness through which the radiation must pass, thus allowing less exposure.[1,4]

8. **(D)** Compression separates overlapping and superimposed areas of glandular tissue and will bring lesions closer to the detector. This action allows visualization of the borders of lesions.[4,5]

9. **(C)** Often, the patient is able to tolerate more compression if the need for compression is explained. Knowledge of the procedure generally alleviates fears, especially fears of the unknown. Any explanation should include a statement on how compression will reduce the radiation dose to help alleviate fears of radiation dangers. Throughout the examination, the patient should be encouraged to relax. Having the patient take a deep breath prior to holding the breath during the exposure is generally contraindicated. The patient may alter her position as the lungs expand, and the expanding ribs and lungs generally contract the pectoral muscles increasing discomfort during the mammogram. The patient should be simply advised to "stop breathing" without moving her body or first taking a deep breath.[1,5]

10. **(A)** Magnification cannot be used to assess lesion size because it gives a magnified image of the area which will not be a true representation of size. Location and density are also not easily assessed using magnification because the magnified image does not include the entire breast, and density comparisons will be difficult if other densities are not present on the image. Magnification is, however, capable of providing accurate assessment of the margins of a lesion (Figure 4-7).[6,7]

11. **(D)** Morphology is the form or structure of the calcification. By magnifying the area of interest, magnification provides images that can be used to assess the morphology, distribution, and number of calcifications.[6]

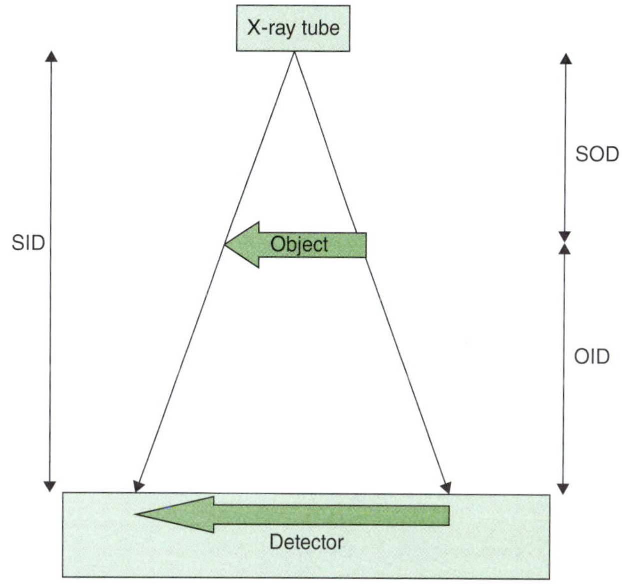

A

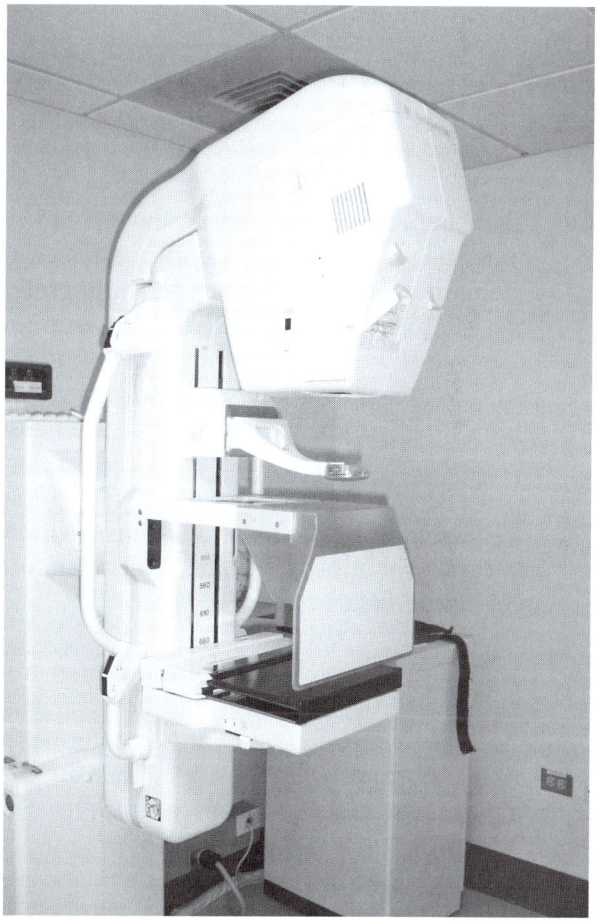

B

Figure 4-7. (A) Schematic diagrams showing the large OID used in magnification mammography. Note the small SOD which places the breast closer to the x-ray source. (B) Actual mammography set up. (C) Normal breast. (D) Magnified breast. (Reproduced with permission from Peart O: Lange Q&A: Mammography Examination, 2nd ed. McGraw-Hill Medical; 2008.)

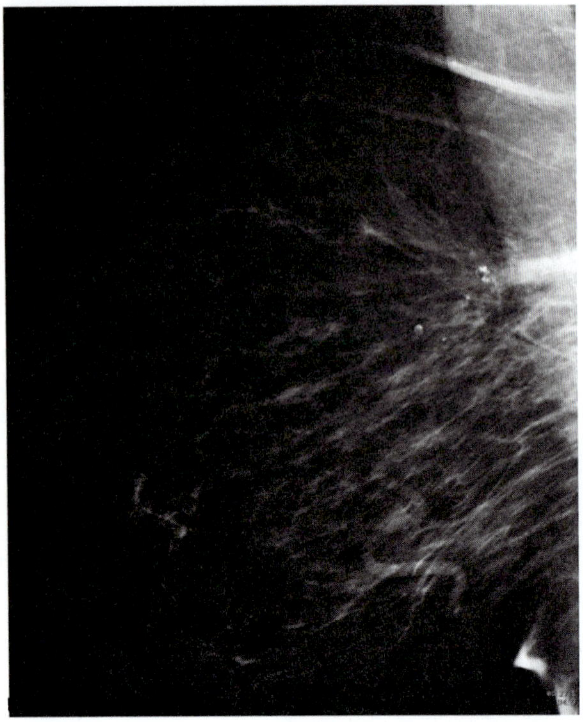

C

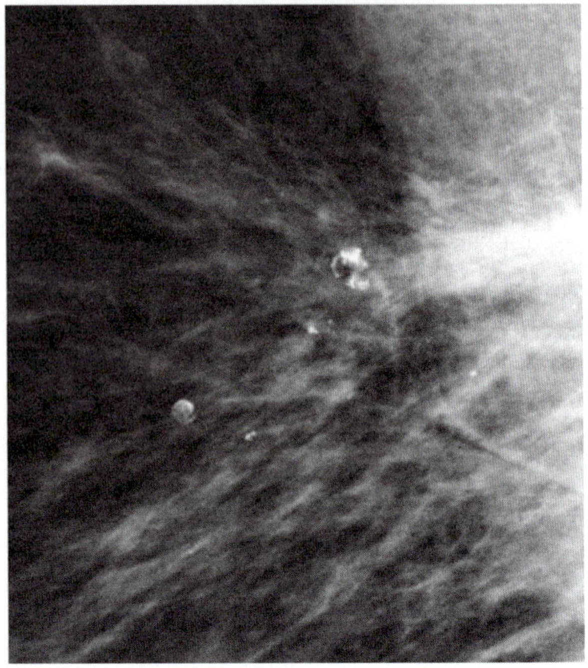

D

Figure 4-7. *(continued)*

12. **(A)** In applying compression, the mammographer needs to be as gentle as possible. The automatic compression should be applied with the mammographer's hand between the breast and the compression plate until the plate touches the back of the hand. Only then should the mammographer remove the hand, pulling the breast out, and applying the final degree of compression slowly. Always apply the last degree of compression using the manual rather than the automatic compression to avoid unnecessary pain to the patient.[5]

13. **(A)** CC projection determines whether the lesion is medial or lateral and how far it is from the nipple. The MLO or ML determines if the abnormality is superior or inferior and its posterior distance from the nipple. The TAN projection skims the area of interest and is best used to determine if a suspected abnormality is located in the breast or the skin of the breast (Figures 4-8 and 4-9).[5]

14. **(A)** The MLO best demonstrates the posterior and upper-outer quadrants of the breast. A good MLO must include both the superior and inferior portions of the breast. However, the medial breast is distorted on the MLO because it is an oblique projection. The CC projection gives a true representation of the medial breast.[5]

15. **(C)** The posterior nipple line (PNL) measures the perpendicular distance from the nipple to the visualized pectoral muscle on the MLO or from the nipple to the edge of the image on the CC. The length of the PNL on the CC view should be within 1 cm of its length on the MLO when the MLO is properly positioned. In approximately 10% of cases, the PNL will be greater on the CC (Figure 4-10).[5]

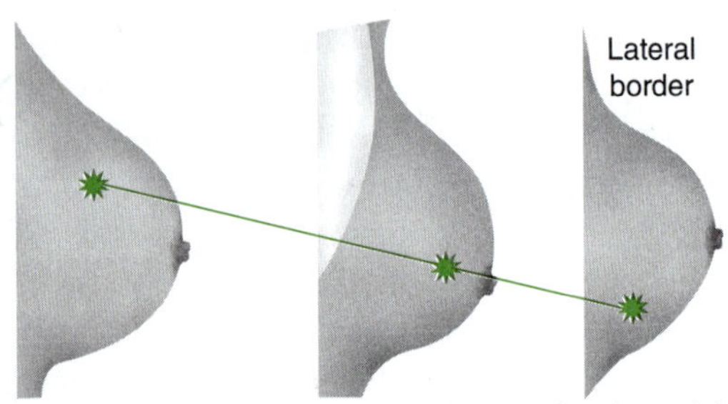

Figure 4-8. A lesion in the medial breast changes position on the MLO and ML.

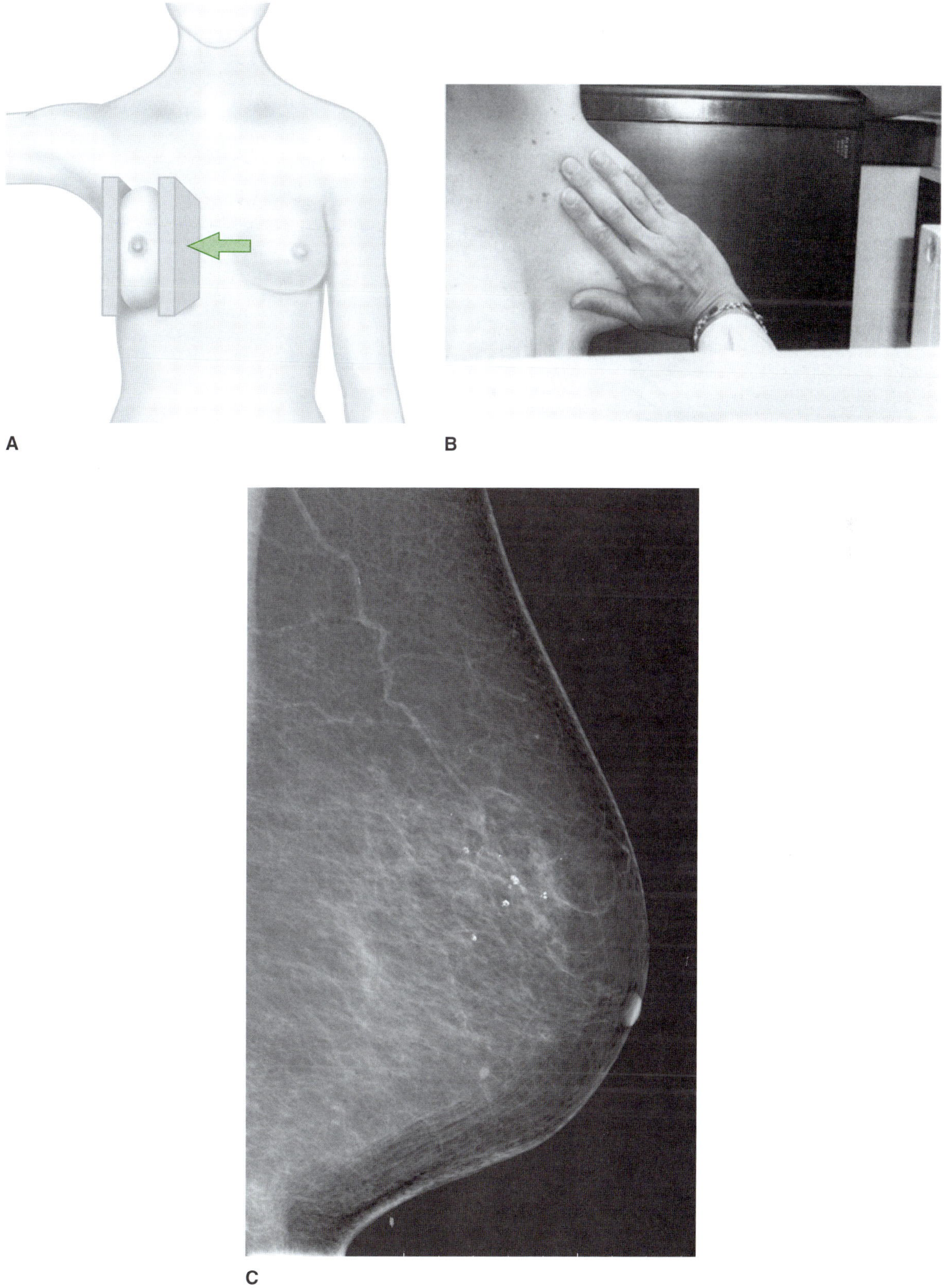

Figure 4-9. Pictogram of projections. Where listed (A) shows a schematic diagram of the position/projection. (B) shows the patient positioning & (C) shows the actual radiograph of the position/projection. (Used with permission from Daniel DiPaolo.)

4-9 (1) 90-degree mediolateral (ML)

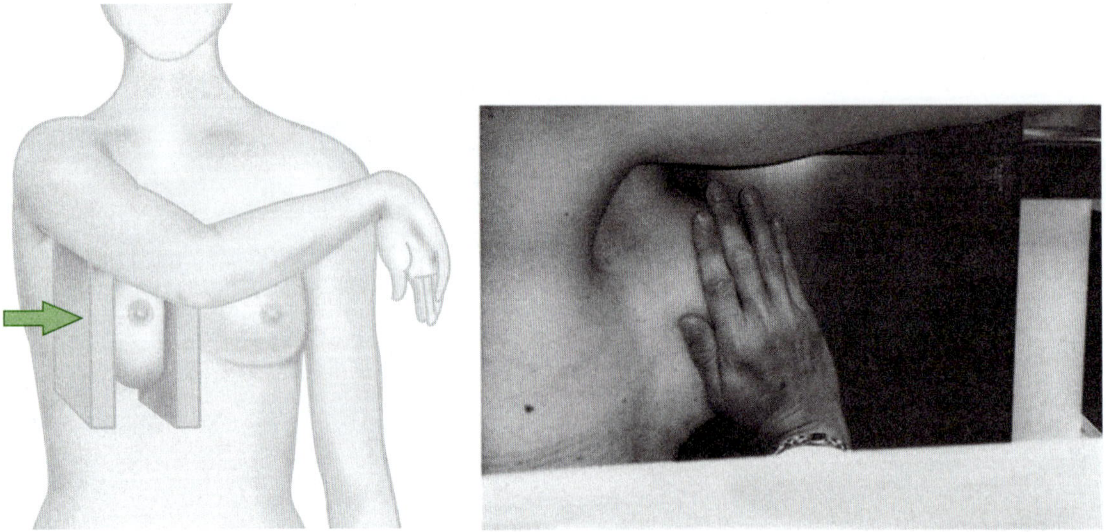

A B

4-9 (2) 90-degree lateromedial (LM)

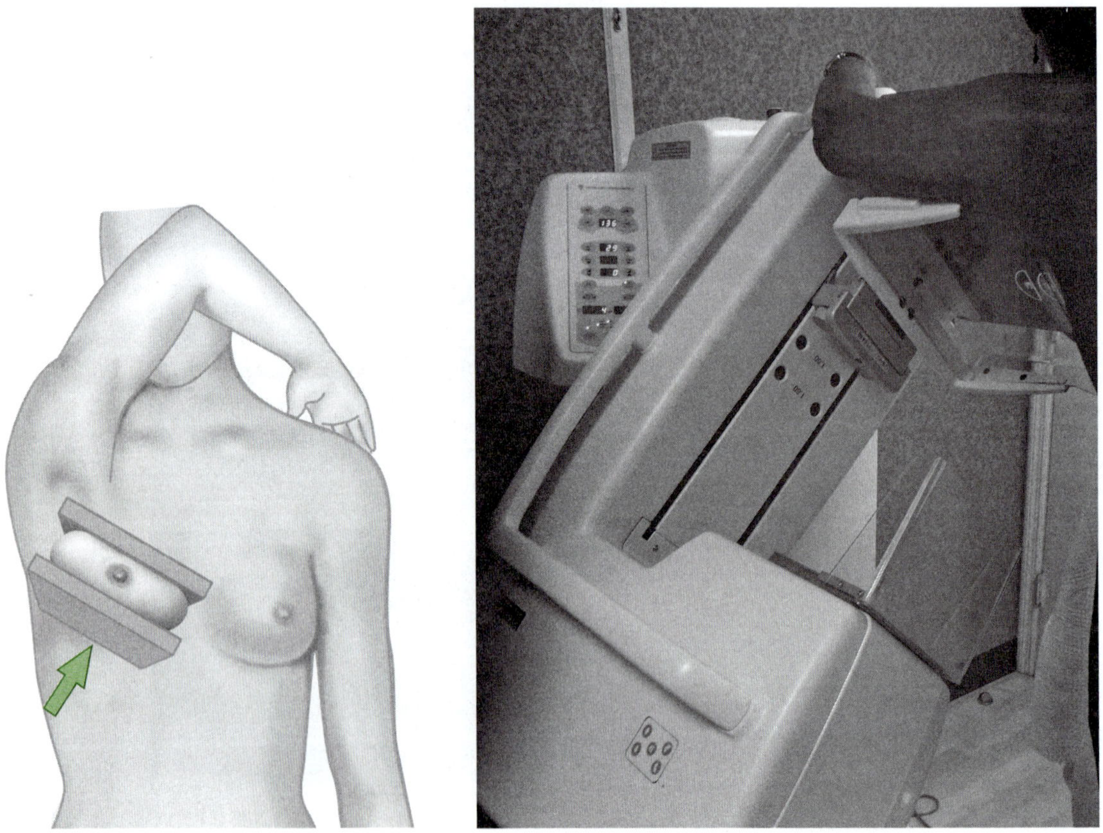

A B

4-9 (3) Lateromedial oblique (LMO)

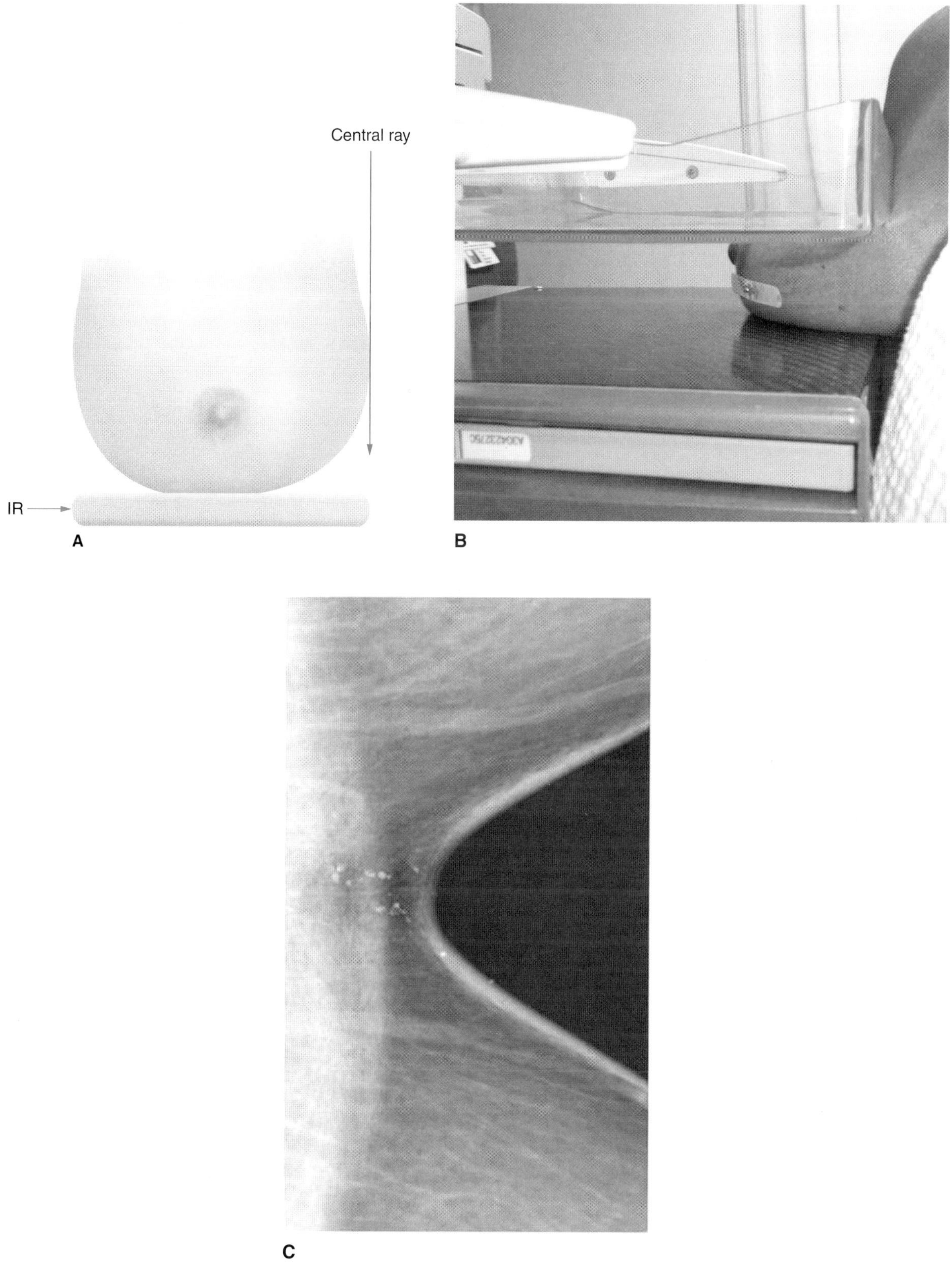

4-9 (4) Tangential projection (TAN)

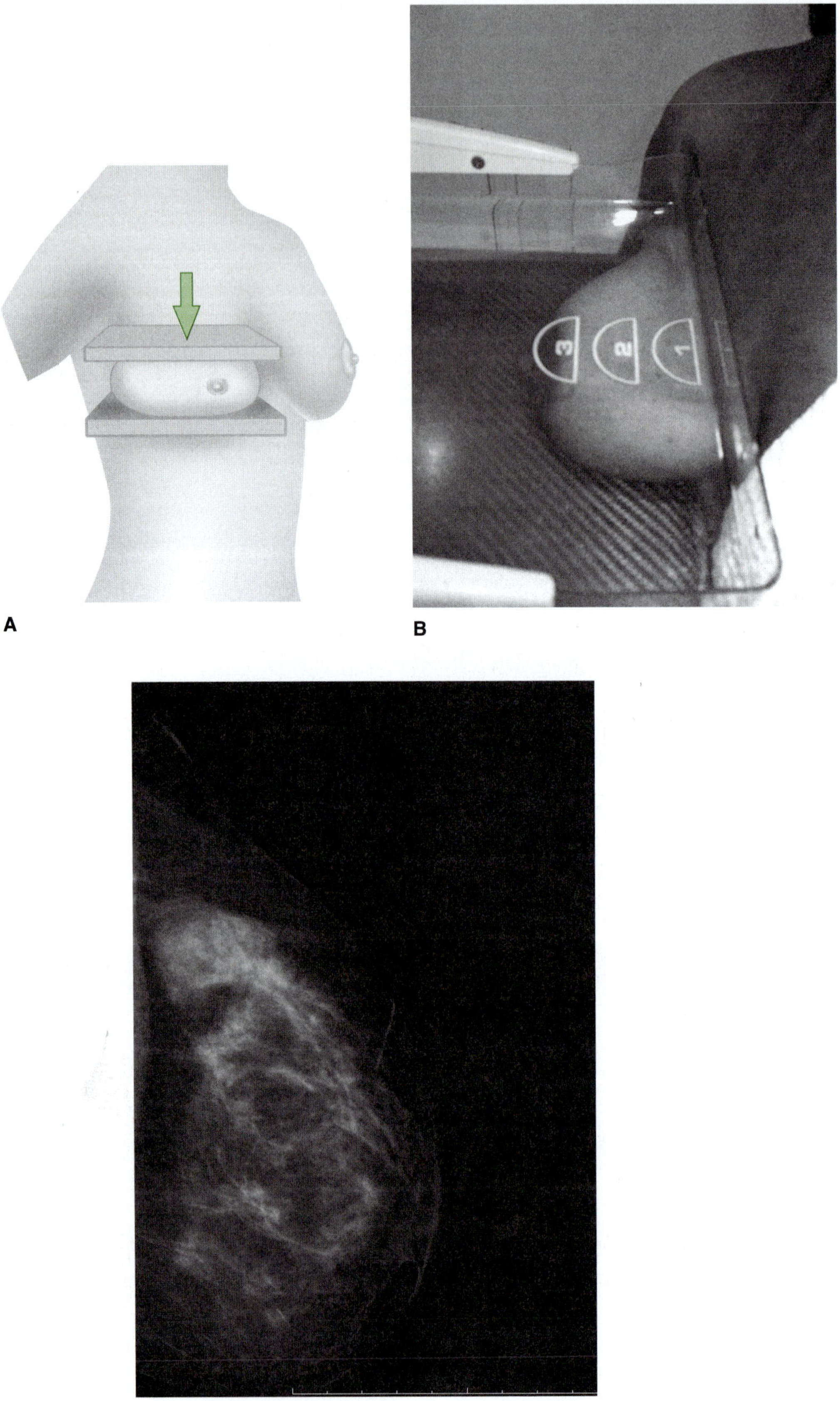

A B C

4-9 (5) Exaggerated craniocaudal lateral (XCCL)

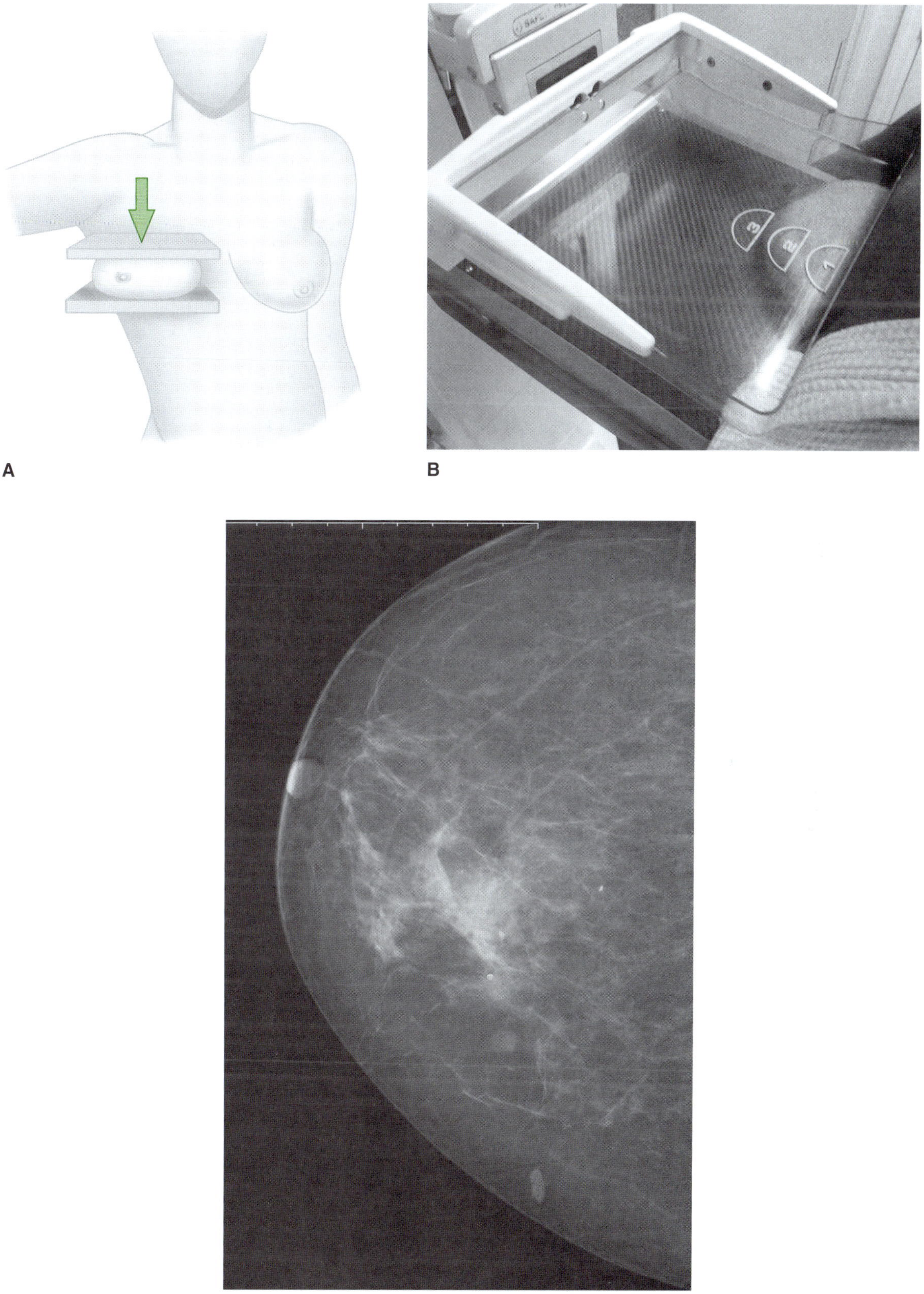

A B C

4-9 (6) Exaggerated craniocaudal medial (XCCM)

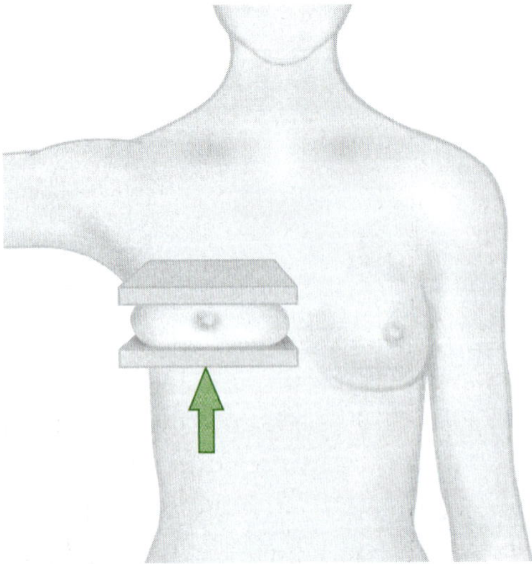

A

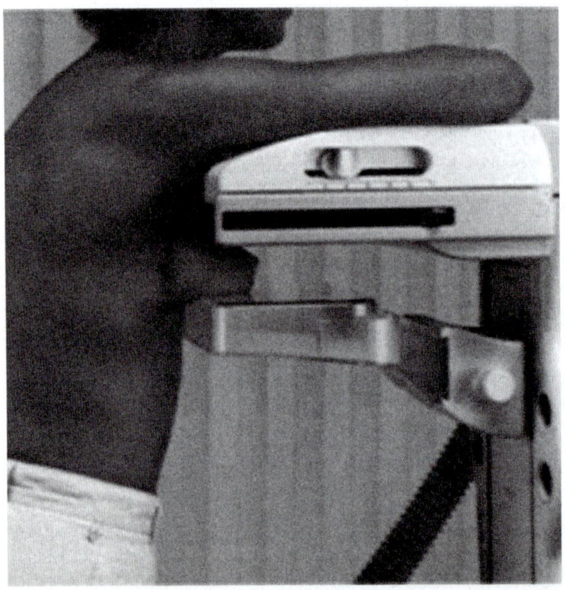

B

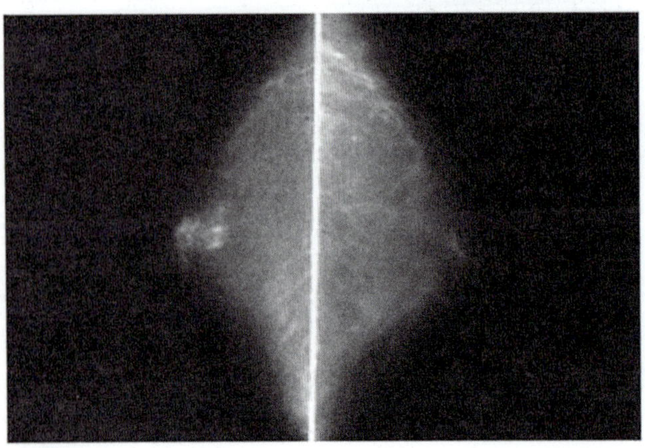

C

4-9 (7) Caudocranial or from below (FB)

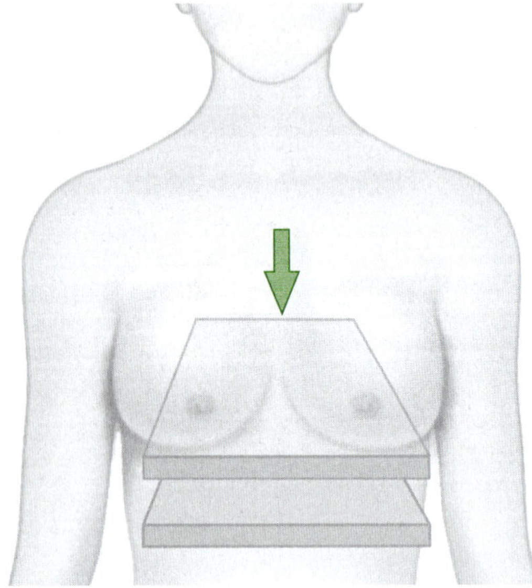

A

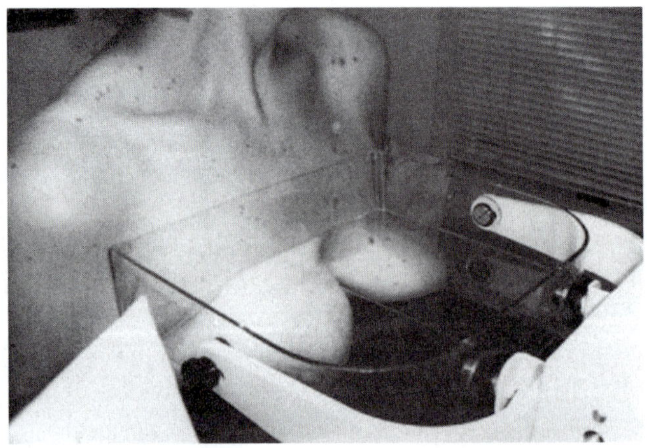

B

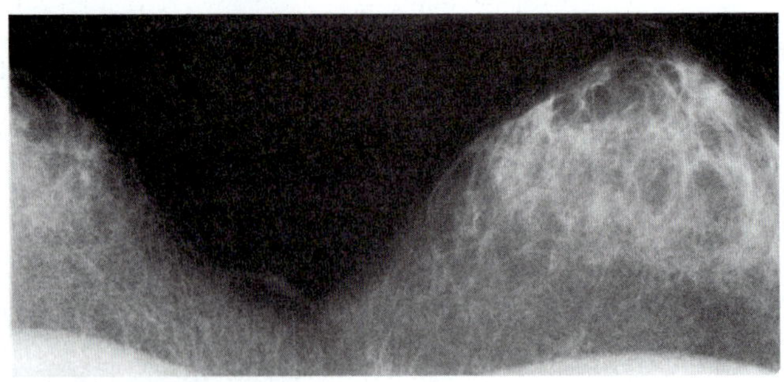

C

4-9 (8) Cleavage or "valley view" (CV)

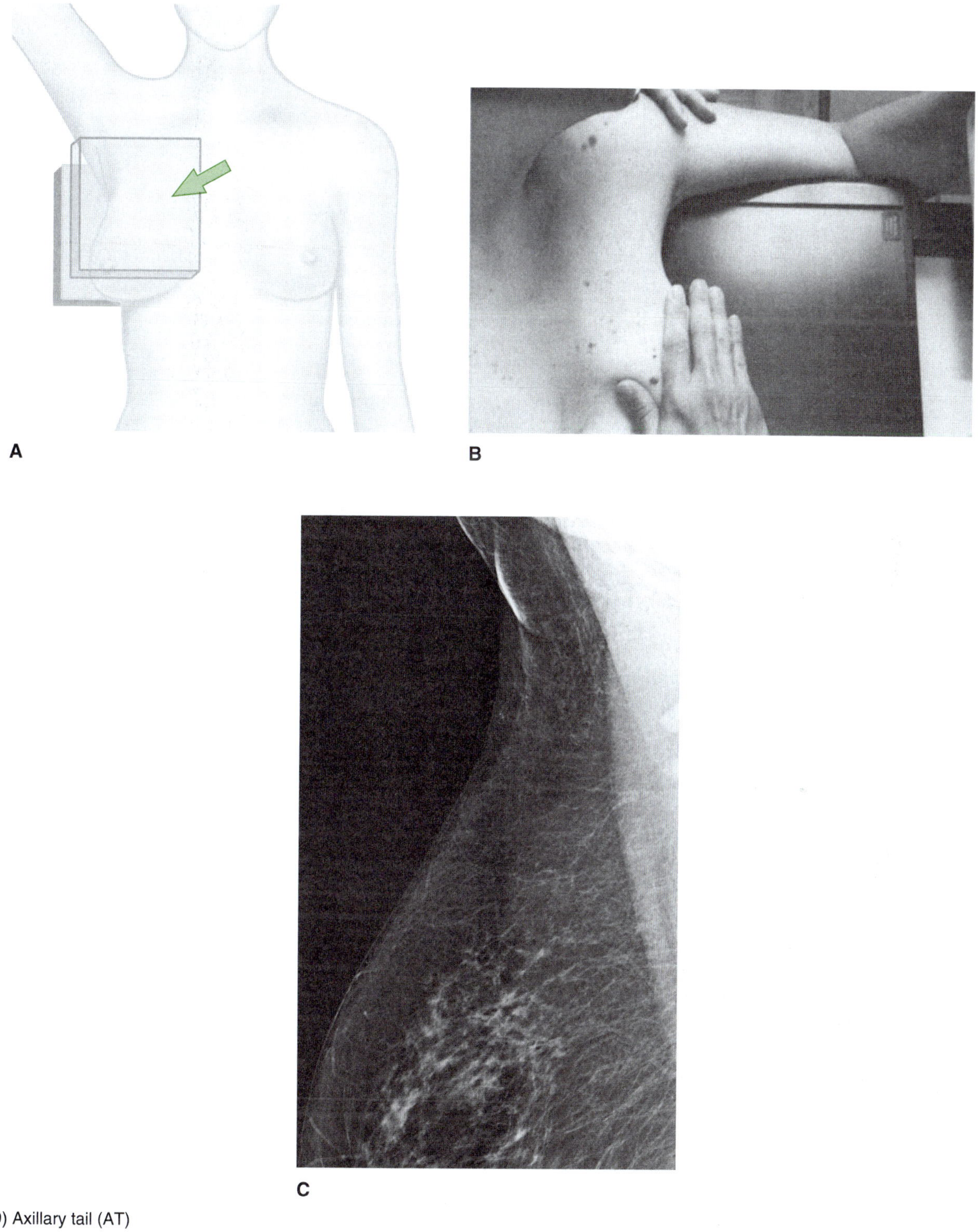

4-9 (9) Axillary tail (AT)

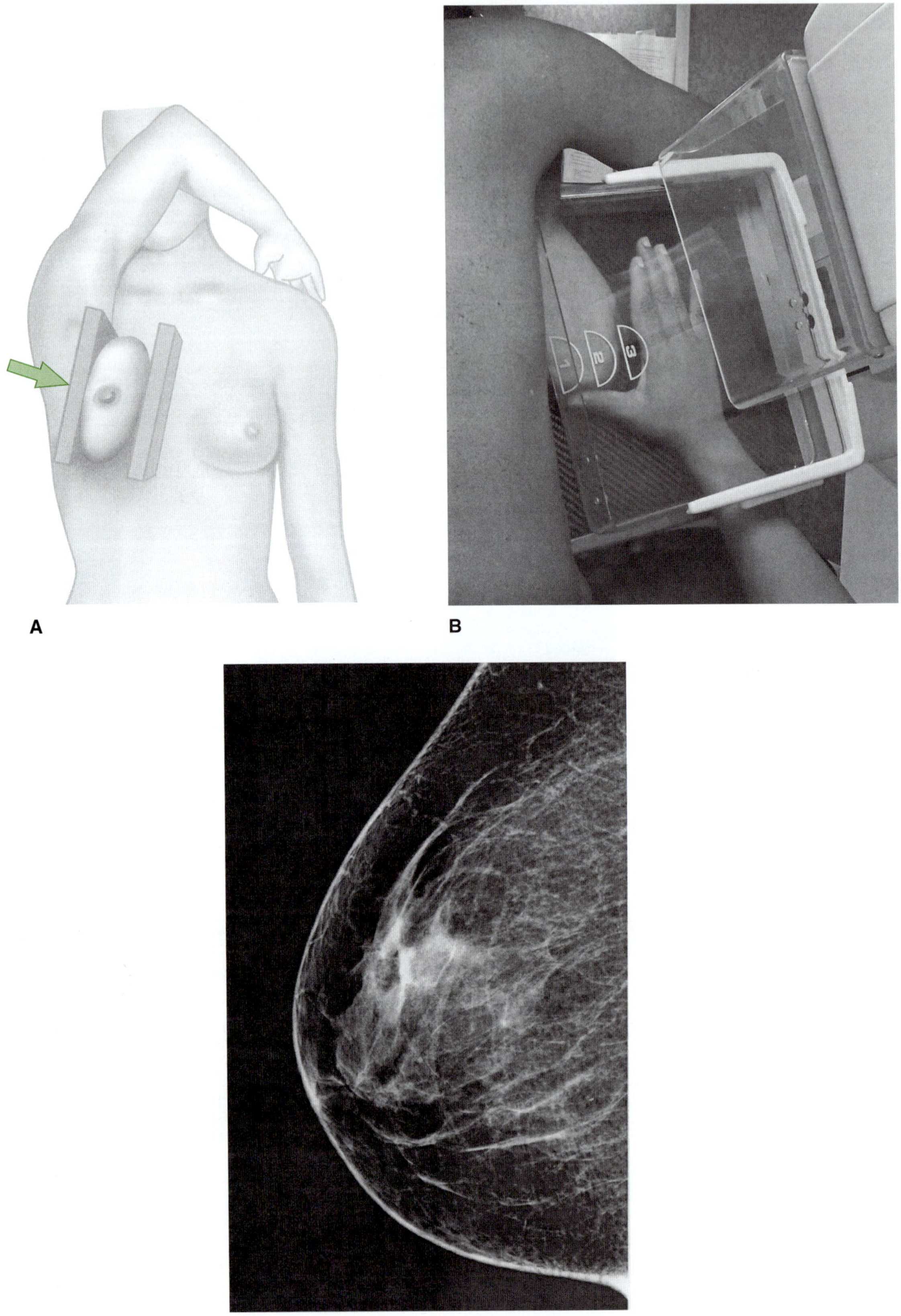

4-9 (10) Superoinferior oblique (SIO)

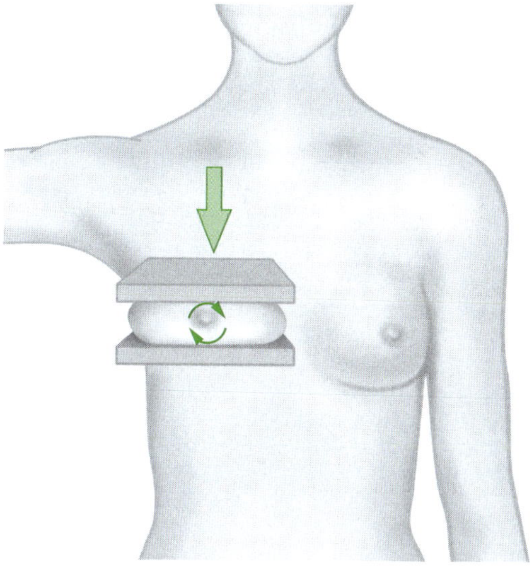

A

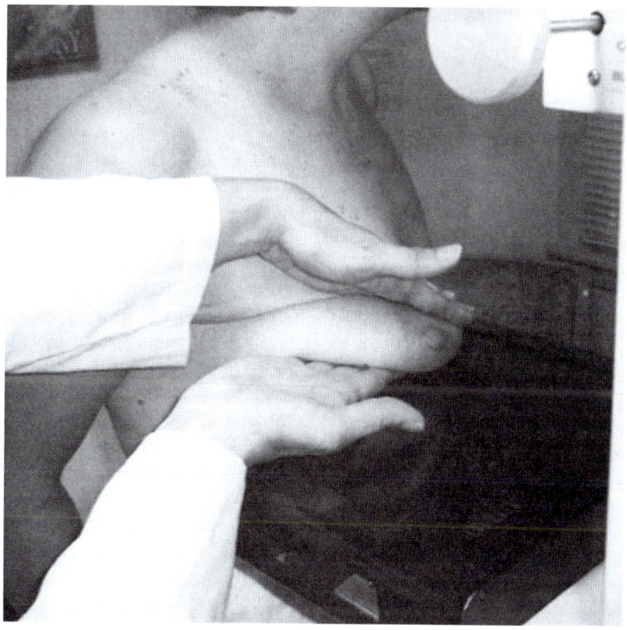

B

4-9 (11) Rolled medial (RM)

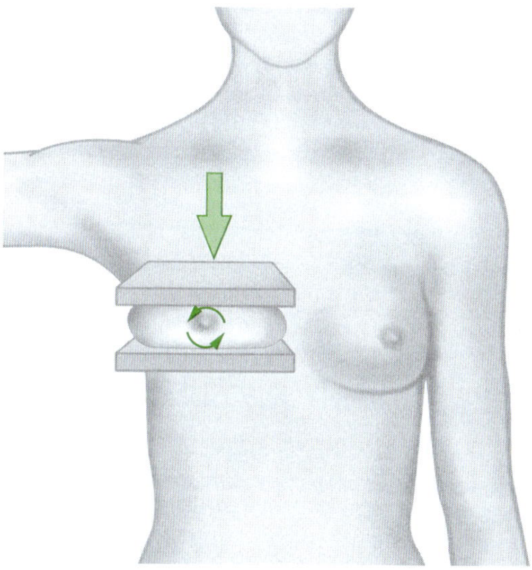

A

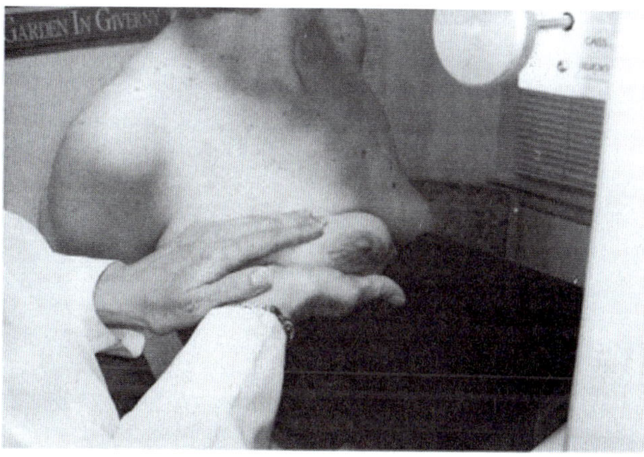

B

4-9 (12) Rolled lateral (RL)

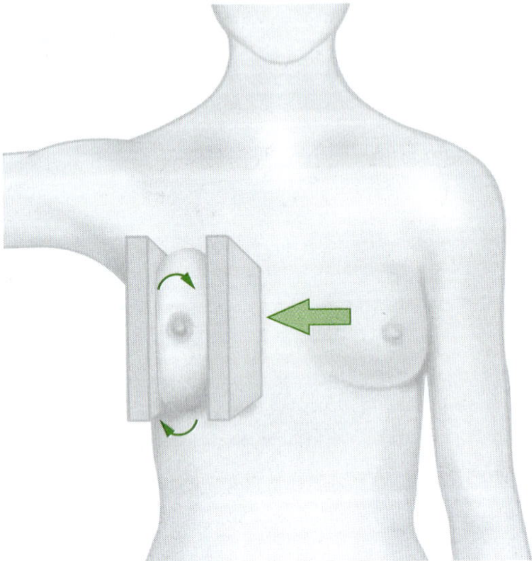

A

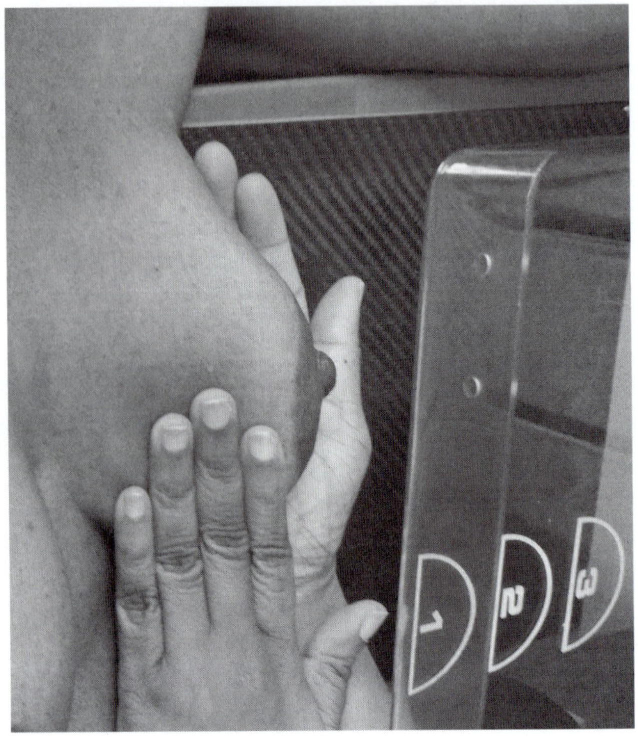

B

4-9 (13) Rolled inferior (RI)

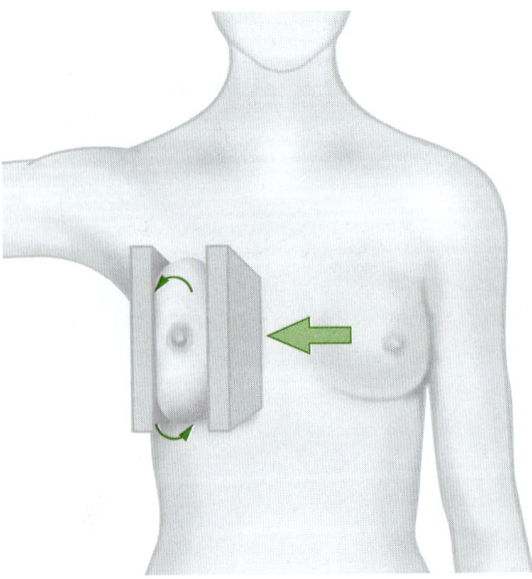

A

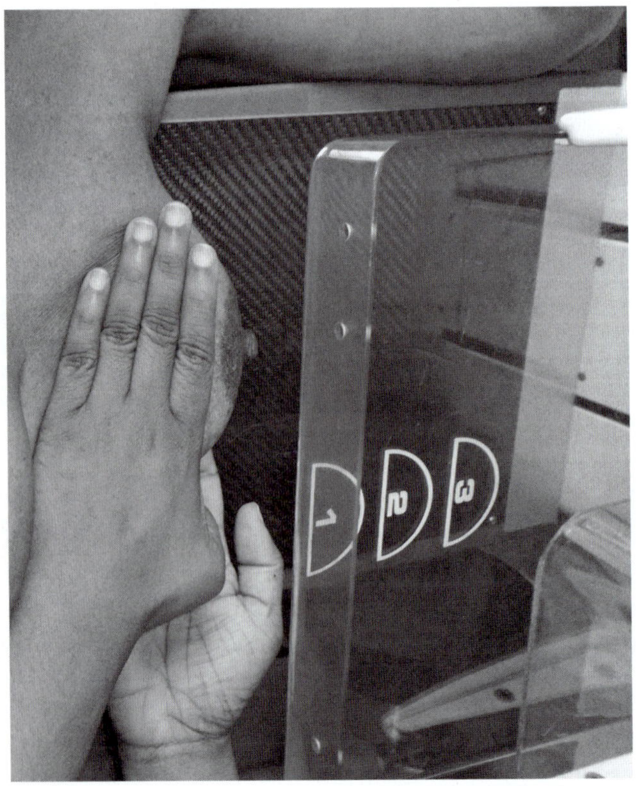

B

4-9 (14) Rolled superior (RS)

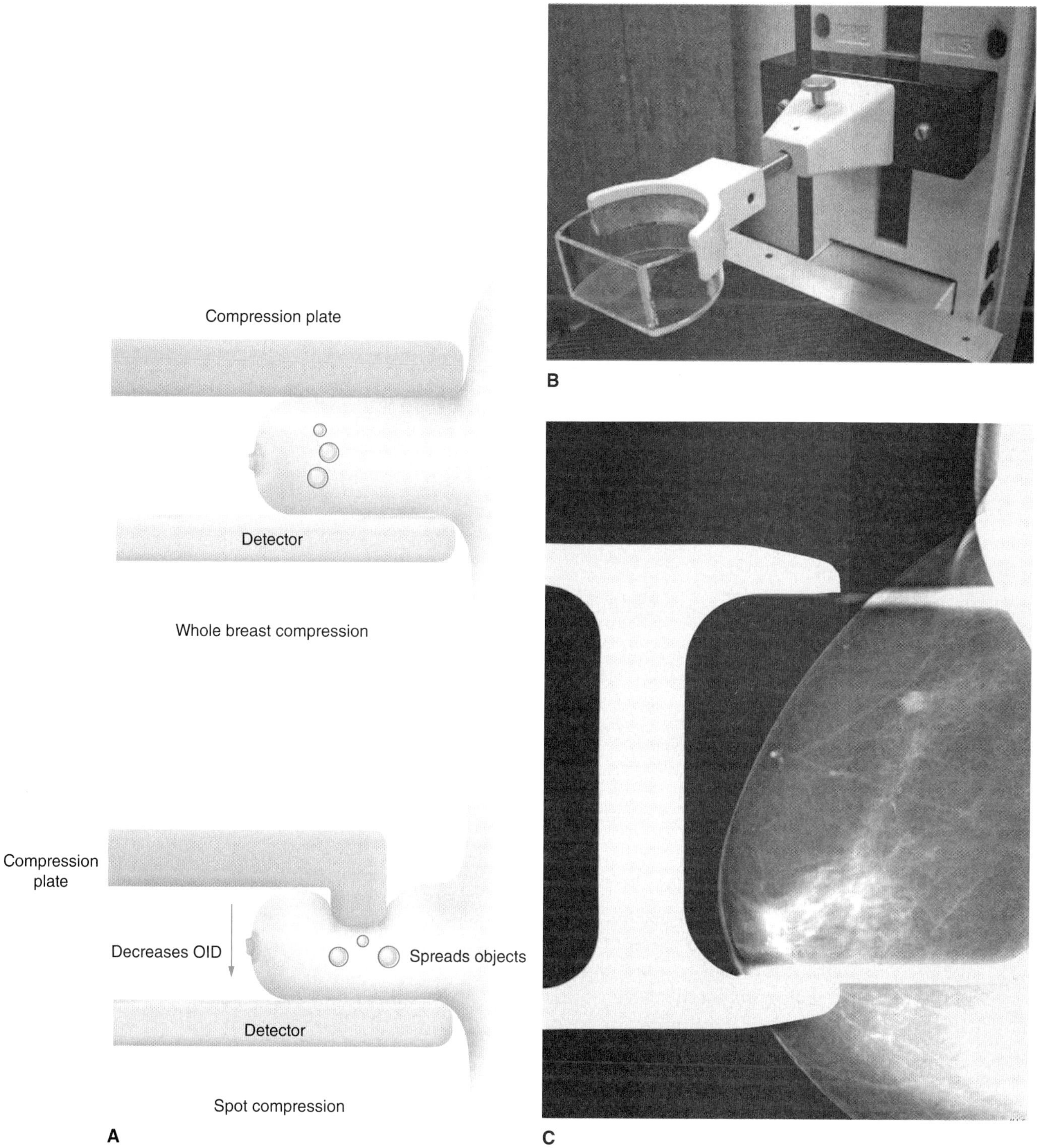

4-9 (15) Spot compression

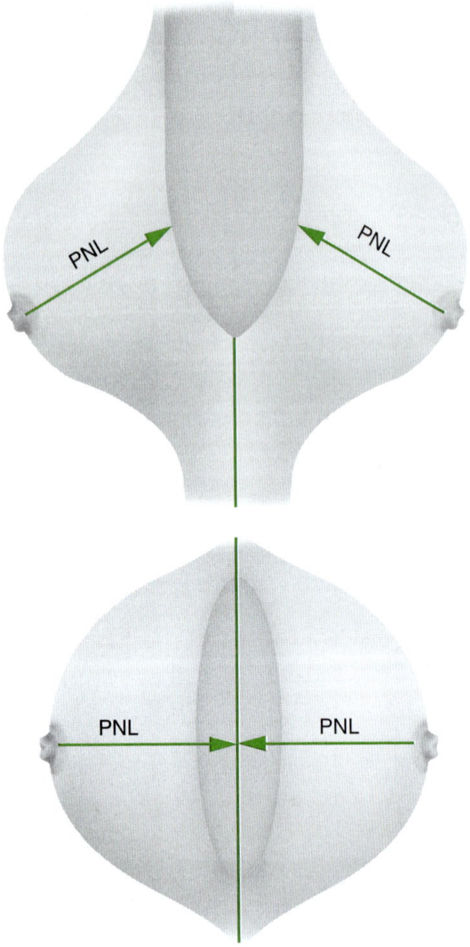

Figure 4-10. Showing the PNL. Measurement of the PNL on the MLO projection should be within 1 cm of the PNL measurement on the CC projection. In about 10% of cases, the PNL will be greater on the CC projection.

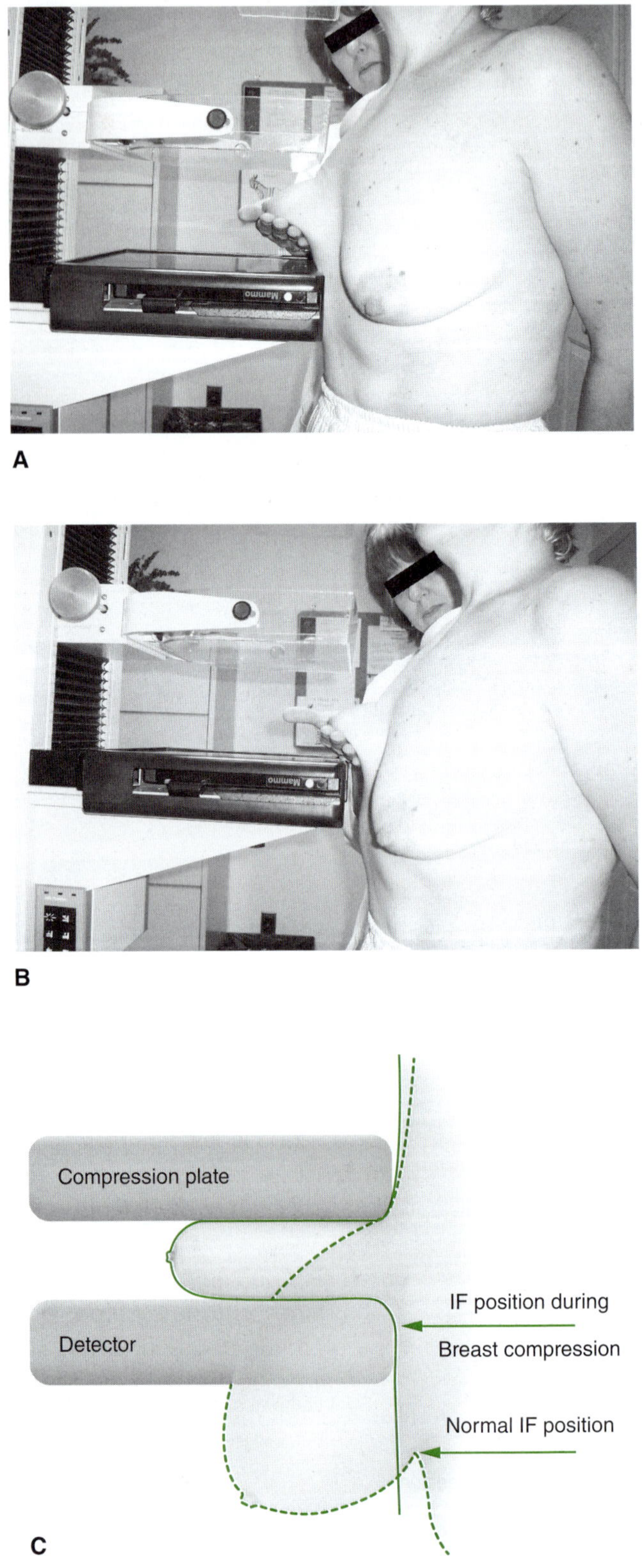

Figure 4-11. Over and under elevation of the IMF on the CC will miss the posterior breast. (A) The IMF raised too high. (B) IMF too low. (C) Movement of the IMF from normal position during the CC positioning.

16. **(D)** In general, guidelines for the MLO include all of these statements. Additionally, the breast should not droop on the image. It may not be possible to meet all these guidelines on all patients. If 1 or more of these guideline elements are missing, the mammographer or radiologist must determine whether a third projection is necessary.[5]

17. **(B)** If the C-arm of the unit is raised too high, the detector will elevate the patient's inframammary fold or crease and the patient will be unable to lean forward and relax. This results in loss of the posterior and inferior breast tissue. If the detector is too low, the breast droops and superior and posterior tissue is lost (Figure 4-11).[5]

18. **(B)** The MLO best visualizes the posterior and upper-outer quadrants of the breast while allowing distortion and overlap of the anterior structures. However, it is the single best projection to visualize a maximum amount of breast tissue. The CC does not image the lateral and posterior lateral breast. The ML does not image the posterior lateral breast. The XCCL will miss the medial breast. (See Figure 4-9.)[5]

19. **(C)** In imaging the MLO, the edge of the detector should be placed parallel to the oblique line formed by pectoral muscle. This oblique line varies in individuals; tall, thin patients require steeper angulations (50-60 degrees), average patients require 40-50 degrees and short, heavy patients 30-40 degrees. The angle is usually the same for both breasts. Male breasts may require even steeper angulations (Figure 4-12).[5]

20. **(B)** The MLO determines if the abnormality is superior or inferior to the nipple and how far posterior it is. The CC or XCCL projections determine whether the lesion is medial or lateral and how far it is from the nipple. The TAN projection skims the area of interest and is best used to determine if a suspected abnormality is located in the breast or the skin of the breast. (See Figure 4-9.)[5]

21. **(A)** The breast is least mobile at the medial and superior aspects and most mobile at the lateral and inferior aspects. To image the maximum amount of breast tissue, the most mobile parts of the breast must be placed adjacent to the detector while applying compression from the least mobile aspect of the breast. In most cases, compression is applied from the superior aspect for the CC projections, to image the maximum amount of superior and posterior breast, and from the medial aspect for the MLO projections, to image the maximum amount of medial and posterior breast.[5]

22. **(A)** The detector must be placed at the level of the elevated IMF or crease. If the detector is raised too high, the patient will be unable to lean forward and relax. This results in loss of posterior and inferior breast tissue. If the detector is at the IMF or is too low, the breast droops and superior and posterior tissues will be lost. (See Figure 4-11.)[5]

23. **(D)** In imaging for the MLO, the edge of the detector is placed parallel to the oblique line formed by pectoral muscle. This oblique line varies in individuals; tall, thin patients require steeper angulations, about 50-60 degrees, average patients require about 40-50 degrees and short, heavy patients needing 30-40 degrees. Males can sometimes require up to 70-degree tube angulation on the MLO. The angle is usually the same for both breasts.[5]

24. **(A)** In the (CC) projection, the beam is directed superiorly to inferiorly, without angulation. The MLO uses tube angulation. The CV shows the medial breast with the patient initially positioned for the CC and the XCCL images the lateral portions of the breast also with the patient initially positioned for the CC. (See Figure 4-1.)[5]

25. **(B)** Having the patient hold the supporting bars with the contralateral hand can stabilize the patient and helps to bring medial breast tissue closer to the detector. This is important because only the CC, in the routine series of MLO and CC, will give a true representation of the medial breast. The patient holding the detector can project body parts in the image (Figure 4-13).[5]

26. **(A)** The right lateromedial oblique (RLMO) is a useful alternative to the right mediolateral oblique (RMLO) in patients with prior pacemaker surgery, open-heart surgery, or any other painful scarring along the sternum where the compression paddle would cause discomfort by pulling on scar tissue. The lateromedial oblique (LMO) projection is a true reverse of the MLO and will demonstrate the same anatomical structures. The ML will not demonstrate adequate posterior breast. Although it provided a limited study, the LM can sometimes be used to replace the MLO in the nonconforming patient.

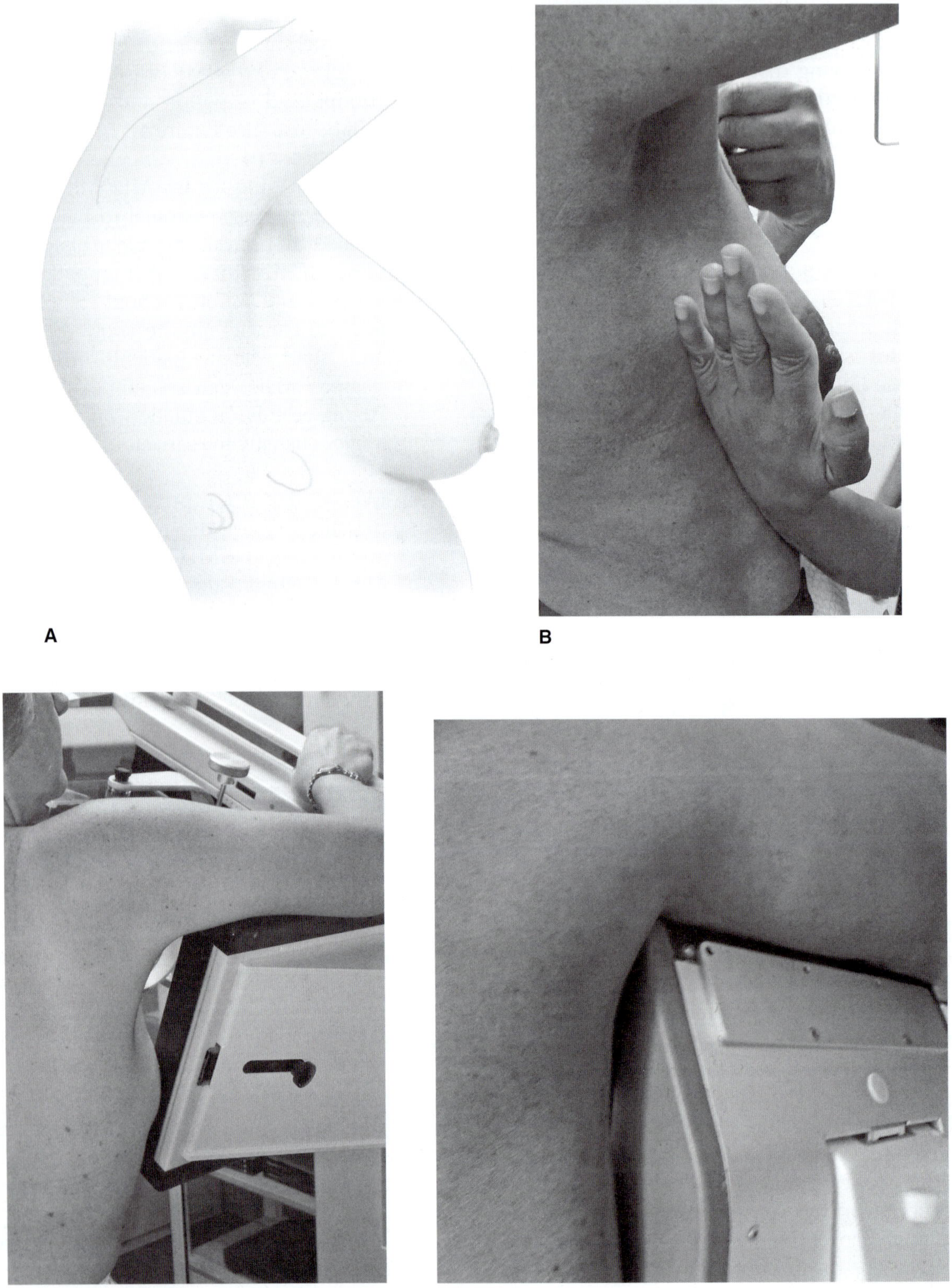

A B C D

Figure 4-12. (A) Determine the angle of the patient midaxillary line. (B) Position the patient's axillary line parallel with the detector. (C) The detector must be placed parallel with the pectoral muscle. Incorrect angulation of the detector can result in poor MLO positioning (D) There should be no gaps between the patient midaxillary line and the detector. (E) Right and (F) Left MLO demonstrating the pectoral muscle to the level of the nipples.

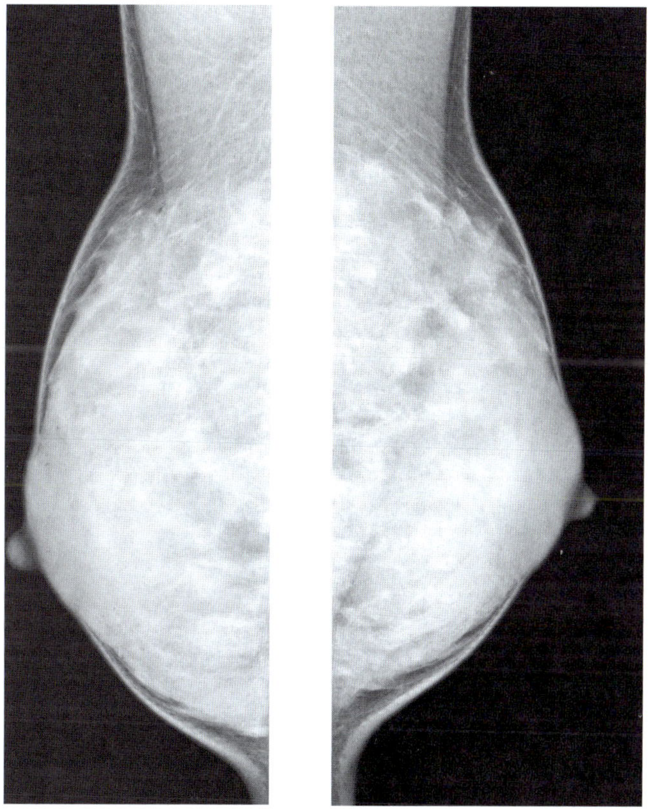

E F

Figure 4-12. *(continued)*

However, in this example a right LM would be needed. (See Figure 4-9.)[5]

27. **(D)** The AT or axillary tail projection demonstrates the axillary contents or tail of the breast, also called the tail of Spence. This projection is especially useful in demonstrating swollen lymph nodes (lymphadenopathy). The AT cannot replace the MLO because it does not image the inferior breast. LMO is the reverse of the MLO with an oblique beam traveling from inferolateral to superomedial. The TAN is used to image lesions in the skin and the LM is a 90-degree lateral, which can be used to image the medial breast. (See Figure 4-9.)[5]

28. **(B)** The TAN projection is used to skim the area of interest. The projection demonstrates skin calcifications and allows visualization of the area of interest free of breast tissue superimposition. The TAN projection also brings the area closer to the detector. Before obtaining a TAN projection, the abnormality must be palpable or visualized on another projection to determine its approximate location. In the LM, the beam travels from lateral to medial at 90 degrees and best images the medial breast. LMO is the reverse of the MLO with an oblique beam traveling from inferolateral to superomedial. The AT or axillary tail projection demonstrates the axillary contents or tail of the breast. (See Figure 4-9.)[5]

29. **(A)** With the nipple in profile, both the ML and the LM are lateral projections that will show the breast structures. With the medial breast closest to the detector, the LM projection is best suited to image medially located abnormalities and will give the best image detail; the ML images lateral abnormalities best. The AT images the tail of the breast and

the TAN best images skin lesion and calcifications. (See Figure 4-9.)[5]

30. **(B)** The XCCL will best image the posterolateral tissue of the breast, which may not be visualized on the CC. The FB is the reverse of the CC with the beam traveling from inferior to superior (caudocranial). The TAN gives a tangential projection of the area of interest and the CV images the medial breast in the CC position. (See Figure 4-9.)[5]

31. **(C)** A patient may present kyphosis, pectus excavatum (sunken chest), barrel chest or pectus carinatum (pigeon breast). With these patients, it is rarely possible to image

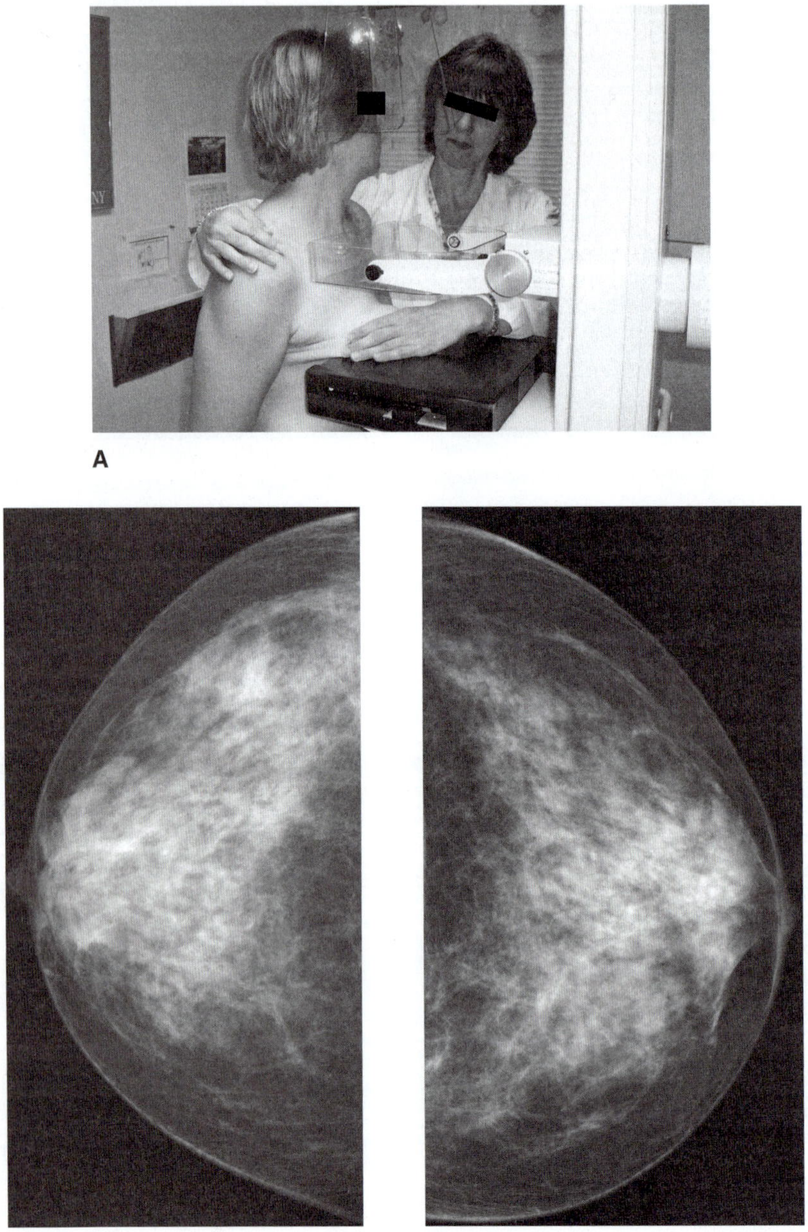

A B C

Figure 4-13. (A) Schematic positioning for CC. The mammographer should stand on the medial side of the patient. (B) Left CC radiograph. (C) Right CC radiograph. (Reproduced with permission from Peart O: Mammography and Breast Imaging PREP: Program Review and Exam Prep. New York, NY: McGraw-Hill Education; 2012.)

the entire breast with the standard 2 projections series. An FB projection in such a situation is often useful. For the FB, the entire mammography unit is rotated 180 degrees and the detector is placed at the superior aspect of the breast. If the FB is not possible, because of limitations of the mammography unit or the patient, the CC and XCCM could be used to image as much medial tissue as possible. Alternatively, the XCCL and XCCM can be used to image both lateral and medial breast tissue respectively. The MLO, LMO, or LM will complete the series. (See Figure 4-9.)[5,8]

32. **(B)** In the triangulation of a lesion, the MLO can be compared to the lateral projection (ML) in search for an abnormality. Medial lesions move up on the lateral projection from their position on the MLO. Lateral lesions move down on the lateral projection from their position on the MLO. Centrally located lesions show little or no movement.[5]

33. **(D)** Milk of calcium deposits are benign calcifications that occur in microcysts as radiopaque particles mixed with fluid. On the CC, XCCL, or FB projections, they will appear as ill-defined calcifications. On a true lateral projection, such as the ML or LM, the radiopaque particles settle to the dependent portion of the cyst, forming crescent- or teacup-shaped calcifications. These may be clustered, scattered, or occur bilaterally (Figure 4-14).[5]

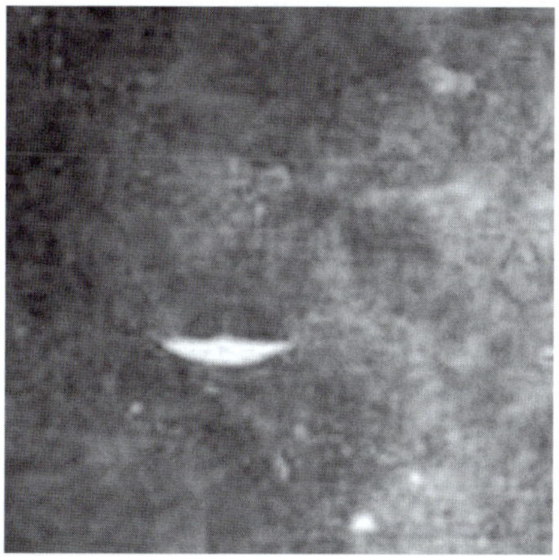

Figure 4-14. Radiograph showing milk of calcium. (Reproduced with permission from Peart O: Mammography and Breast Imaging PREP: Program Review and Exam Prep. New York, NY: McGraw-Hill Education; 2012.)

34. **(B)** The TAN projection can be used to skim the area of interest. The projection demonstrates skin calcification or any area free of breast tissue superimposition. The TAN projection also brings the area closer to the detector. The CV images the medial breast, and both the LMO and the AT are oblique projections. (See Figure 4-9.)[5]

35. **(D)** The axillary tail (AT) projection is an oblique projection used to visualize the axillary area or tail of the breast. In the ML, the beam travels from medial to lateral at 90 degrees and best images the lateral breast. The XCCL images the lateral portions of the breast and the FB is a caudocranial projection that best images the superior breast tissue. (See Figure 4-2.)[5]

36. **(B)** The XCCL can be used to image the extreme posterolateral tissue missed on the CC. As with the CC projection, the beam is directed superiorly to inferiorly. The CV images the medial breast and the MLO and AT are oblique projections.[5]

37. **(A)** The From Below (FB) or caudocranial projection is the reverse of the CC and can be used to image nonconforming patients, such as those with extreme kyphosis. The FB also places superior lesions that are high on the chest wall closer to the detector, providing more detail of the lesion. Inferior lesions are imaged furthest from the detector.[5]

38. **(C)** The LM projection gives a true representation of breast structure in relation to the nipple. The LM places medially located lesions close to the detector. For the LM, the beam is directed laterally to medially. The CV shows the medial breast from the CC position. In the ML, the beam travels from medial to the lateral at 90 degrees and best images the lateral breast. The MLO is a routine projection with the beam traveling from superomedial to inferolateral. (See Figure 4-3.)[5]

39. **(C)** The MLO projection gives a distorted and overlapping image of the anterior and medial structures of the breast because it is

an oblique projection. However, it is the single best projection used to image the breast in its entirety. The MLO is also best at visualizing the posterior and upper-outer quadrants of the breast. The ML is poor at visualizing the most posterior and lateral parts of the breast.[5]

40. **(D)** The CV projection is the best at imaging the extreme medial aspect of the breast with the beam directed CC. The CC is a routine projection and will image medial breast tissue, but does not always capture posteromedial breast tissue. The MLO distorts the medial breast and the ML often misses the medial breast.[5]

41. **(A)** The rolled image helps to separate superimposed breast structures assisting the radiologist in determining whether a suspected lesion is real. The breast is rolled in equal and opposite directions through physical manipulation of the patient's breast. For the RM, the breast is first positioned for the CC projection. The superior (upper) surface is then rolled medially and the inferior (lower) surface is rolled laterally. For the RL, the superior (upper) surface is rolled laterally and the inferior (lower) surface is rolled medially. "M" indicates magnification and ML is a 90-degree lateral projection. (See Figure 4-9.)[5]

42. **(C)** The LMO is a reverse of the MLO and results in a similar image. For the LMO, the beam is directed from the inferolateral (lower outer) aspect of the breast to the superomedial (upper inner) aspect In the LM, the beam travels from lateral to medial at 90 degrees and best images the medial breast. The ML is also a true lateral, with the beam traveling from medial to lateral. The MLO is a routine projection with the beam traveling from superior-medial to inferolateral.[5]

43. **(B)** The CV is a CC projection used to image the extreme medial aspect of the breast. (See Figure 4-4.)[5]

44. **(C)** In the rolled image, the breast is rolled in equal and opposite directions via physical manipulation of the patient's breast. For the RL, the patient is positioned for the CC projection. The superior (upper) surface of the breast is then rolled Laterally and the inferior (lower) surface is rolled medially. For the RM, the patient is also positioned for the CC projection. The superior (upper) surface of the breast is rolled medially and the inferior (lower) surface is rolled laterally. The MLO is a routine projection with the beam traveling from superomedial to inferolateral. The CV shows the medial breast. (See Figure 4-5.)[5]

45. **(B)** Magnification mammography (M) is especially useful in assessing or finding breast calcifications, or to better outline the borders of masses. The other projections will image the calcification but do not provide a magnified image of the area of concern. The MLO is a routine projection with the beam traveling from superior-medial to inferolateral. The CV shows the medial breast. (See Figure 4-9.)[5]

46. **(A)** In the rolled image, the breast is rolled in equal and opposite directions via physical manipulation of the patient's breast. For the RM, the patient is positioned for the CC projection. The superior (upper) surface of the breast is then rolled medially and the inferior (lower) surface is rolled laterally. For the RL, the patient is also positioned for the CC projection. The superior (upper) surface is rolled laterally and the inferior (lower) surface is rolled medially. (See Figure 4-6.)[5]

47. **(D)** With magnification, the breast may be magnified up to twice its original size; therefore, the entire breast is rarely imaged. The patient's skin dose increases because the breast is closer to the radiation source. Magnification can be used to image specimens and lesions and to assess the borders of lesions, or to assess calcifications (see Figure 4-14).[4,5]

48. **(C)** For the rolled superior (RS) from the ML position, thc medial portion of the breast is rolled superiorly and the lateral portion of the breast is rolled inferiorly. For the rolled inferior (RI) from the ML lateral position, the

medial portion of the breast is rolled inferiorly and the lateral portion of the breast is rolled superiorly. (See Figure 4-9.)[5]

49. **(D)** For the RM, the patient is positioned for the CC projection. The upper (superior) surface of the breast is rolled medially and the lower (inferior) surface is rolled laterally. For the RL, the patient is positioned for the CC projection. The upper (superior) surface is rolled laterally and the lower (inferior) surface is rolled medially. (See Figure 4-9.)[5]

50. **(D)** A patient with pectus excavatum has a sunken or depressed sternum and rib cage, which make imaging the medial and lateral breast tissue difficult on the routine CC projection. Extensive pectoral muscle is mainly a problem when imaging males in the MLO projection. In barrel chest, the chest protrudes and the kyphotic patient has exaggerated thoracic curvature or rounded shoulders.[5]

51. **(A)** In the modified ID projections, the prosthesis is displaced posteriorly and superiorly against the chest wall while gently pulling the breast tissue anterior away from the prosthesis, onto the detector. The implant or prosthesis is held in place posteriorly, with the compression device (Figure 4-15).[5]

52. **(D)** The routine series for an implant patient includes the routine CC, routine MLO, CC with ID, and MLO with ID. It may be difficult to displace the implant on some patients, especially if the implant is encapsulated. If it cannot be adequately displaced, another projection, such as the 90-degree lateral with the implant included, could be added to the routine CC and MLO projections of the implant. Imaging the patient in 3 projections ensures visualization of all quadrants of the breast. The TAN best images skin lesions or skin calcifications. Another useful projection to image encapsulation is the SIO (Figure 4-16).[5]

53. **(D)** The spot compression projection focuses the compression on a single area to improve resolution and evenly spread out the breast tissues. This is sometimes useful in eliminating pseudomasses. The TAN best images skin lesions or skin calcifications. The CV images the medial breast and the AT images the axillary tail. (See Figure 4-9.)[5]

54. **(D)** The routine series for an implant patient includes the routine CC, routine MLO, CC with ID, and MLO with ID. The total projections per patient would therefore be 8.[5]

55. **(C)** Radiation-induced changes in the breast usually begin to decline at 6 months after treatment, but changes may exist for up to 1 year. Initially, the breast may exhibit erythema and edema, or it may harden. The breast may also be extremely sensitive and distorted because of surgery. Although the timing of the mammography examination must be adapted for each patient, a mammogram is not recommended earlier than 6 months after radiation treatment.[9]

56. **(A)** Spot compression focuses compression on a single area to improve resolution and evenly spread out the breast tissues. This is sometimes useful in eliminating pseudomasses. Spot compression can be taken with or without magnification and in any projection. XCCL, AT, and CV are all specific supplementary projections with set central ray directions and tube orientations. (See Figure 4-9.)[5]

57. **(C)** With postlumpectomy imaging, it is no longer possible to make a comparison between 2 "mirror-image" breasts. Therefore, an additional projection will give the radiologist a better opportunity to diagnose cancer. The ML or LM is often the preferred additional projection. The CC and the MLO are routine projections and the CV shows the medial breast from the CC position.[9]

58. **(A)** Caution should be used when compressing implants to avoid implant rupture. Compression should therefore be used for immobilization only and not to separate breast tissue structures. The TAN best images

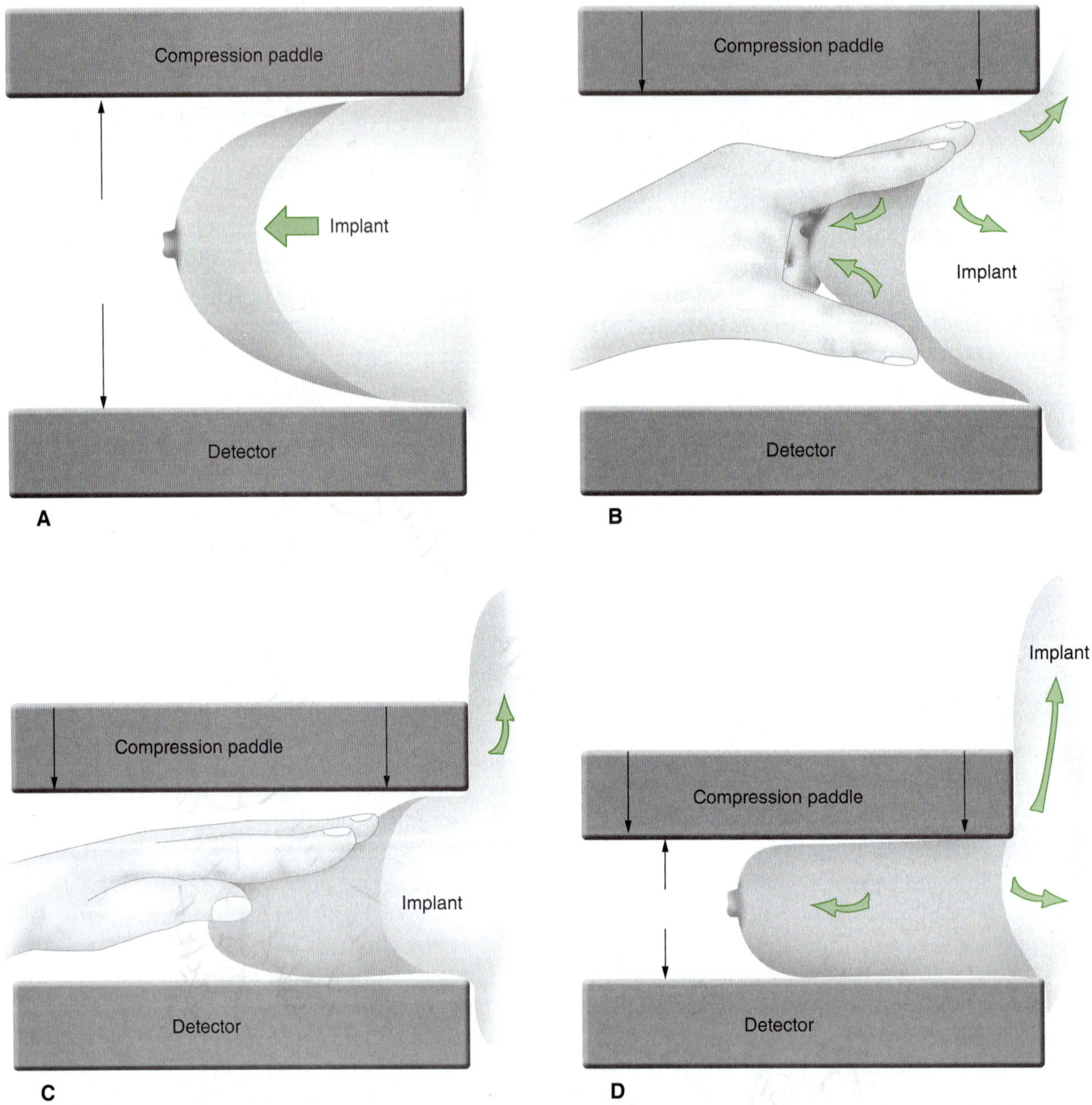

Figure 4-15. Diagram showing the ID or Eklund method of imaging. The ID or implant-displaced technique or Eklund method for implants displaces the implant posteriorly and superiorly to image the breast tissue free of the implant. (A) Normal compression. (B and C) Displacing the implant posteriorly and superiorly prior to compression. (D) Compression of the breast tissue free of implant. (E) CC and MLO projections of the breast with minimum compression. (F) The ID or implant-displaced technique or Eklund method for implants displaces the implant posteriorly and superiorly to image the breast tissue free of the implant. (Reproduced with permission from Peart O: Mammography and Breast Imaging PREP: Program Review and Exam Prep. New York, NY: McGraw-Hill Education; 2012.)

skin lesions or skin calcifications and magnification could be used to evaluate the borders of lesions and calcifications. The implant displaced (ID) compression technique is used to apply vigorous compression when imaging portions of the breast that would not be visualized because of superimposition of the implant.[5]

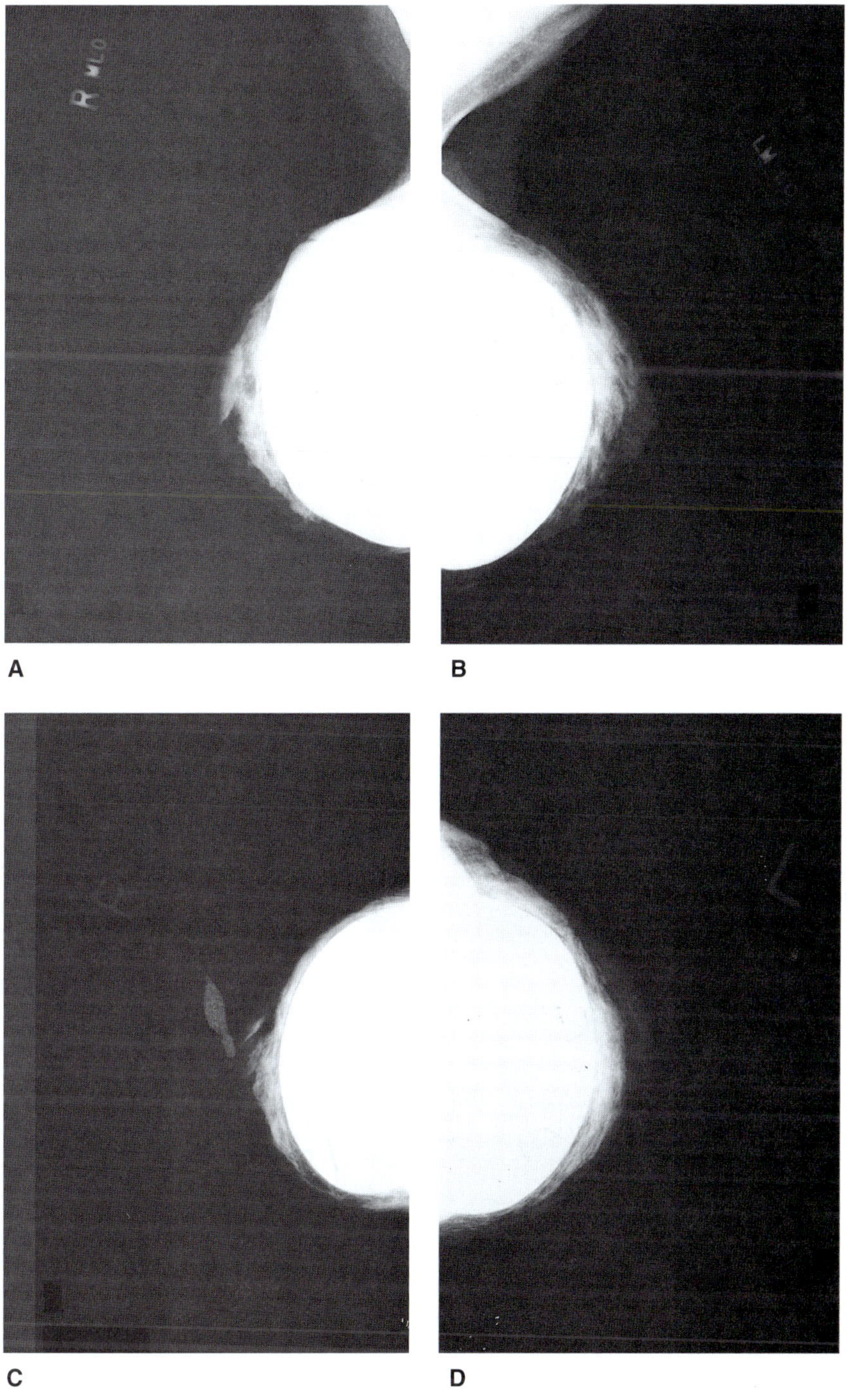

Figure 4-16. Radiographs of Implant series. (A–D) Shows MLO and CC imaging with limited compression. (E–H) Shows MLO and CC implant displaced (ID) projections. The ID or Eklund method for implants displaces the implant posteriorly and superiorly to image the breast tissue free of the implant. (Reproduced with permission from Peart O: Lange Q&A: Mammography Examination, 2nd ed. New York, NY: McGraw-Hill Education; 2008.)

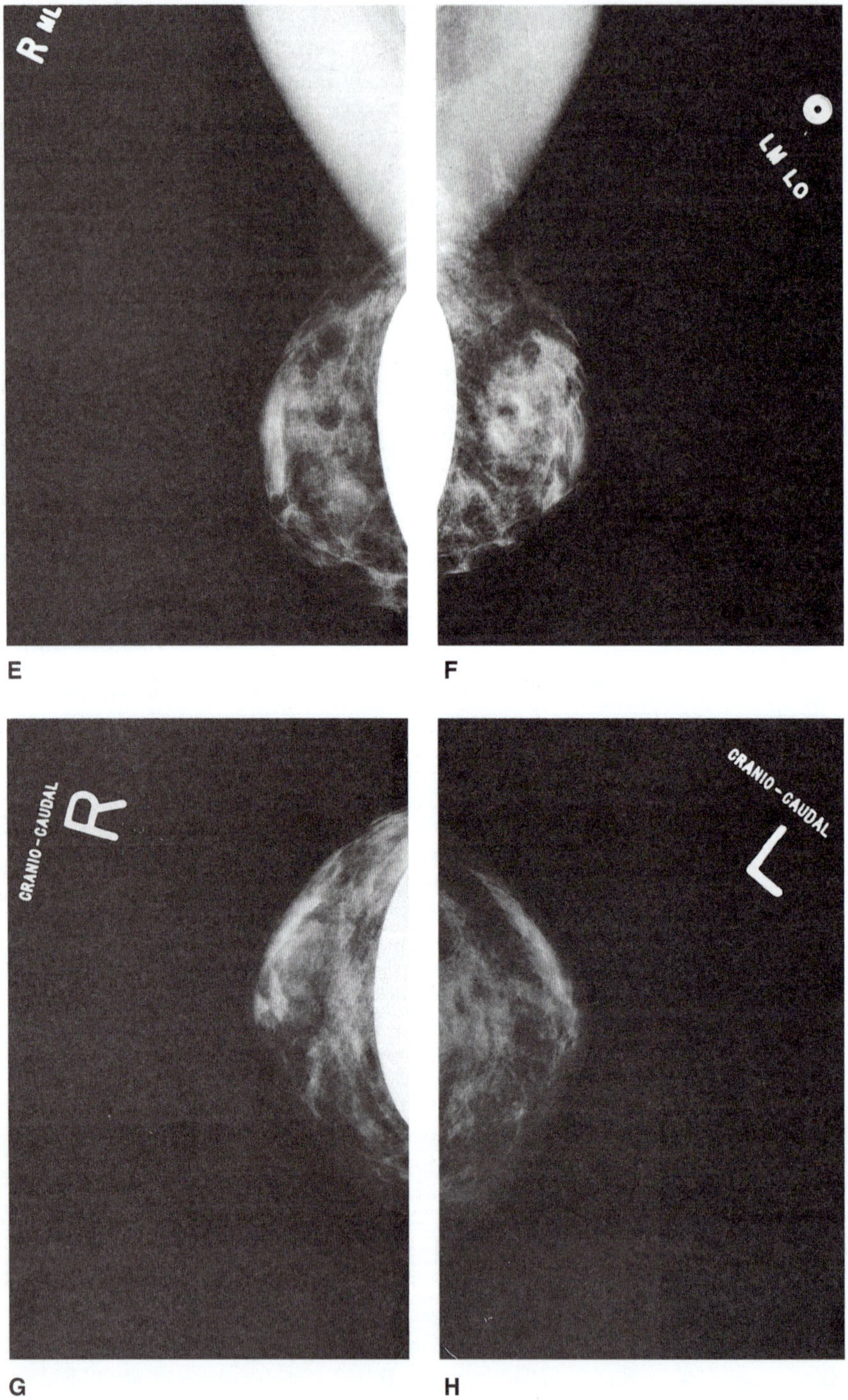

E F G H

Figure 4-16. (*continued*)

References

1. Peart O. Patient education and assessment. In: *Mammography and Breast Imaging: Prep*. New York, NY: McGraw-Hill; 2012:23-64.
2. FDA U.S. Food And Drug Administration. Policy Guidance Help System. http://www.fda.gov/Radiation-EmittingProducts/MammographyQualityStandardsActandProgram/Guidance/PolicyGuidanceHelpSystem/default.htm#Quality. Last Update March 20, 2013. Accessed March 22, 2014.
3. Papp J. Mammography quality standards. In: *Quality Management in the Imaging Sciences*. 3rd ed. St. Louis, MO: Mosby; 2006:195-229.
4. Bushong SC. Advanced x-ray imaging. In: *Radiologic Science for Technologists—Physics, Biology and Protection*. 10th ed. St. Louis, MO: Mosby; 2004:371-384.
5. Peart O. Breast imaging mammography. In: *Mammography and Breast Imaging: Prep*. New York, NY: McGraw-Hill; 2012:213-262.
6. Tabár L, Dean PB. Calcifications in the mammogram In: *Teaching Atlas of Mammography*. 4th ed. New York, NY: Thieme; 2011:149-238.
7. Peart O. Breast benign and malignant diseases of the breast. In: *Mammography and Breast Imaging: Prep*. New York, NY: McGraw-Hill; 2012:263-332.
8. Venes D, Biderman A, Adler E. *Taber's Cyclopedic Medical Dictionary*. 21st ed. Philadelphia, PA: F.A. Davis; 2005:1-2518.
9. Peart O. Treatment options. In: *Mammography and Breast Imaging: Prep*. New York, NY: McGraw-Hill; 2012:397-432.

CHAPTER 5

Diagnostic, Interventional, and Treatment Procedures

Summary of Important Points

INTERVENTIONAL OPTIONS

The first step in the fight against breast cancer is detection. However, after a lesion is discovered the next step is a histologic or cytologic analysis to definitely confirm or rule out malignancy. A finding can be palpable or nonpalpable, microcalcifications, mass densities, or an area of enhancement, but only by removing a sample of the tissue or cells in question and examining the removed sample using microscopic analysis, can a definitive diagnosis be made.

Cytologic Analysis

The microscopic examination of cell samples

Histological Analysis

The microscopic examination of tissue samples

Aspiration or FNA

Fine-needle aspiration (FNA) is removal of the content of a cyst for testing or analysis.

Stereotactic Breast Biopsy

- If a lesion is nonpalpable stereotactic imaging is an option to determine its exact location before it can be biopsied.
- The stereotactic equipment uses angled images to triangulate the depth of a lesion within the breast, and to calculate its position in 3 dimensions.
- The tube is angled 15 degree to the left and right along the X axis for 2 scout images, used for calculations of the depth (Z axis). The stereotactic calibrations are then used to position a biopsy probe within the breast at the calculated coordinates.
- This procedure can be performed either using a standard mammographic unit with an "add-on" attachment, or with a dedicated prone biopsy system. Some mammography units are capable of serving dual roles as an imaging unit and a biopsy system.

Advantages/Disadvantages of the Add-On Stereo Units

Advantages

- The patient is imaged in the upright position.
- The unit is relatively inexpensive when compared to the prone units.
- The units do not require a dedicated biopsy room.
- After use the unit can revert to use as a mammography unit.
- Imaging the posterior and axilla area of the breast is often easier using the add-on units.

Disadvantages

- There is less work space.
- The patient is upright with a greater risk of vasovagal reactions.
- Patient motion can be a problem.

Advantages/Disadvantages of the Dedicated Prone Stereo Units

The prone units are dedicated procedure units where the patient lies prone with the breast of interest extending through a hole near the middle of the table. The mammography unit and needle guidance device are under the table. The table can be raised or lowered to suit the radiologist's preference.

Advantages

- There is less chance for a vasovagal reaction.
- The patient lies in relative comfort during the procedure.

Disadvantages

- The unit is more expensive.
- Although these units can be used for needle localization, their major function as a biopsy unit will be underutilized if there is a low biopsy volume.

Preoperative Needle Localization for Excisional Biopsy

- If stereotactic technology is not available the preoperative needle localization technique can be used to locate any nonpalpable lesion or calcification within the breast. This procedure is done prior to a surgical excisional biopsy.
- The localization wire can be placed in the breast using either mammographic or sonographic guidance.
- Since this is a prelude to a surgical biopsy the patient should be scheduled for needle localization only after review of images and coordination of plans with a surgeon.
- The lesion is located and needle is placed directly in the lesion. It needle is removed leaving at least 5 mm of the wire guide within the lesion. The hook of the wire should be approximately 1 cm beyond the lesion.
- Any approach to the lesion should be parallel to the chest wall to minimize complications.
- In general, the shortest approach is used however sometimes an inferior approach will produce better cosmetic results.
- After the procedure, the relevant images, with the lesion clearly marked, should be sent to the surgeon. The wire should be carefully anchored in place after the localization because inaccurate placement or displacement of the wire can result in a missdiagonosis
- Some radiologists also provide the surgeon with line diagrams or a brief description, showing or telling the approximate distance from the breast skin surface to the lesion.

Breast Biopsy

Breast biopsy is the taking of a sample specimen for cytologic or histological analysis.

- The type of biopsy performed depends on a number of factors such as how suspicious is the abnormality, size, shape, and the location of the abnormality or the number of abnormalities present.
- Other relevant factors include the patient's medical history, patient's preference, training of the radiologist or surgeon, and the facility or equipment available.

Fine-Needle Biopsy

This technique is used to obtain cellular material from the area in question for cytologic analysis.

- Fine-needle biopsy (FNB) can be used to diagnose both cystic and solid lesions such as fibroadenomas. If the lesion is not palpable the needle can be guided to the lesion under ultrasound guidance or mammographically under stereotactic breast localization.
- FNB can reduce the necessity for a surgical breast biopsy but the accuracy of FNB is dependent on the individual performing the procedure—the radiologist or surgeon—and the ability of the cytologist.

Core Biopsy

- The core biopsy is the most commonly performed minimally invasive technique. The procedure can be performed under ultrasound, mammography, or MRI guidance.
- It is inexpensive, easy to perform, and highly accurate for many lesions.
- Core biopsy removes a sample of tissue versus FNB which removes only fluid and cells.
- The tissue samples are obtained using an 11-14 gauge or larger needle.
- Modality-based core biopsy is needed if a lesion is found only with 1 modality.

Automatic or Mechanical Core "Gun"

For this procedure the skin is numbed and a small cut (less than ¼ inch) is made. The gun needles have an inner needle with a trough extending within it. One end is covered by a sheath and attached to a spring-loaded mechanism. The device is inserted into the lesion. When the mechanism is activated, the needle moves forward, filling the trough with breast tissue. The outer sheath instantly moves forward to cut into the lesion and keep it in the trough. The gun-needle combination is designed to move a cutting needle rapidly through the breast. To yield adequate specimens a minimum of approximately 5 core samples are needed when assessing a lesion and at least 10 for an assessment of calcifications.

Vacuum Core Biopsy

For this procedure the skin is numbed and a small cut (less than ¼ inch) is made. A hollow probe is inserted and guided to the area of interest. A cylinder of tissue is then suctioned out and pulled into the probe through a hole in its side. A rotating knife inside the probe cuts the tissue sample from the rest of the breast.

Ultrasound Core Biopsy

Ultrasound can provide a highly accurate way to evaluate suspicious masses within the breast that are visible on ultrasound, whether or not they can be felt on the breast self-examination or the clinical breast examination. The procedure precludes the need to remove tissue surgically, plus it is faster than mammographically guided stereotactic biopsies and uses no ionizing radiation.

MRI-Guided Needle Biopsy

If a suspicious area is detected only on MR imaging or is not well seen on ultrasound or mammography, the radiologist may recommend an MR-guided breast biopsy. MR-guided biopsy requires only a topical anesthetic. Like ultrasound or mammographic minimally invasive biopsies, the MR biopsy is less costly than surgical biopsy, will leave little to no scarring, and can be performed in less than an hour.

Advantages of a Minimally Invasive Biopsy

- Can be performed as an outpatient procedure.
- Less visible scarring.
- Fewer complications and no anesthesia is involved.
- Less pain and usually less bleeding.
- Less costly since patients are sent home the same day and normally will not require an overnight stay in the hospital.

Open Surgical Biopsy

This is a major surgical procedure that will involve anesthesia and sometimes a hospital stay.

- **Incisional** biopsy is used to remove parts of a lesion.
- **Excisional biopsy** is used to remove the entire lesion.

Comparison of the Various Biopsy Methods

Complications and severity of side effects of a biopsy will depend on the method used and the quality of the care team.

- The open surgical biopsy has the lowest false-negative rates, less than 0.5% but is the most invasive and has the highest complication rate.
- The core biopsy has a reported 4%-10% false-negative rate but the most common error in core is understating the multifocality of the cancer, for example, a ductal carcinoma in situ could be diagnosed on a core but invasion found at excisional biopsy.
- FNB is less expensive, less invasive, and faster than core biopsy although it is more likely to lead to error due to insufficient sampling. The false-negative rate for the FNB can range from 5% to 20% and is higher for less experienced operators.
- The most substantial limitation for FNB is the high rate of insufficient sampling.
- Ultrasound-guided biopsy performed using any of the biopsy methods is faster and less expensive than stereotactic biopsy. It also does not involve ionizing radiation.
- Ultrasound also offers real-time visualization of the needle, which means the motion of the biopsy needle can be followed.
- Most palpable lesions are best biopsied under ultrasound guidance, whereas calcifications are best biopsied stereotactically with mammography guidance.

Specimen Radiography

The specimen is the breast tissue removed during a biopsy. A specimen radiograph should be performed after every biopsy to confirm that the lesion was removed and that the margins are clean.

- In imaging the specimen, speed, and efficiency are important since the patient may be under anesthesia.
- The mammographer should always use compression and magnification is recommended for calcifications.
- If microcalcifications are present in a specimen they should be counted and noted.
- The radiologist should indicate where the pathology is located on the specimen, as this will help the pathologist in evaluating the lesion.
- If the tumor is close to the margins of the specimen or if the margins are positive for cancer, additional tissue must be excised before the incision is closed.

Ductography or Galactography

- Ductography can be performed to evaluate a suspicious nipple discharge. The discharge can be spontaneous, bilateral or unilateral and may be clear, serous, or bloody.
- The technique can only be performed if nipple discharge is present.
- Ductography can detect abnormalities such as filling defects, wall irregularity, duct expansion, or abrupt cutoff of a duct; however, the procedure is rarely performed today because ultrasound can now be used to identify and localize duct abnormalities or filling defects.

Pathology Review

- The final stage of any interventional process is the pathology review. There should be good communication among the radiologist, the surgeon, and the pathologist.
- Most facilities now have a system in place to track all positive pathologic findings.
- A tracking system is required to comply with the *Mammography Quality Standards Act* (MQSA).
- Regular reviews and medical audits will help the facility to identify areas of concern including high false-negative or false-positive rates. By identifying possible problem areas, the facility can improve service and enhance breast cancer detection and screening.

Mammoplasty

- Mammoplasty is the general term used when describing reshaping of the breast. The breast can be lifted to reduce a sagging breast, enlarged (augmented), or reconstructed after the removal of a tumor.

Cosmetic Interventional

- Cosmetic interventional includes any reconstruction of the breast that is not related to medical reasons. This can include reduction or augmentation. Over the years, breasts will lose their shape and firmness from pregnancies, nursing, and the aging process. Cosmetic intervention can improve self-confidence or improve appearance.
- Surgery and reconstruction after breast cancer does not fall under the heading of cosmetic intervention.

Breast Reduction

- The process reduces the overall size of the breast. It can be done for cosmetic or medical reasons. Some of the breast tissue is removed and the nipple area often relocated higher on the breasts for better cosmetic results.

Breast Augmentation

- A technique to increase breast size. It can be performed for cosmetic or medical reasons.
- Implants can be placed in front of the pectoral muscle (*subglandular* or *retromammary* implants) or behind the pectoral muscle (*subpectoral* or *retropectoral* implants).

BREAST CANCER TREATMENT OPTIONS

Surgical Options

Mastectomy is the surgical removal of the entire breast. There are different types of mastectomy.

- **Radical mastectomy** removes the entire breast, lymph nodes, and chest wall muscles under the breast. It is rarely performed today because the modified mastectomy is just as effective plus the modified is less debilitating and deforming.
- **Modified radical mastectomy** removes the entire breast including the nipple/areolar region and some of the underarm lymph nodes.
- **Prophylactic mastectomy** removes a healthy breast when the individual has a high risk factor for developing breast cancer. All the breast

tissue including the nipple/areolar region may be removed. Alternatively, nipple sparing mastectomy may be performed.

- **Lumpectomy** removes the breast cancer tumor and surrounding margins of the normal breast tissue.
  - Lumpectomy is often combined with other therapy options such as radiation treatment, chemotherapy or hormonal treatment.
  - If followed by radiation therapy, the patient is usually given 6 weeks of radiation therapy to ensure that all cancer cells in the remaining breast have been destroyed. Radiation treatment usually begins 1 month after surgery after giving the breast time to heal. However, there are newer radiation treatment options that begin and end earlier.
  - Lumpectomy can be followed by chemotherapy to control the systemic spread of breast cancer or treatment with the drug Tamoxifen.
  - Breast conservation should only be performed if the treatment provides a cure rate equal to that obtained from a mastectomy.

Surgical Complications

- Wound infection.
- Hematoma or microhematoma.
- Seroma—clear fluid trapped in the wound.
- Lymphedema if the lymph nodes are removed during the operation.
- Numbness in the upper arm and skin—can be caused by the removal of lymph nodes and the resulting edema.
- Phantom breast pain/sensations. These symptoms can include unpleasant itching, pins and needles, pressure and throbbing often associated with small nerves between the breast tissue and skin, which were cut during surgery. The neural connection in the brain is undergoing a process of reorganization called neural plasticity. This results in the spontaneous firing of electrical signals from the ends of the cut or injured nerves causing the phantom sensations. Phantom pain can be relieved by massage and or pain medication.

Axillary Node Dissection

This procedure removes the underarm lymph nodes during a mastectomy or lumpectomy. A common complication of axillary node dissection is lymphedema or chronic swelling of the arm due to the accumulation of lymphatic fluids. Lymphedema is exaggerated when axillary node dissection is combined with radiation therapy.

Sentinel Lymph Node Biopsy

This is a more conservative process and involves the removal of only 1-3 sentinel lymph nodes in the axillary area. Prior to a sentinel node biopsy the sentinel node or first nodes in the lymphatic chain must be identified using any of the adjunctive detection options. If cancer is discovered in the sentinel nodes more nodes are usually removed.

Breast Cancer Staging

Staging determines the nature of the cancer whether it is invasive or noninvasive including its size, its location, if there is lymph node involvement and if the cancer has spread to other parts of the body. Staging results are important in determining prognosis and treatment options. The American Joint Committee on Cancer (AJCC) has a standardized staging system based on "T," "N," and "M" where "T" is related to the tumor size, "N" denotes lymph node spread, and "M" assesses distant metastasis.

RADIATION THERAPY

Radiation treats breast cancer with high-energy radiation to destroy cancer cells in the chest wall, axilla, and the breast. Radiation therapy is often used in conjunction with other treatment options to remove the remaining cancer cells in the breast, chest wall, and axilla area and can also be used before surgery to shrink the size of the tumor.

External beam radiation usually begins 1 month after surgery after giving the breast time to heal. Treatment time is typically 15-30 minutes given 5 times per week for 5-8 weeks. The procedure itself is painfree and the patients are generally outpatients. During treatment patients will be monitored via closed circuit television.

Internal Radiation

Internal beam radiation or *brachytherapy* involves applying the radiation from the inside out. Treatment can be reduced from 8 weeks to 5-9 days.

Advantages of Internal Beam Radiation (Brachytherapy)

- Reduction in the time of treatment from 6 weeks to 7-9 days.
- Less irritation of healthy breast tissue.
- Less delay before the start of treatment—the treatment can start immediately after a lumpectomy.
- Fewer skin reactions such as redness, rashes, or irritation.

Side Effects of Radiation Treatment

Most side effects will disappear after 6-12 months. The breast will sometime remain firm. On rare occasions the breast may become enlarged due to fluid buildup or smaller due to tissue changes. The skin can become more or less sensitive. Other side effects can include:

- Fatigue—extreme tiredness.
- Swelling of the breast.
- Heaviness in the breast.
- Sunburn-type appearance of the breast skin.
- Loss of appetite.

DRUG AND HORMONAL OPTIONS

Chemotherapy is an adjuvant therapy and involves the use of drugs to treat cancer that may have spread beyond the breast. *Neoadjuvant chemotherapy* is given before surgery to help shrink the cancerous tumor. *Adjuvant chemotherapy* is given in addition to another breast cancer treatment, for example, mastectomy.

- Chemotherapy regimens are tailored for the individual patient and can vary tremendously. The type of treatment will depend on the patient's age, overall health, stage and grade of the cancer, past or future treatment, and other health problems.
- Chemotherapy is often a combination of drugs. Most physicians prefer a combination of lower doses of individual drugs versus a high dose of 1 powerful drug. Lower dose drugs are also associated with fewer side effects.
- Chemotherapy is a systemic treatment and because the drug is distributed throughout the body it will affect all the cells, tissues and organs in the body. Many chemotherapy drugs work to kill actively reproducing cells; however, some drugs will work on cells in a particular phase of the cell cycle.

Method of Chemotherapy Administration

- The chemotherapy is often administered through a semipermanent catheter (port-a-cath) implanted into a large vein in the arm or hand or the subclavian vein near the clavicle. Some chemotherapy drugs are given orally as tablets or liquids. Chemotherapy can also be given as an intramuscular injection, topically, or injected directly into the cancer area.
- Chemotherapy courses can be given daily, weekly, monthly, or other scheduling options depending on the patient's response to the drug.
- The treatment lasts 3-6 months. Most long chemotherapy sessions include built-in rest cycles to give the healthy cells recovery time.

Hormonal Treatment

This often involves the use of a class of drugs called selective estrogen receptor modulators or SERMs. They are used to shrink or stop the recurrence of breast cancer or to lower the risks of breast cancer recurrence in postmenopausal women.

Tamoxifen Treatment

- Tamoxifen is an antiestrogen drug that blocks estrogen and can lower the risk of breast cancer recurrence in postmenopausal women after surgery.
- Some cancers have estrogen receptors (ER positive) on the surface of their cells. These cancers rely on a supply of estrogen to grow. Tamoxifen prevents estrogen from latching onto tumor cell receptors and directing them to multiply.
- Tamoxifen is also used to shrink large tumors.
- Tamoxifen by itself is recommended for 5 years. Some studies now suggest that it offers added protection after 5 years. The benefits of Tamoxifen are thought to outweigh the risks.

Rolaxifene

- Works similar to Tamoxifen but is less toxic.

Herceptin

- Can be used to treat HER2-positive metastatic breast cancer.

Aromasin

- Carries fewer side effects than Tamoxifen. Aromasin suppresses blood levels of estrogen by blocking aromatase, the enzyme that helps the body produce it.

Pain medication is available for patients in severe pain from cancer. Newer pain medications are even more potent than morphine.

Postbreast Cancer—Breast Reconstruction

Breast reconstruction aims to restore the appearance of the breast.

- Options include reconstruction using saline or silicone implants. Modern techniques (subpectoral or retropectoral placement) place the implants behind the pectoral muscle. Older techniques (subglandular or retromammary placement) placed the implants in front of the pectoral muscle.
- Flap surgery removes skin and fat from the abdomen, back, or buttock and uses it to form a new breast. Flap techniques can be *pedicle flap*, where the flap remains attached to its original blood supply and it is tunneled under the skin to the breast area, or *free flap*, where the flap is completely removed and microsurgery is needed to recreate a blood supply when the flap is positioned as a breast mold. The recovery time for most flap reconstruction is 4-6 week. Patients are usually required to have a drain for 1-2 weeks.

Questions

1. The surgical specimen is radiographed to
   (A) confirm that the entire lesion was removed
   (B) compare various needle localization techniques
   (C) magnify the lesion to assess any possible microcalcifications
   (D) check the position of the lesion

2. The specimen is compressed to reduce
   (A) motion unsharpness
   (B) radiation exposure
   (C) tissue thickness
   (D) magnification factor

3. Which procedure is performed to obtain cellular material from a suspicious area for cytological analysis?
   (A) ductography
   (B) needle localization
   (C) pneumocystogram
   (D) fine-needle biopsy (FNB)

4. Preoperative localization will
   1. direct the surgeon to the area requiring biopsy
   2. help the surgeon to excise a smaller specimen
   3. ensure that the correct area is removed

   (A) 1 and 2 only
   (B) 2 and 3 only
   (C) 1 and 3 only
   (D) 1, 2, and 3

5. Core biopsy techniques developed as an alternative to surgical biopsy because this technique provided a larger sample of the area of suspicion and thus more information than
   (A) ductography
   (B) needle localization
   (C) pneumocystogram
   (D) FNB

6. An ultrasound of a lesion showed a spherical mass with smooth regular borders, anechoic interior, and acoustic enhancement. The lesion is likely to be a
   (A) fibroadenoma
   (B) abscess
   (C) simple cyst
   (D) ductal carcinoma

7. In ultrasound, the term acoustic enhancement refers to
   (A) a structure without internal echoes
   (B) a structure with internal echoes
   (C) the amount of sound passing through an anechoic structure
   (D) few echoes within a structure

8. A procedure whereby the lactiferous duct is cannulated and a small amount of contrast agent is injected into the duct is termed
   (A) ductography
   (B) needle localization
   (C) pneumocystogram
   (D) FNA

9. A patient had an ultrasound, which confirmed the presence of a cyst in the breast. The radiologist wished to assess the contents of the cyst. What additional study could be recommended?

(A) ductography
(B) needle localization
(C) pneumocystogram
(D) FNA

10. Biopsy performed using a 14-gauge needle to remove tissue samples from the breast is termed

(A) core biopsy
(B) cytology
(C) ductography
(D) aspiration

11. Stereotactic breast localization is used to

(A) obtain 2-dimensional information on palpable breast lesions
(B) calculate the vertical position of nonpalpable lesions
(C) obtain a 3-dimensional image of the breast
(D) calculate the horizontal, vertical, and depth position of nonpalpable lesions

12. A cyst aspiration can only be performed

(A) under ultrasound guidance
(B) using mammographic imaging
(C) using MRI guidance
(D) none of the above

13. Which of the following biopsy techniques is most accurate?

(A) FNB
(B) open surgical biopsy
(C) core biopsy
(D) MRI core biopsy

14. In general, the optimal duration of Tamoxifen treatment is

(A) 2 years
(B) 3 years
(C) 4 years
(D) 5 years

15. Lumpectomy describes the process of

(A) removing the entire breast including the nipple
(B) removal of the breast cancer tumor and surrounding margins of normal breast
(C) making a small incision over or near the site of the breast lesion
(D) removing benign lumps from the breast

16. Radiation therapy can be used

1. with other treatment options
2. to kill any remaining cancer cells in the breast, or chest wall area
3. to shrink the size of a tumor before surgery

(A) 1 and 2 only
(B) 2 and 3 only
(C) 1 and 3 only
(D) 1, 2, and 3

17. Chemotherapy is a class of drugs that can be used to

(A) kill cancer cells in other parts of the body
(B) block estrogen from cancer cells
(C) reduce estrogen levels in the body
(D) kill cancer cells by using high-energy radiation

18. Breast reconstruction can involve the placement of small fluid-filled sacs behind the pectoral muscle. Two common types of such implants are

(A) saline and flap surgery
(B) TRAM flap and silicone implant
(C) silicone or saline implants
(D) saline-filled implant and latissimus dorsi flap implant

19. Chemotherapy
    (A) involves the use of drugs to treat cancer that may have spread
    (B) is the destruction of cancer cells using estrogen receptor drugs
    (C) involves mapping the area around a tumor with the injection of a radioactive tracer
    (D) is the removal of the cancerous tissue from the breast

20. A process of removing tissue and fat from the abdomen and transferring that tissue to reconstruct the breast is called
    (A) deep inferior epigastric perforators (DIEP) flap
    (B) latissimus dorsi flap
    (C) TRAM flap
    (D) TUG flap

21. Antiestrogen drugs such as Tamoxifen can be used to
    1. slow or stop the cancer's growth
    2. prevent breast cancer in high-risk women
    3. prevent the recurrence of breast cancer

    (A) 1 and 2 only
    (B) 2 and 3 only
    (C) 1 and 3 only
    (D) 1, 2, and 3

22. MRI imaging
    (A) uses complex magnetic properties of elements
    (B) explores the behavior of liquids or solids in metal
    (C) images the patient in less than 15 minutes
    (D) is less sensitive than a mammogram

23. Most of the risk of MR imaging of the breast are associated with
    (A) the magnetic properties of the patient
    (B) ferromagnetic metals
    (C) technologist errors
    (D) radiologist errors

24. In breast cancer staging the patient was rated N1. This means that
    (A) the cancer has not spread beyond the breast
    (B) the cancer is confined to 1-2 lymph nodes
    (C) the patient has a small tumor
    (D) the is no evidence of metastasis

25. Cyst aspiration describes the removal of
    (A) a sample of the content of a cyst for biopsy
    (B) cell samples taken from a cyst for analysis
    (C) fluid from a cyst
    (D) any mass from the breast

26. If a breast lesion is seen only on the breast ultrasound, which modality should be used when performing a biopsy of the lesion?
    (A) mammogram
    (B) ultrasound
    (C) MRI
    (D) nuclear medicine

27. The pathology review is
    (A) a method of tracking and reviewing all positive findings
    (B) a process of eliminating all positive findings
    (C) a method of tracking cosmetic intervention
    (D) a process of identifying all mammoplasty

28. The technique used where by contrast is injected into the ducts to check for an abnormality is called
    (A) augmentation
    (B) ductography
    (C) biopsy
    (D) mammoplasty

29. Cosmetic intervention could be considered
   (A) breast reconstruction after treatment for breast cancer
   (B) surgical reconstruction of the breast to increase its firmness
   (C) breast biopsy to check a suspicious lesion
   (D) breast reduction to relieve back pain

30. A process by which the breast size is increased using implants is called
   (A) augmentation mammoplasty
   (B) ductography
   (C) needle biopsy
   (D) needle aspiration

31. The removal of 1-3 axillary nodes for testing is included in a/an
   (A) axillary node dissection
   (B) sentinel node mapping
   (C) sentinel node biopsy
   (D) lumpectomy

32. Specimen radiography confirms that
   (A) a biopsy is not necessary
   (B) the patient has no malignancy
   (C) the patient needs a mastectomy
   (D) the suspected lesion is in the tissue that was removed

33. Which of the following are side effects of radiation treatment?
   1. loss of appetite
   2. fatigue
   3. heaviness of the breast

   (A) 1 and 2 only
   (B) 2 and 3 only
   (C) 1 and 3 only
   (D) 1, 2, and 3

34. A big advantage of brachytherapy over traditional radiation therapy treatments is
   (A) reduced time of treatment
   (B) the ability of brachytherapy to treat larger tumors
   (C) more radiation can be given to healthy tissue
   (D) it is more convenient because of the longer treatment times

35. Side effects of chemotherapy include
   (A) nausea and or vomiting
   (B) reduced white cell count
   (C) none of the above
   (D) A and B

36. What is Tamoxifen?
   (A) an adjuvant therapy using drugs to reduce the risk of certain cancers
   (B) a drug regimen that will effectively block hormones in the body
   (C) an external method of killing cancer cells
   (D) the removal of all cancer cells from the body thereby reducing cancer risks

37. Which of the following biopsy techniques is the most accurate?
   (A) FNB
   (B) core biopsy
   (C) stereotactic breast biopsy
   (D) open surgical biopsy

38. Which of the following is the least expensive and least invasive method of breast biopsy?
   (A) FNB
   (B) core biopsy
   (C) open surgical biopsy
   (D) stereotactic breast biopsy

39. A technique used to assess and evaluate nipple discharge by checking for defects or wall irregularity is called
   (A) ductography
   (B) interventional radiography
   (C) aspiration biopsy
   (D) lumpectomy

40. Neoadjuvant chemotherapy refers to treatment
    - (A) before surgery to help shrink the size of cancerous tumors
    - (B) after mastectomy to slow the growth of cancer
    - (C) before surgery utilizing an antiestrogen drug
    - (D) after surgery that involves radiation

41. Preoperative localization is
    - (A) stereotactic breast localization of a palpable abnormality
    - (B) used to locate palpable breast lesions
    - (C) a technique use to locate nonpalpable lesions
    - (D) a check of the tissue for malignancy

42. A biopsy technique that often requires the presence of a cytologic technologist describes
    - (A) open surgical biopsy
    - (B) core biopsy
    - (C) stereotactic breast biopsy
    - (D) fine-needle biopsy

43. Cosmetic intervention describes
    1. breast reconstruction after treatment for breast cancer
    2. surgical reconstruction of the breast at the patient's request
    3. breast augmentation for personal reasons
    - (A) 1 and 2 only
    - (B) 2 and 3 only
    - (C) 1 and 3 only
    - (D) 1, 2, and 3

44. The side effects of chemotherapy are related to the effect of the drug on
    - (A) all tissues and organs in the body
    - (B) cancer cells only
    - (C) the growth of cancer
    - (D) hair follicles only

45. Any size tumor with cancer spread to chest wall and/or skin of breast and up to 10 axillary or claviclar lymph nodes is describes as stage
    - (A) 1
    - (B) 2
    - (C) 3
    - (D) 4

46. Which of the following would be contraindicated for lumpectomy?
    1. women with previous lumpectomy
    2. women with multiple cancer sites in 1 breast
    3. large tumors in small breast
    - (A) 1 and 2 only
    - (B) 2 and 3 only
    - (C) 1 and 3 only
    - (D) 1, 2, and 3

47. The staging of a cancer will determine
    1. if the cancer is invasive
    2. the exact tumor size
    3. if the cancer has spread to distant sites
    - (A) 1 and 2 only
    - (B) 2 and 3 only
    - (C) 1 and 3 only
    - (D) 1, 2, and 3

48. In breast cancer staging the patient was rated T1. This means that
    - (A) the cancer has not spread beyond the breast
    - (B) the cancer is confined to 1-2 lymph nodes
    - (C) the patient has a small tumor
    - (D) there is no evidence of metastasis

ANSWERS

1. **(A)** The specimen is radiographed to ensure that the lesion was removed for surgical biopsy or sufficiently sampled for core biopsy. The lesion should be circled on the specimen radiograph and all the borders checked to confirm that the entire lesion was removed. The specimen can be magnified, especially if calcifications are present, to count and confirm that all the calcifications have been removed (**Figure 5-1**).[1]

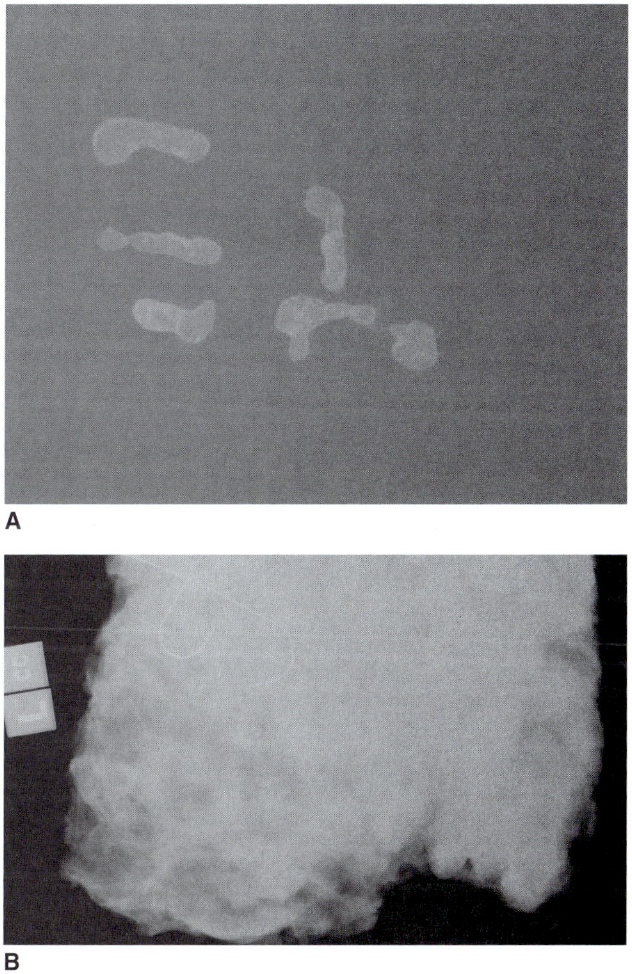

Figure 5-1. Specimen imaging (A) core sample, (B) open biopsy sample.

2. **(C)** Compression of the specimen reduces tissue thickness, thus improving subject contrast. Structures are spread out, and tissue density is uniform with less superimposition of structures. The specimen can also be magnified to image microcalcifications. The overall effect is improved visualization and a more uniform density. Motion unsharpness and radiation reduction are not an issue in specimen imaging. Compression will improve visualization of structures in the magnified specimen but will not alter the magnification factor.[1]

3. **(D)** FNB obtains cellular material for cytological analysis. FNB uses small-gauge needles (23 gauge), which limits the amount of cells that can be aspirated. The accuracy of the procedure depends on the radiologist performing the examination and the cytologist interpreting the results. Ductography cannulates a duct to introduce a contrast agent. Needle localization positions a guide wire in a nonpalpable lesion for surgical removal. Pneumocystogram injects air in a cyst for analysis of the inner lining of the cyst (**Figure 5-2**).[1]

4. **(D)** Preoperative localization is performed on nonpalpable lesions or suspicious areas that are identified only mammographically. The radiologist assists the surgeon by placing a wire in the suspicious area as a guide for the surgeon. The surgeon is then able to excise only the lesion and surrounding margins rather than a larger area of the breast. Once excised, the wire with the specimen radiograph confirms that the correct area was removed (**Figure 5-3**).[1]

5. **(D)** Core biopsy provides a larger sample of breast tissue for histological study. The

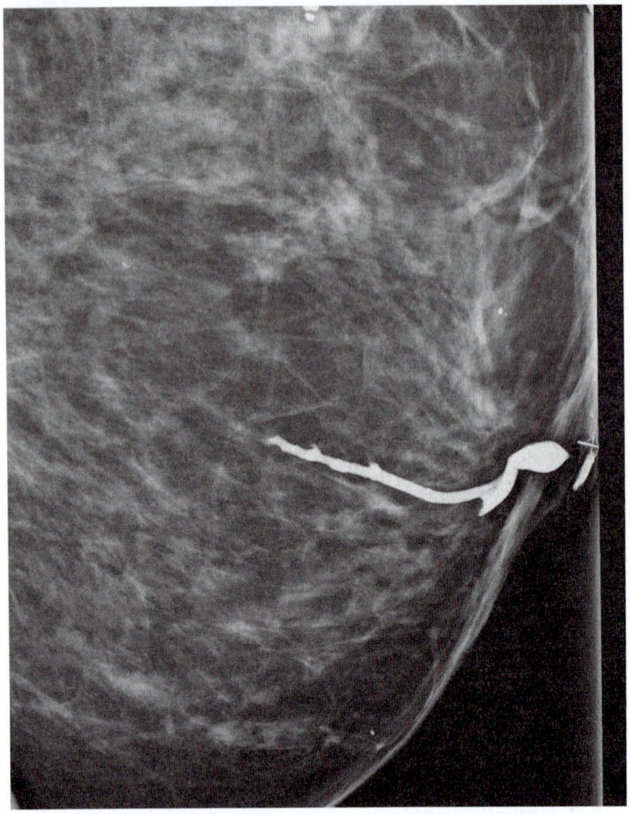

Figure 5-2. Ductogram imaging showing blocked ducts.

larger sample (generally an 8- to 14-gauge needle is used) offers a more definitive diagnosis when compared with FNB. Ductography cannulates a duct to introduce a contrast agent. Needle localization positions a guide wire in a nonpalpable lesion for surgical removal. Pneumocystogram injects air in a cyst for analysis of the inner lining of the cyst (**Figure 5-4**).[1,2]

6. **(C)** A cyst is usually fluid filled with smooth walls that allow transmission of sound. Sound traveling through a fluid-filled structure is barely attenuated; the structures distal to a cystic lesion appear to have more echoes than neighboring areas. This process is referred to as distal echo enhancement. It is rare for calcifications in a cyst wall or debris within the cyst to present through transmission. A fibroadenoma usually has low-level internal echoes and the borders may be smooth, round, or lobulated. An abscess will be fluid filled and usually has some internal echoes. Their borders are generally well defined, but irregular. Ductal carcinomas typically are taller than they are wide—benign masses spread out horizontally. Cancers have a spiculated outline with alternating echopenic and echogenic straight lines radiating from the surface of the mass (echopenic means there are few echoes within a structure; echogenic describes a structure that produces echoes; anechoic means no internal echoes) (**Figure 5-5**)[1,2]

7. **(C)** If the sound traveling through a cyst is barely attenuated then the structure distal to the cyst appears to have more echoes than neighboring areas. The phenomenon is referred to as acoustic enhancement or through transmission.[2,3]

8. **(A)** Ductography or galactography can be performed on patients with nipple discharge. A small amount of contrast agent is injected into the duct and radiographs are taken in the cranio-caudal and lateral positions. The contrast agent outlines the ducts to visualize any pathology. Needle localization positions a guide wire in a nonpalpable lesion for surgical removal. Pneumocystogram injects air in a cyst for analysis of the inner lining of the cyst. FNA removes fluid from a cystic lesion for cytologic analysis. (See Figure 5-2.)[1,2]

9. **(D)** FNA can be used to remove the content of a cyst. A pneumocystogram is not a common procedure. It may be performed in conjunction with cyst aspiration. Air is injected into the cyst, which has been emptied. The inner walls of the cyst can then be assessed. In general, the air is reabsorbed by the body within a week. Ductography examines the ducts and the needle localization is used to locate nonpalpable lesions.[1,2]

10. **(A)** Breast biopsy is the taking of a sample specimen of breast cells or tissue for cytological or histological analysis. In a core biopsy, a large-gauge (8-14 gauge) needle is used to remove tissue samples. The core biopsy needles can be mechanical, an automatic core "guns" with an inner needle, or a vacuum core system. The needle gun

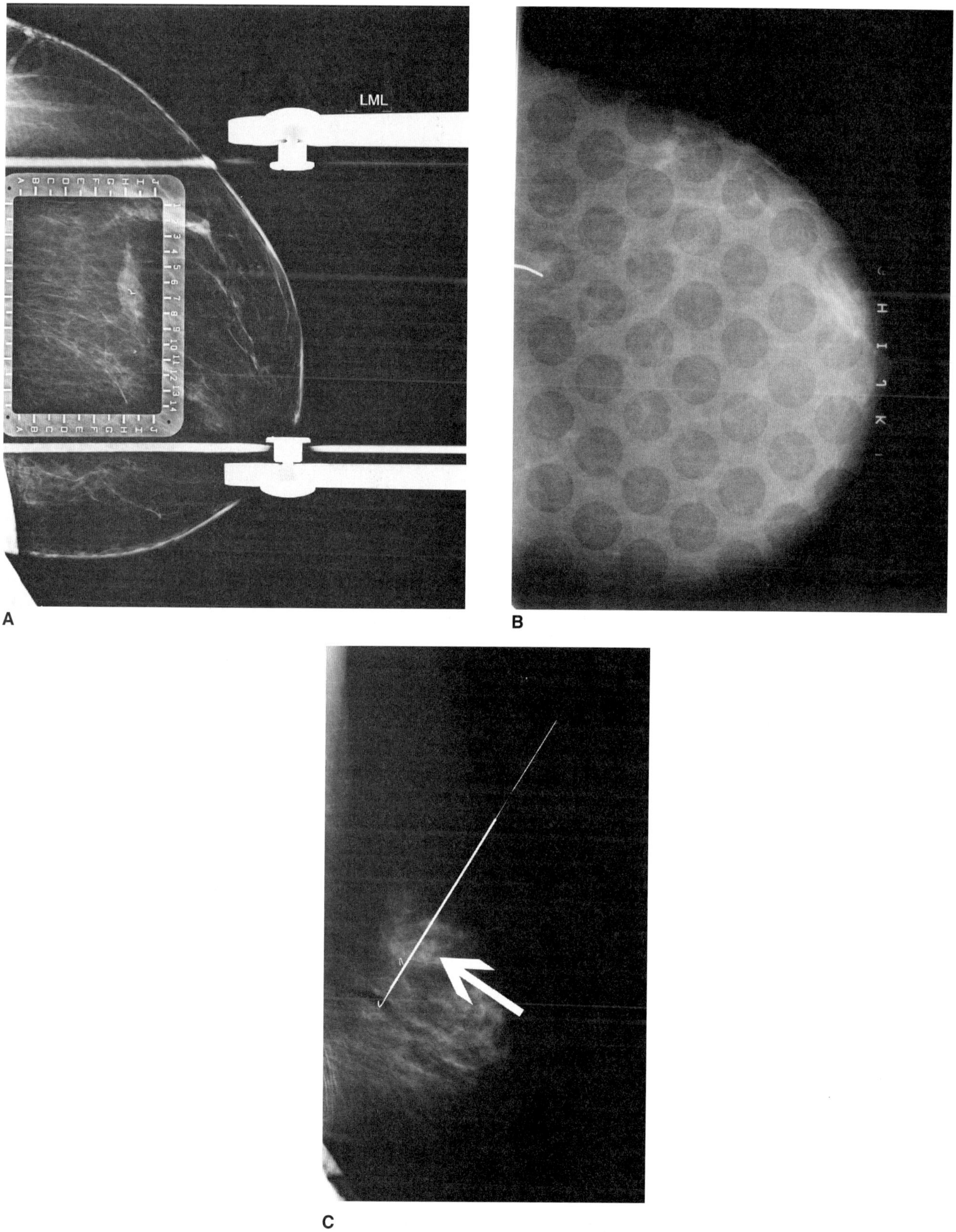

Figure 5-3. In the wire needle localization procedure, the radiologist assists the surgeon by placing a hook wire in the suspicious area as a guide for the surgeon (A) open localization compression plate, (B) grid localization compression plate, (C) hook wire in place through lesion (indicated by arrow).

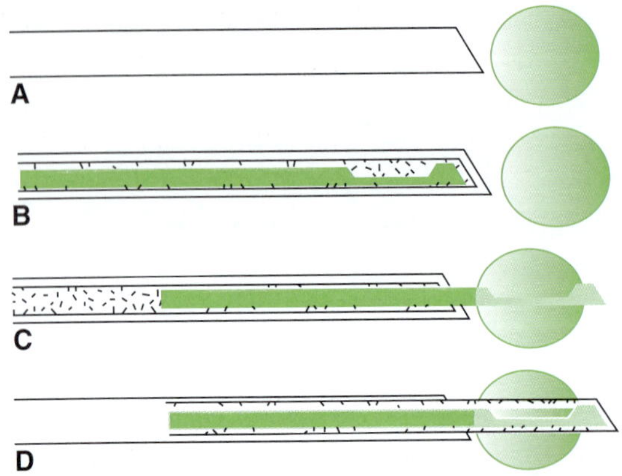

Figure 5-4. Core biopsy gun (A) prefire; (B) trough without the needle; (C) postfire into the lesion—the needle moves forward, filling the trough with breast tissue; and (D) postfire—the outer sheath moves forward to cut the tissue and keep it in the trough. (Reproduced with permission from Peart O: Mammography and Breast Imaging PREP: Program Review and Exam Prep. New York, NY: McGraw-Hill Education; 2012.)

combinations are designed to move a cutting needle rapidly through the breast to obtain a tissue sample. Core biopsies can be performed under mammography, ultrasound, or MRI guidance. Cytology refers to the study of cells. Ductography is used to evaluate patients with abnormal nipple discharge. The lactiferous duct is cannulated and a small amount of contrast agent is injected before the area is imaged. Aspiration is a method of removing fluid from a cyst using a needle (see Figure 5-4).[1,4]

11. **(D)** Stereology is the science of determining the 3-dimensional location of an object based on 2-dimensional images. Stereotactic breast localizations can be used to locate the horizontal, vertical, and depth position of nonpalpable lesions. A computer performs the necessary calculations therefore if the input information is inaccurate, errors in localization will result (Figure 5-6).[1,2]

12. **(D)** Cyst aspiration removes the contents of a cyst for analysis. Although the technique is often done with ultrasound guidance, nonpalpable lesions can be aspirated under mammographic guidance and large palpable lesions can be assessed clinically without imaging guidance. MRI aspirations are not common because often cysts, if not visualized on the mammogram, are visualized on ultrasound. The needle size used depends on the

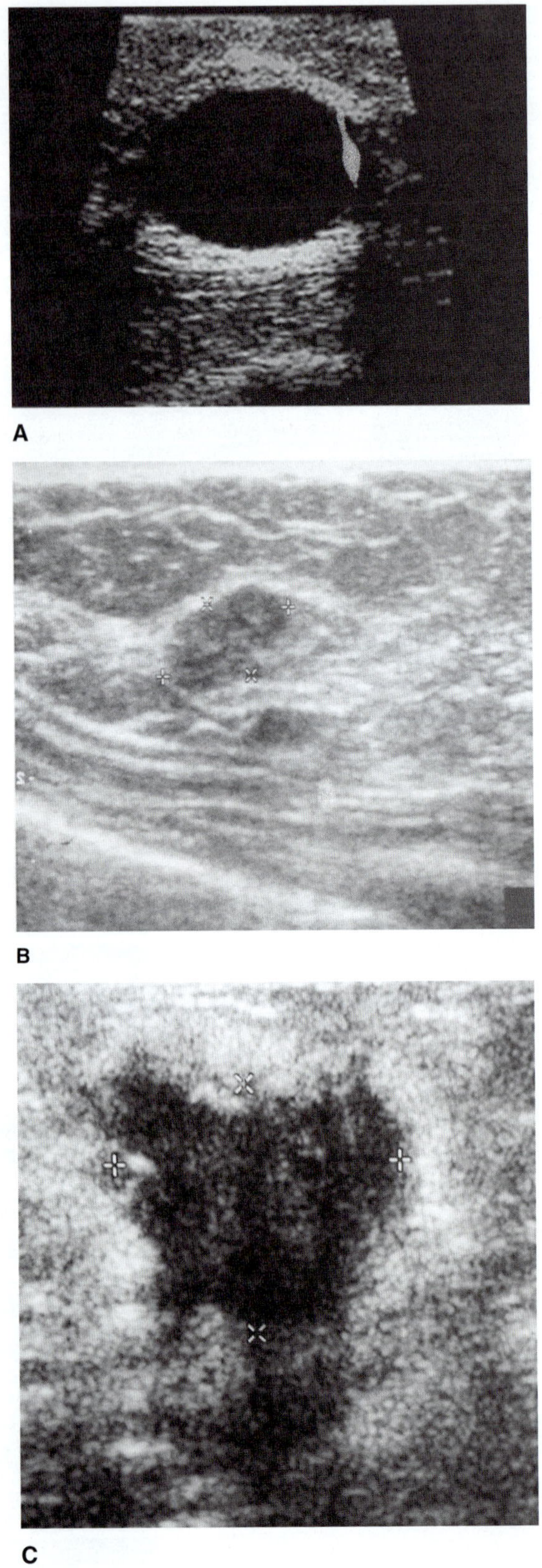

Figure 5-5. Ultrasound images showing (A) cyst, (B) fibroadenoma, and (C) malignancy. (Figure 5-5 B, C: Reproduced with permission from Peart O: Mammography and Breast Imaging PREP: Program Review and Exam Prep. New York, NY: McGraw-Hill Education; 2012.)

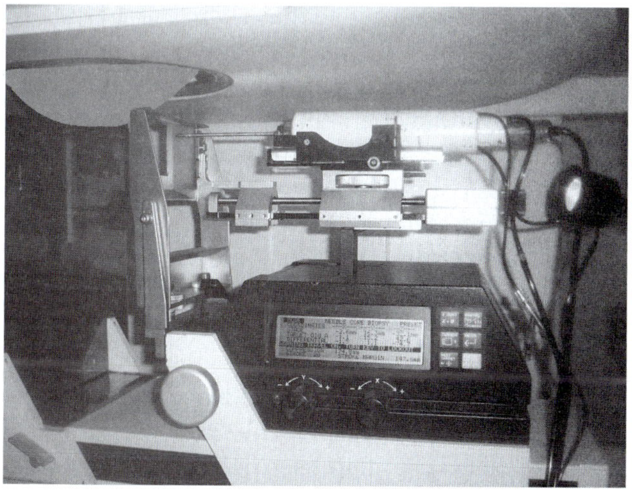

Figure 5-6. The stereotactic system will calculate the exact coordinates of the lesion. Stereo localization of a lesion.

viscosity and thickness of the fluid content of the cyst but generally a small gauge (e.g., 21 gauge) is used to reduce patient discomfort.[1,2]

13. **(B)** The open surgical biopsy is the most invasive procedure, but it has the lowest false-negative rate. Open surgical biopsies will need more hospital time, require anesthesia, and will leave visible scars on the breast. These factors can all contribute to a higher complication rate with open biopsy when compared with the other minimally invasive procedures. FNB is the least expensive but least accurate biopsy method. The main cause is insufficient samples because of the small-needle gauge used. Core biopsy has a lower false-negative rate than FNB, but again insufficient samples can reduce the accuracy. MRI-guided biopsy is usually used for lesions seen only on MR imaging. The technique involves the removal of core samples and is considered a minimally invasive procedure.[1,4]

14. **(D)** The optimal duration of Tamoxifen in postmenopausal women is 5 years although recent studies have suggested added benefits with longer use. Tamoxifen will react with the estrogen receptor in other areas of the body, such as bone and the lining of the uterus. With the cells in these areas, Tamoxifen acts like estrogen to promote growth, leading to increased bone density and a higher risk of uterine cancer. Other side effects of Tamoxifen include endometrial cancer, pulmonary embolism, stroke, and deep vein thrombosis. Tamoxifen can also cause milder reactions such as tiredness, dizziness, weight gain, and visual problems such as blurred or reduced vision.[5]

15. **(B)** Lumpectomy is a breast-conserving surgery whereby the breast tumor and surrounding margin of normal tissue are removed. Removing a benign lump is not called a lumpectomy. The main advantage of a lumpectomy is that it cosmetically preserves most of the breast. Factors that can affect the choice of lumpectomy over mastectomy include past lumpectomy, tumor size, tumor type, and cancer stage.[1,2,5,6]

16. **(D)** Radiation will kill both normal and cancerous cells. In any radiation treatment, the cell cycle is important because radiation usually works best on cells that are actively or rapidly dividing but does not work well on cells that are in the resting phase (G_0) or are dividing slowly. Radiation is often used after surgery and in conjunction with other treatment options to remove any remaining cancer cells in the breast, chest wall, and axilla area but can be used before surgery to shrink the tumor and allow a better cosmetic surgical result (Table 5-1).[1,5]

17. **(A)** Chemotherapy is an adjuvant therapy and involves the use of drugs to kill cancer cells and treat cancer that may have spread

Table 5-1. THE CELL CYCLE

G_0 phase (resting stage): Cells have not yet started to divide. Cells spend much of their lives in this phase. Depending on the type of cell, this step can last for a few hours to many years. When the cell is signaled to reproduce, it moves into the G_1 phase.

G_1 phase: During this phase, the cell starts making more proteins to get ready to divide. This phase lasts about 18-30 hours.

S phase: In the S phase, the chromosomes that contain the genetic code (DNA) are copied so that both of the new cells formed will have the right amount of DNA. This phase lasts about 18-20 hours.

G_2 phase: The G_2 phase is just before the cell starts splitting into 2 cells. It lasts from 2-10 hours.

M phase: (mitosis): In this phase, which lasts only 30-60 minutes, the cell actually splits into 2 new cells.

beyond the breast. The drug is distributed throughout the entire body via the blood stream and tends to attack cells that are rapidly dividing, whether they are cancerous or not. Drugs that block estrogen from latching onto cancer cells are antiestrogen drugs such as Tamoxifen and Raloxifene. Another class of drugs—aromatase inhibitors—that suppress blood levels of estrogen are also available in the fight against breast cancer. Radiation therapy uses high-energy radiation to destroy cancer cells.[1,5,7]

18. **(C)** Breast reconstruction can involve the placement of saline or silicone-filled sac either in front of or behind the pectoral muscle. Implants placed behind the pectoral muscle (subpectoral or retropectoral placement) are becoming more popular than the older method of placing the implants in front of the pectoral muscle (subglandular or retromammary placement). Subpectoral placement allows easier imaging of the breast mammographically and is less prone to encapsulation. Flap surgery uses skin, fat, or muscle from other parts of the body to form a natural-looking breast mound (Figure 5-7).[1,5,6]

19. **(A)** Chemotherapy involves the use of drugs to treat kill cancer cells that may have spread beyond the breast. It can also be used to slow the growth of cancer or to relieve the symptoms of cancer. The chemotherapy treatments may last 3-6 months depending on the intensity of the chemotherapy drug and how far the cancer has spread. Generally, chemotherapy treatment is given in cycles, with a period of treatment followed by a recovery period.[1,5]

20. **(A)** In the DIEP flap procedure, skin and fat from the abdomen are used to reconstruct a natural breast after mastectomy. Unlike the TRAM flap, the DIEP flap does not take any abdominal muscles. However, because the tissue is completely removed, microsurgery is needed to connect blood vessels. Transverse rectus abdominus myocutaneous flap (TRAM flap) procedure uses tissue and muscle from the lower abdominal wall to create a breast shape. There are 2 types of TRAM flaps: the *pedicle flap* where the flap is left with its original blood supply and tunneled under the skin to the breast area; and the *free flap* where the tissue from the abdomen is completely removed from its original location. This process requires microscopic surgery to reconnect a blood supply. The TRAM flap procedures leave weak abdominal muscle and are no longer popular. Latissimus dorsi flap involves the removal of muscle and skin from the upper back to create a breast shape. The transverse upper gracilis (TUG) flap uses tissue from the inner upper thigh, near the crease of the groin as well as some muscle to create breast tissue. This is not a common procedure and it is only performed if the patient does not have adequate tissue in the abdomen or buttock region. Other flap techniques are the superficial inferior epigastric artery (SIEA) flap that uses fat, blood vessels, nerves, and skin from the lower abdomen to create breast tissue. It does not require blood vessels going through or around the abdominal muscles but this technique is possible only on 15% of all patients. The superior gluteal artery perforator (SGAP) flap uses tissue from the top of the buttocks to create breast tissue.[1,5,8,9]

21. **(D)** Tamoxifen belongs to a class of drugs called SERMs or selective estrogen receptor modulators. Normally, the estrogen receptor molecules in cancer cells will react with estrogen in the body, allowing the cells to grow. Antiestrogen drugs work by attaching to the estrogen receptor molecule in breast cancer cells that would normally react with estrogen. This prevents the estrogen receptor cancer cells from interacting with body estrogen and can slow or stop the cancer's growth. It can also be used to prevent breast cancer or the recurrence of breast cancer at local sites or distant metastasis after a lumpectomy or radiation treatment.[1,7]

22. **(A)** Breast MRI examinations are extremely sensitive. They are conducted using high magnetic fields and dedicated breast coils. The way the body's activities respond to

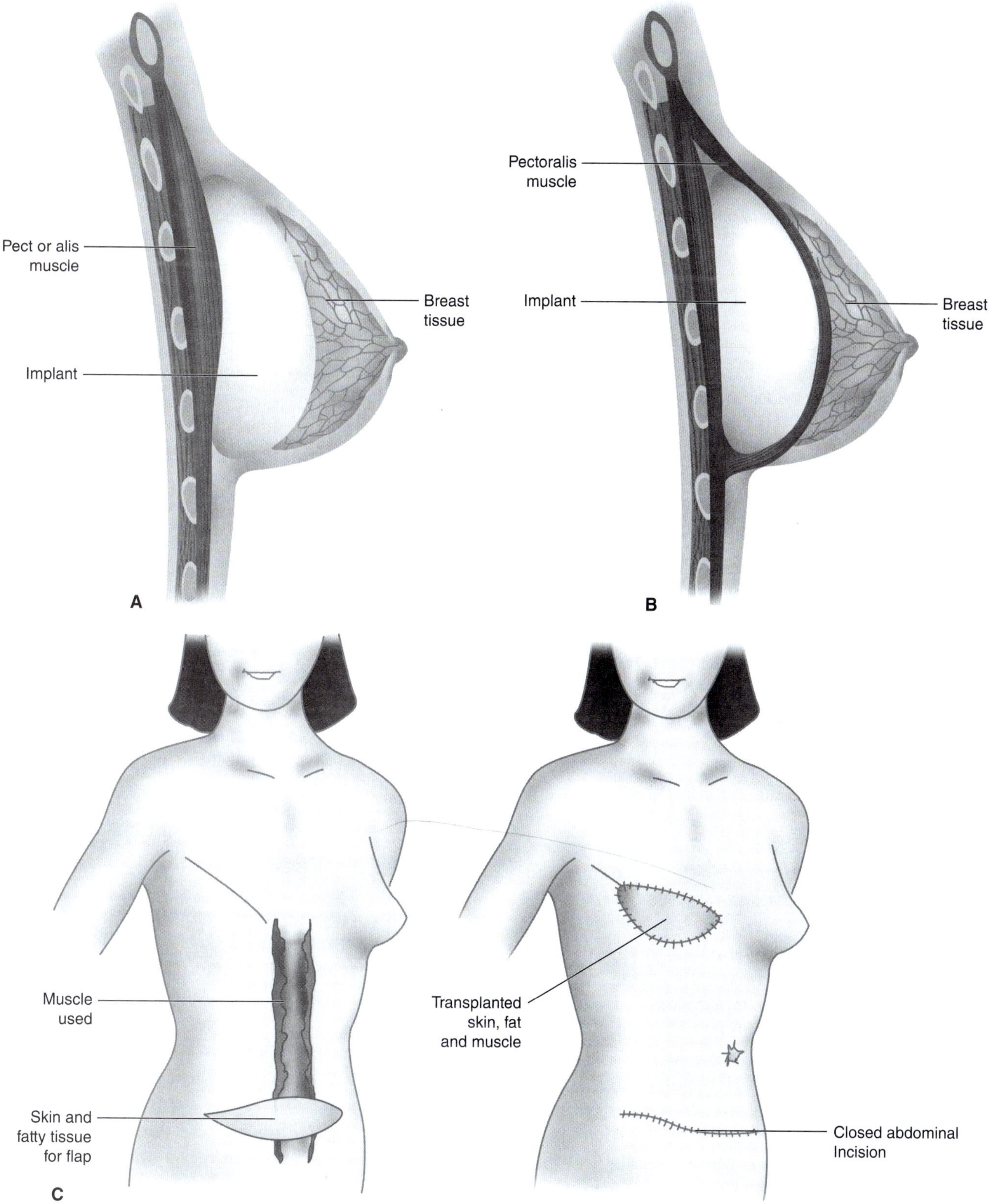

Figure 5-7. Breast reconstruction. (A) Subglandular implant placement, (B) subpectoral implant placement, (C) TRAM flap technique. (Reproduced with permission from Peart O: Mammography and Breast Imaging PREP: Program Review and Exam Prep. New York, NY: McGraw-Hill Education; 2012.)

magnetic fields and how they relax in the magnetic field is used to analyze and record structures in the breast. Each image compiled by the computer will represent a different area of the breast. The actual examination can take up to 45 minutes[3,5] (**Figure 5-8**).

23. **(B)** During the MRI examination, the patient is placed within a powerful magnetic field. Patients are therefore required to give detailed medical history for any examination because any metal objects can potentially be extremely dangerous inside or around the MRI unit.[1,3]

24. **(B)** In breast cancer staging, the cancer can be classified by the letters T, N, or M. A 'T" grade would only describe the tumor size and spread to the skin or chest wall under the breast. Tumors are graded from 0 to 4 with higher numbers indicating a larger or wider spread tumor. The letter N is graded from 0 to 3 and indicates cancer spread to the lymph nodes in the axilla and would indicate the number of lymph nodes affected. The letter M is graded from 0 or 1 and indicates cancer spread to distant organs.[6]

25. **(C)** A cyst aspiration removes the content of the cyst. A breast biopsy is the taking of the sample specimen for cytologic or histologic analysis. Cytologic analysis analyzes cell samples while the histologic analysis analyzes tissue samples. A core or vacuum biopsy removes tissue samples for histologic analysis.[1,2]

26. **(B)** Before any biopsy, the lesion must be localized. If it is not seen on a modality it cannot be localized on that modality.[1]

27. **(A)** The pathology review will assess whether the initial diagnosis matches the confirmed findings. Facilities must have a medical audit in place to track all positive pathological findings. This tracking is required to comply with US MQSA, but a regular review of the medical audit will help the facility identify areas of concern including high false-negative or false-positive rates.[10,11]

28. **(B)** Ductography is used to evaluate nipple discharge, detects duct filling irregularities, duct expansions, or duct defects. Contrast media is introduced to the ductal system via the ducts exiting at the nipple. A breast biopsy is the taking of the sample specimen for cytologic or histologic analysis. Breast augmentation will increase the size of the breast. Mammoplasty is a procedure whereby the breast is reconstructed for cosmetic or therapeutic reasons (see Figure 5-2).[1,2]

29. **(B)** Cosmetic intervention is selective treatment requested by the patient for a variety of reasons. Treatment can be augmentation or reduction. Required treatment due to medical problems or breast cancer is not considered cosmetic intervention.[1,2]

30. **(A)** In the process of breast augmentation silicone or saline filled sacs are inserted into the breasts to increase breast size. Needle biopsy takes cell or tissue samples from the breasts for testing. Needle aspiration removes fluid from cyst for testing. Ductography evaluates the ducts immediately behind the nipple using contrast media.[1,9]

31. **(C)** Sentinel node mapping is the injection of a radiopharmaceutical into the subareolar lymphatic plexus (or lesion). The tracer travels to the sentinel node—identifying that node for dissection and eliminating the need for extensive lymph node dissection. Sentinel node biopsy is the removal of the sentinel lymph node plus 2-3 more adjacent nodes for testing. Lumpectomy is the removal of the tumor plus surrounding margins. Axillary node dissection is the removal of most of the lymph nodes from the axilla for testing.[5,7]

32. **(D)** A specimen can be removed during a core biopsy procedure or an open surgical biopsy. Specimens should be imaged after the biopsy to confirm that the lesion was removed or adequately sampled. The specimen can also confirm that the margins are clean if a total excision is being performed.[1]

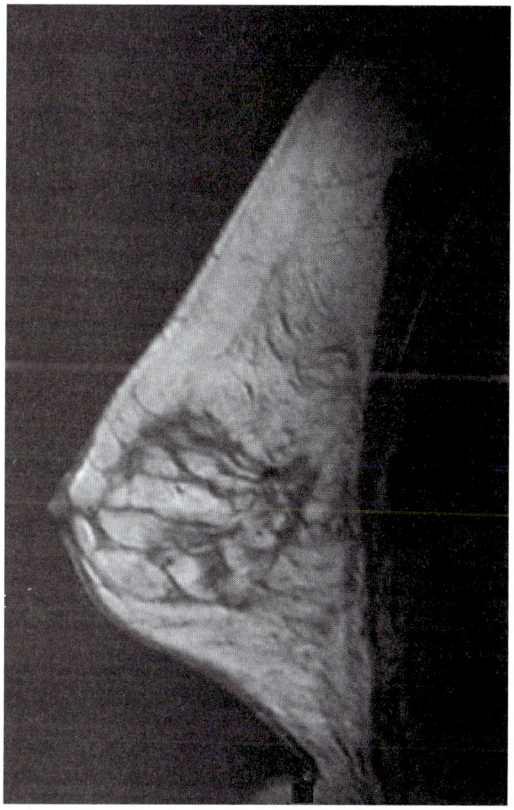
A

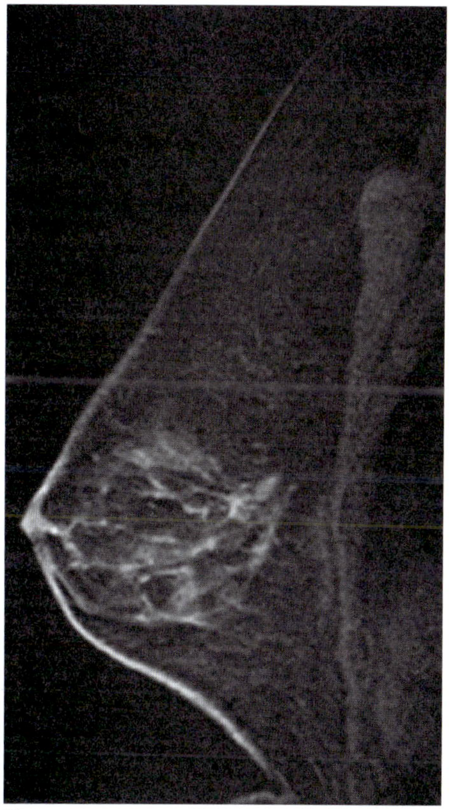
B

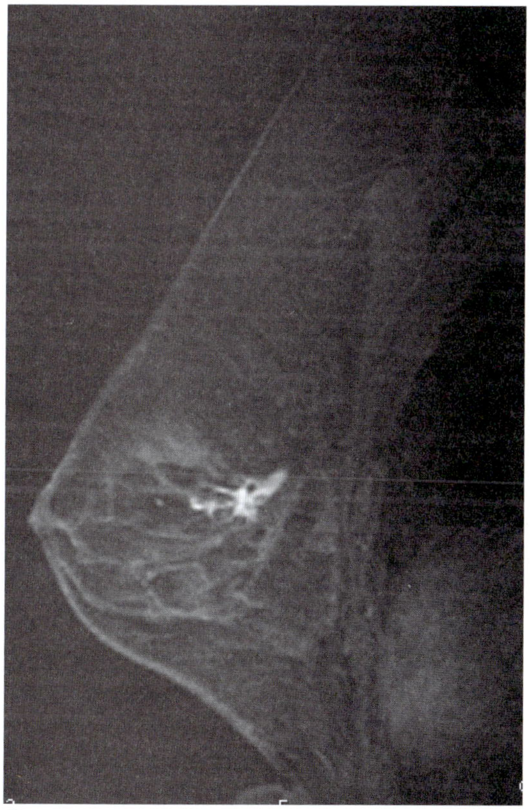
C

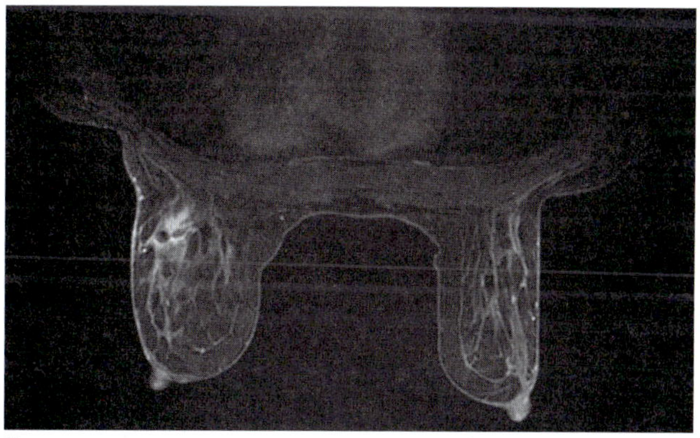
D

Figure 5-8. (A) Nonfat saturated T_2 weighted imaging (T2 NON FAT SAT), (B) spoiled gradient (SPGR) precontrast, (C) SPGR FAT SAT postbiopsy showing DCIS, (D) Axial SPGR FAT SAT postcontrast. (Reproduced with permission from Peart O: Mammography and Breast Imaging PREP: Program Review and Exam Prep. New York, NY: McGraw-Hill Education; 2012.)

33. **(D)** The side effects of radiation are often temporary and can include: fatigue, swelling of breast, heaviness in the breast, sunburn-type appearance of the breast skin, and loss of appetite and neutropenia which is a decrease in white blood count. Most side effects will disappear after 6-12 months.[5]

34. **(A)** Brachytherapy can deliver a high dose of radiation to small areas. Instead of radiation coming from outside the body, the active source is temporarily placed directly in the body or tumor cavity. There are 2 methods. One involves seed implantation brachytherapy with the placement of the radioactive seeds directly in the breast tissue next to the cancer. First 10-20 plastic catheters are surgically placed into the breast tissues. Radioactive pellets—Iridium-192—are inserted into the catheters. The catheters are connected to a high-dose rate brachytherapy machine 9 or more times in a week for about 10 minutes. The catheters are removed after treatment. In this method the source radiation remains in the patient's body between treatments. Other methods involve surgically implanting an inflatable balloon catheter device at the site of the tumor. The device remains in place for the duration of the treatment but at each treatment session a tiny radioactive bead attached to a wire is threaded into the inflated balloon. The wire device is moved to various places inside the inflated balloon delivering different levels of radiation. After completion of treatment the balloon is deflated and the system is removed. This method has no source of radiation remaining in the patient's body between treatments. The patients are treated for 5-9 days versus the 6-8 weeks of external radiation treatments.[5]

35. **(D)** Side effects from chemotherapy will vary depending on the strength of drugs used, the dosage and the duration of treatment. Some patients experience few side effects; others experience many of the common side effects, which include:

- Hair loss, *alopecia,* is generally temporary and occurs because in some women the hair follicles are weakened by the chemotherapy drug causing hair to fall out at a much faster rate than normal hair growth. Most hair loss will not begin until after the second chemotherapy session and grows back at the end of treatment—sometimes with a change in texture.
- Irritation of the lining of the stomach or intestine can cause nausea and vomiting.
- Mouth sores and taste changes.
- Decreased appetite, diarrhea, or constipation.
- Infertility or premature menopause. The closer the woman is to menopause when she undergoes chemotherapy the more likely she is to experience premature menopause.
- Birth defects if taken when pregnant.
- Tingling or burning sensations and numbness in hands and or feet.
- Skin irritations—redness, itching, peeling, or acne.
- Dark brittle or cracked fingers and/or toenails.
- Low blood cell counts (white, red, or platelet). A low white cell count will make the body more susceptible to infections. A reduction in red blood cells causes anemia, which is associated with fatigue, dizziness, headaches, irritability, and increased heart rate or breathing. Low platelet count is referred to as thrombocytopenia. Symptoms include the tendency to bruise easily or to develop large and small bruises, increased clotting time, nosebleeds, or bleeding gums. Severe cases can cause internal bleeding. Extreme low blood cell count whether white, red, or platelet may require transfusion.[5]

36. **(A)** Tamoxifen has been used since the 1970s to treat patients with estrogen receptor positive breast cancer. It is considered an anti-estrogen drug that blocks estrogen and can lower the risk of breast cancer recurrence in postmenopausal women.[5]

37. **(D)** The open surgical biopsy is the most accurate biopsy method, but has the most complications. The fine-needle biopsy (FNB) is the fastest, has the least complications but is the least accurate. Stereotactic biopsy and core biopsy removes samples for histological analysis. The result is not as accurate as the open surgical biopsy but it is better than a fine-needle biopsy.[1,2]

38. **(A)** The FNB is the least invasive and the most cost-effective. The open surgical biopsy is the most expensive biopsy option. Stereotactic and core biopsies are not as expensive as the open surgical biopsy.[1,2]

39. **(A)** Ductography can be used to evaluate nipple discharge, to detect duct filling irregularities or duct expansions and duct defects. Lumpectomy is the removal of the tumor plus the surrounding margins. An aspiration removes the content of a cyst to relieve pain or to assess content. It is often performed under ultrasound guidance.[1,2]

40. **(A)** Neoadjuvant chemotherapy is given before surgery to slow or shrink the size of the cancerous tumor. Adjuvant chemotherapy is given in addition to other treatments.[1,2]

41. **(C).** Preoperative localization is performed on nonpalpable lesions or suspicious areas that are identified only on imaging. The radiologist assists the surgeon by placing a wire in the suspicious area as a guide for the surgeon. The surgeon is then able to excise only the lesion and surrounding margins rather than a larger area of the breast. Once excised, the wire with the specimen radiograph confirms that the correct area was removed.[1]

42. **(D)** The FNB is the least invasive and the most cost-effective. It removes cell samples which can be easily contaminated by serous fluid or blood. It is recommended that a cytotechnologist confirms accuracy of the sample before the patient leaves the department. The other techniques remove tissue, core samples, for histological analysis.[1]

43. **(B)** Cosmetic intervention is selective treatment requested by the patient for a variety of reasons. Treatment can be augmentation or reduction. Required treatment due to medical problems or breast cancer is not considered cosmetic intervention.[5]

44. **(A)** Chemotherapy is an adjuvant therapy and involves the use of drugs to treat cancer that may have spread beyond the breast. The drug is distributed throughout the entire body via the blood stream and tends to attack cells that are rapidly dividing, whether they are cancerous or not. Side effects of chemotherapy will vary depending on the strength and type of the drugs used, the dosage and the duration of treatment.[2,5]

45. **(C)** Breast cancer is staged according to tumor size, lymph node status, and the presence or absence of distant metastases. Other considerations before treatment include estrogen-receptor and progesterone-receptor levels in the tumor tissue, human epidermal growth factor receptor 2 (*HER2/neu*) status, menopausal status, and the general health of the patient.[6]

Stage	
O	Carcinoma in situ
IA	Tumor ≤ 2 cm; axillary node negative
IB	Tumor ≤ 2 cm; axillary node negative With cancer cell in lymph node ≤ 2 cm
IIA	Tumor 2-5 cm with 1-3 positive nodes or tumor > 5 cm without positive lymph nodes
IIB	Tumor 2-5 cm with positive nodes 0.2-2 mm
IIIA	Tumor > 5 cm or no tumor with 1-3 positive nodes or any size tumor with 4-9 positive nodes
IIIB	Any size tumor with cancer spread to chest wall and/or skin of breast and up to 9 lymph nodes
IIIC	Any size tumor with cancer spread to chest wall and/or skin of breast and up to 10 axillary or claviclar lymph nodes
IV	Cancer has spread to other organs, i.e., there is distant metastasis (e.g., to bone, lungs)

46. **(D)** Lumpectomy is only possible with small cancers and there are a number of critical considerations. Women with large cancers in small breasts will have poor cosmetic results or breast deformity. The type and stage of the cancer could be a contraindication for lumpectomy. Other contraindications can include: multifocal cancers located at multiply sites within a single duct; multicentric cancers located within multiple ducts; women who have already undergone radiation in the breast/chest area cannot have additional radiation treatment; women whose previous lumpectomy did not completely remove the cancer; women with

connective tissue diseases such as scleroderma, osteoarthritis, or rheumatoid arthritis, may have tissues that are sensitive to radiation; women who are pregnant, if radiation therapy is indicated.[1,2]

47. **(D)** Staging finds out how widespread the cancer is. Breast cancer is staged according to tumor size, lymph node status, and the presence or absence of distant metastases.[6]

48. **(C)** In breast cancer staging the cancer can be classified by the letters T, N, or M. A "T" grades the tumor size and spread to the skin or chest wall under the breast. It is graded from 0 to 4 with higher numbers indicating a larger or wider spread tumor. The letter N is graded from 0 to 3 and indicates cancer spread to the lymph nodes near the breast plus the number of lymph nodes affected. The letter M is graded from 0 to 1 and indicates cancer spread to distant organs.[6]

References

1. Peart O. Interventional procedures. In: *Mammography and Breast Imaging: Prep*. New York, NY: McGraw-Hill; 2012:363-396.
2. Venes D, Biderman A, Adler E. *Taber's Cyclopedic Medical Dictionary*. 21st ed. Philadelphia, PA: F.A. Davis; 2005:1-2518.
3. Peart O. Breast imaging emerging modalities. In: *Mammography and Breast Imaging: Prep*. New York, NY: McGraw-Hill; 2012:333-262.
4. Fostbinder R, Orth D. Magnetic resonance imaging. In: *Essentials of Radiologic Science*. Philadelphia, PA: Lippincott Williams & Wilkins; 2012:271-285.
5. Peart O. Treatment options. In: *Mammography and Breast Imaging: Prep*. New York, NY: McGraw-Hill; 2012:397-432.
6. American Cancer Society. How is breast cancer staged? http://www.cancer.org/cancer/breast-cancer/detailedguide/breast-cancer-staging. Last Reviewed 1/31/14. Accessed March 25, 2014.
7. American Cancer Society: Early Detection, Diagnosis, and Staging. Can breast cancer be found early? http://www.cancer.org/cancer/breastcancer/detailedguide/breast-cancer-detection. Last Review 01/31/2014. Accessed March 14, 2014.
8. Tortora GJ, Derrickson B. The reproductive systems. In: *Principles of Anatomy and Physiology*. 12th ed. New York, NY: John Wiley & Sons; 2009:1110-1112.
9. ACS-Types of breast reconstruction. http://www.cancer.org/cancer/breastcancer/moreinformation/breastreconstructionaftermastectomy/breast-reconstruction-after-mastectomy-types-of-br-recon.
10. Papp J. Mammography quality standards. In: *Quality Management in the Imaging Sciences*. 3rd ed. St. Louis, MO: Mosby; 2006:195-229.
11. http://www.fda.gov/Radiation-EmittingProducts/MammographyQualityStandardsActandProgram/Guidance/PolicyGuidanceHelpSystem/default.htm#Quality. Last Update March 20, 2013. Accessed March 22, 2014.

CHAPTER 6

Practice Test 1

Questions

1. Radiation therapy is a treatment that utilizes
   (A) drugs to treat cancer that may have spread
   (B) high-energy radiation to destroy cancer cells
   (C) radioactive tracers to track the path of cancer to the lymph nodes
   (D) potent pain medication to treat the severe pain from cancer

2. Between ages 20 and 30 an asymptomatic woman should be having a mammogram every
   (A) year
   (B) 2 years
   (C) 3 years
   (D) none of the above

3. Medical history may include questions on hormone use because
   (A) synthetic hormones such as hormone replacement therapy (HRT) will always cause breast cancer
   (B) the use of reproductive hormones can increase risk factors for breast cancer
   (C) family history of hormone use predisposes a woman to cancer
   (D) personal history of hormone use decreases a woman's risk for breast cancer

4. In imaging implants some of the projections taken will include an image of the implant. In these projections the compression is used
   (A) to allow a uniform density
   (B) for immobilization only
   (C) to separate the breast tissue
   (D) to separate and spread out the implant

5. The glandular dose is a measure of
   (A) the radiation dose to the skin of the breast
   (B) the dose to the radiosensitive cells of the breast
   (C) the significant background dose recorded in United States
   (D) the radiation dose to the gonads

6. Which of the following is true of screen-film systems?
   (A) Screen-film systems have a higher spatial resolution than digital systems.
   (B) Screen-film systems have a wide latitude and dynamic range than digital systems.
   (C) When compared to a digital system screen-film systems help to increase workflow.
   (D) Screen-film systems typically result in less repeats due to exposure errors when compared to digital systems.

7. In digital imaging, a graph of the density range to the log of relative exposure is a
   (A) shallow sloping curve
   (B) steep sloping curve
   (C) linear response
   (D) curvilinear response

8. In the American College of Radiology (ACR)-approved accreditation phantom, the total number of fibers, speck groups, and masses are
   (A) 5 fibers, 5 speck groups, and 5 masses
   (B) 5 fibers, 6 speck groups, and 5 masses
   (C) 6 fibers, 5 speck groups, and 5 masses
   (D) 5 fibers, 5 speck groups, and 6 masses

9. The circular pigmented area around the nipple is called the
   (A) skin
   (B) areola
   (C) Montgomery gland
   (D) ampulla

10. A keratosis is demonstrated mammographically as a
   (A) sharply outlined multilobulated lesion
   (B) sharply outlined lesion with a halo
   (C) mixed-density circular lesion with a radiolucent center
   (D) mixed-density oval lesion

11. Figure 6-1 indicates
   (A) mammographically benign calcifications
   (B) malignant calcifications
   (C) keratosis
   (D) fibroadenomas

12. The advantages of a quality assurance program such as the MQSA includes all of the following *except*
   (A) increased efficiency
   (B) cost-effectiveness
   (C) allows manipulation of the final image
   (D) improved patient satisfaction

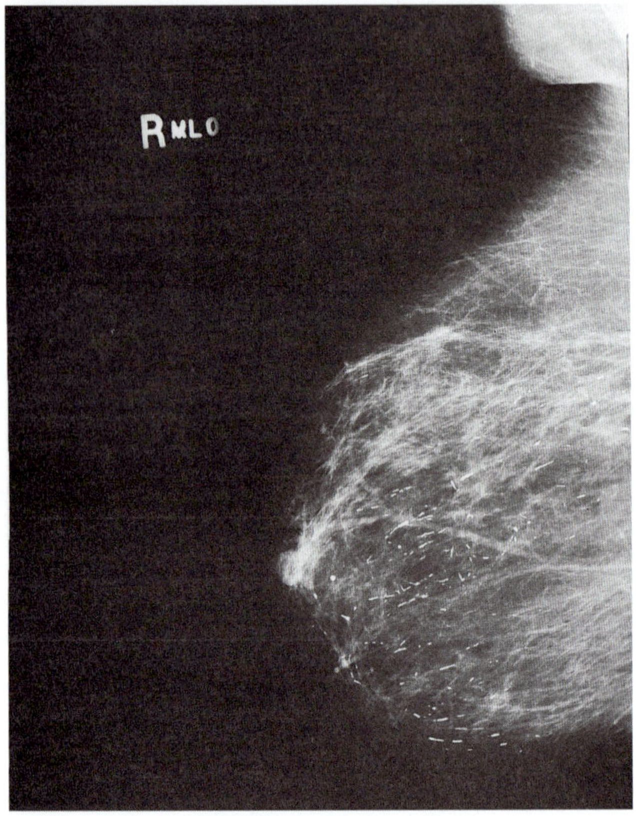

Figure 6-1.

13. In magnification, what immediate role does the large object-to-image receptor distance (OID) play in reducing scattered radiation?
   (A) It allows the use of lower peak kilovoltage (kVp) values.
   (B) There is increased SOD which allows for absorption of the scattered radiation.
   (C) Most of the scattered radiation misses the detector.
   (D) The larger OID utilizes a smaller SID.

14. Using a small focal-spot size is recommended for magnification
   (A) to reduce the resultant loss of image detail
   (B) because of increased patient dose
   (C) to compensate for the small OID
   (D) to compensate long exposure times

15. What is the best placement for the needle wire during needle localization?
    (A) The needle wire should pass immediately below the lesion.
    (B) The needle wire should pass immediately above the lesion.
    (C) The needle wire should pass through the lesion.
    (D) The needle wire should pass immediately beside the lesion.

16. Although it may mean losing some of the lateral breast tissue, in imaging for the craniocaudal (CC) projection, most experts agree that all efforts should be made to maximize imaging of the medial breast tissue. Why?
    (A) Medial breast is imaged best on the CC.
    (B) Medial breast is imaged only on the CC.
    (C) Most cancers are found in the medial breast.
    (D) The lateral breast is generally distorted on the CC.

17. Which is true when positioning for all tangential (TAN) projections?
    (A) The patient is always in the CC position.
    (B) The central ray is always directed vertically.
    (C) The central ray is always parallel to the plane of the breast.
    (D) The central ray is always parallel to the skin surface.

18. In the rolled medial (RM) position, the inferior (lower) surface of the breast is rolled in which direction?
    (A) laterally
    (B) medially
    (C) inferiorly
    (D) superiorly

19. A radiopaque implant that is used in breast reconstruction and can be adjusted for cup size after surgical placement in the breast is the
    (A) silicone gel implant
    (B) flap implant
    (C) silicone liquid implant
    (D) saline implant

20. In addition to the routine CC and mediolateral oblique (MLO), a routine series for a postmastectomy patient could also include the
    (A) axillary tail (AT)
    (B) ML
    (C) TAN
    (D) lateromedial oblique (LMO)

21. Men with a family history of breast cancer will
    (A) have a greater risk for breast cancer
    (B) have a minor risk for breast cancer
    (C) have no significantly increased risk for breast cancer
    (D) always get breast cancer

22. The clinical breast examination (CBE) should be performed
    (A) at or near the time of the annual mammogram
    (B) only by the radiologist
    (C) monthly, preferably at the same time of the month
    (D) at least twice a year

23. The absorbed dose in mammography is generally _______ the entrance skin exposure (ESE).
    (A) significantly higher than
    (B) significantly lower than
    (C) about the same as
    (D) slighter higher than

24. In the compression test required by The Mammography Quality Standards Act (MQSA), the maximum compression for the initial power drive should not exceed

(A) 100 N
(B) 200 N
(C) 400 N
(D) 500 N

25. Collimation should not extend beyond any edge of the detector by more than

(A) 1% of the SID
(B) 2% of the SID
(C) 3% of the SID
(D) 4% of the SID

26. Inherent filtration will include filtration by all of the following *except*

(A) exit port of the tube
(B) compression paddle
(C) molybdenum filters
(D) mirror assembly

27. The MQSA standards were enacted

(A) because mammography was overregulated
(B) to address the inconsistent quality mammograms that were available
(C) to enforce continuing education for radiologic technologist
(D) to enforce continuing education for radiologist

28. Grids in mammography are utilized

(A) during normal imaging
(B) during magnification imaging only
(C) only if requested by the radiologist
(D) to reduce radiation dose to the patient

29. Breast tissue can extend medially to the

(A) latissimus dorsi muscle
(B) midsternum
(C) retromammary space
(D) inframammary crease

30. Which of the following hormones has the most influence on the normal physiological changes of the breast?

(A) estrogen and prolactin
(B) estrogen and progesterone
(C) prolactin and estrogen
(D) progesterone and prolactin

31. Which of the following is (are) considered a first-degree relative?

(A) mother and aunt
(B) first cousin and mother
(C) aunt and sister
(D) sister and mother

32. A woman should perform breast self-examination (BSE) monthly to

(A) become familiar with both of her breasts
(B) excise cancerous lumps
(C) determine skin versus breast tissue calcifications
(D) monitor nipple discharge

33. The breast of a woman below age 35 is

(A) not related to radiation sensitivity
(B) less sensitive to radiation
(C) less sensitive to low-dose radiation
(D) more sensitive to radiation

34. In the low kVp range using a molybdenum target tube, what type of photon interaction predominates?

(A) photoelectric
(B) Compton
(C) Bremsstrahlung
(D) coherent

35. In digital imaging a repeat analysis test is

(A) unnecessary—digital imaging automatically corrects exposure mistakes
(B) necessary—digital imaging cannot correct for overexposure
(C) unnecessary—digital imaging corrects unsharpness by altering the spatial display
(D) necessary—digital imaging cannot correct factors such as motion unsharpness

36. The same mammographer should view the phantom images because

(A) subjective judgment about images is always difficult
(B) it is not wise to have different individuals handling the phantom
(C) not all mammographers know the MQSA regulations
(D) given set values, different mammographers will calculate the densities differently

37. The from below (FB) projection utilizes a beam directed

(A) perpendicular to the detector
(B) horizontally
(C) tangentially
(D) parallel to the detector

38. Changes in the breast due to radiation therapy include

(A) erythema
(B) edema
(C) hardening
(D) all of the above

39. Scanning the breast to locate a cancer based on the vast amount of glucose/sugar utilized by cancer cells is the technique used in

(A) scintigraphy
(B) PEM imaging
(C) MRI
(D) lymphoscintigraphy

40. Which of the following projections could be used to replace the MLO in patients where the MLO is not possible?

(A) ML
(B) LM
(C) RL
(D) AT

41. Which of the following does *not* describe mammography filtration?

(A) It shapes the emerging beam by absorbing low-energy x-rays that would only be absorbed by the superficial tissue and contribute to patient dose.
(B) It will affect the HVL of the emerging x-ray beam.
(C) Filtration makes the emerging beam compatible with the breast characteristics.
(D) The filtration used in mammography imaging is never aluminum.

42. The best time for a woman to perform a BSE is

(A) before the start of menstruation
(B) immediately, at the start of menstruation
(C) within 5-10 days after the start of menstruation
(D) anytime

43. Evaluations such as the mammography equipment evaluation (MEE) is performed by the

(A) radiologic assistant
(B) mammographer
(C) medical physicist
(D) radiologist

44. The test pattern used to measure the resolution of a digital system

(A) SNR
(B) SMPTE
(C) CNR
(D) MTF

45. Which of the following tests are performed monthly?

    (A) phantom images
    (B) repeat/reject analysis
    (C) compression check
    (D) visual checklist

46. On a reject/repeat analysis, the rate was lower than 5% but one category of the reject/repeat analysis is significantly higher than others. What should be done?

    (A) Although the rate is below 5%, that one area should be targeted for improvement.
    (B) If the other categories are within normal limits, that area can be disregarded.
    (C) Because the rate was more than 2%, the entire department needs to be reassessed.
    (D) With an overall rate lower than 5%, one high rate is statistically meaningless.

47. Typically, grid ratios in mammography range from

    (A) 7:1 to 8:1
    (B) 6:1 to 7:1
    (C) 4:1 to 6:1
    (D) 3:1 to 5:1

48. Positron emission tomography/mammography (PET or PEM) imaging is useful in staging tumors because

    (A) the positron emitting isotopes are radioactive
    (B) PET or PEM imaging can display the extent and location of the tumor
    (C) the positron emitting isotopes will destroy the tumor bed
    (D) PET or PEM imaging tracks the increased blood flow from the cancerous tumor

49. Medical history is important in

    (A) assessing risk factors for breast cancer
    (B) preventing breast cancer
    (C) evaluating treatment options
    (D) more than 1 of the above

50. Unlike general radiography x-ray tubes, some mammography tubes are tilted 6-24 degrees from the horizontal. The effect of this is to

    (A) allow the use of smaller focal-spot size
    (B) minimize the heel effect
    (C) increase resolution
    (D) all of the above

51. The retromammary space describes the area

    (A) between the breast and pectoral muscle
    (B) separating the skin of the breast from the deep fascia
    (C) separating the skin from the superficial fascia
    (D) between the glandular tissue and the inframammary fold

52. In which of the following are breast cysts least common?

    (A) young women in their early 20s
    (B) premenopausal woman
    (C) postmenopausal woman on estrogen therapy
    (D) women aged 70

53. The CC shows a circumscribed oval radiolucent lesion. There was a definite halo surrounding the lesion. It is most likely to be a

    (A) fibroadenoma
    (B) galactocele
    (C) cyst
    (D) hematoma

54. The indirect effect of breast compression on Compton interaction is

    (A) The absolute number of Compton interactions increases.
    (B) The absolute number of Compton interactions decreases.
    (C) Compression has no affect on Compton interactions.
    (D) Compression affects Compton interaction only above 70 kVp.

55. Visual inspection done during CBE involves

(A) feeling for changes in the breast
(B) looking for changes in the breast
(C) palpating the breast
(D) examining areas under the armpit

56. Grids with strips that are linear, but slanted to match the divergence of the x-ray beam are _____ grids.

(A) parallel
(B) crossed
(C) focused
(D) moving

57. Fatty tissue is generally radiolucent and will show on the mammogram as

(A) glandular areas
(B) high-optical density areas
(C) low-optical density areas
(D) white or gray areas

58. The mammogram of a woman age 50 who has recently started estrogen replacement therapy is likely to show a breast that is

(A) more fibroglandular than her past mammographic study
(B) more fatty than her previous mammogram
(C) less fibrous and less glandular than her previous studies
(D) unchanged from her previous mammograms

59. The mammogram shows an oval-shaped lesion with mixed density. The lesion has a central radiolucent area and is freely movable. This lesion is most likely to be a

(A) fibroadenoma
(B) hematoma
(C) lymph node
(D) galactocele

60. The method of locating the lymph node/s through which cancer is leaving the breast is called

(A) scintigraphy
(B) PEM imaging
(C) MRI
(D) lymphoscintigraphy

61. The change in OID could cause loss of image detail in magnification mammography. What factor/s helps to compensate for this loss of image detail?

(A) decreased OID and breast compression
(B) increased focal-spot size and breast compression
(C) decreased focal-spot size and compression of the part
(D) increased OID and compression of the part

62. What does the actual focal-spot size measure?

(A) the area on the anode exposed to electrons
(B) the area projected on the patient
(C) the area projected on the detector
(D) the nominal focal-spot size

63. The mammography report has an assessment finding of breast imaging reporting and data system (BIRAD) 0. This means that

(A) the mammogram is negative
(B) there is a high probability of a benign finding
(C) additional imaging is needed
(D) the findings are suspicious

64. Differentiate between repeat and reject images.

(A) Repeat is the percentage of repeats from a specific cause. Reject is the percentage of repeats from multiple causes.
(B) Rejects are all images that are discarded. Repeat are images that resulted in extra radiation dose to the patient.
(C) Repeats are all images that are discarded. Rejects are images that resulted in extra radiation dose to the patient.
(D) Rejects are images discarded after any QC testing. Repeats are any images thrown out.

65. What is epithelial hyperplasia?
   (A) a calcified hematoma resulting from trauma
   (B) an oil cyst within the breast
   (C) an overgrowth of cells in the ducts or lobules
   (D) an epidermoid cyst on the skin of the breast

66. Figure 6-2 shows a (an)
   (A) ruptured implant
   (B) encapsulated implant
   (C) herniated implant
   (D) implant removal

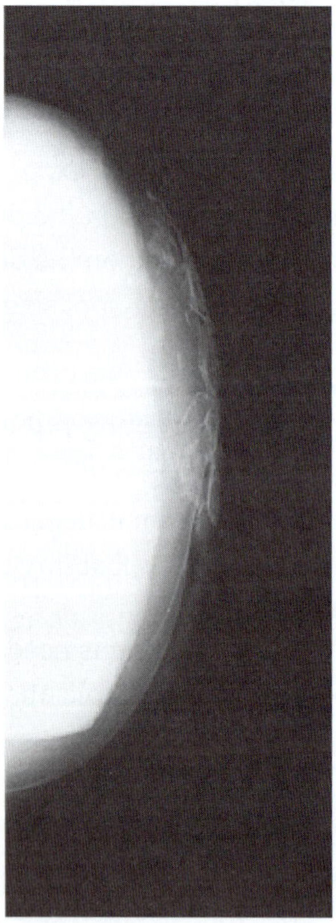

Figure 6-2. (Reproduced with permission from Peart O: Lange Q&A: Mammography Examination, 2nd ed. New York, NY: McGraw-Hill Education; 2008.)

67. After a 4-projection mammogram, calcifications are visualized superior to the nipple but only on the MLO projection. What additional projection would best be used to locate the position of the lesion?
   (A) exaggerated craniocaudal (XCCL)
   (B) cleavage (CV)
   (C) ML
   (D) AT

68. Approximately how much contrast agent is injected into the breast during ductography?
   (A) approximately 1 cc
   (B) 15-25 cc
   (C) 30-40 cc
   (D) approximately 50 cc

69. What does the glandular dose measure?
   (A) the average dose to the patient's skin
   (B) the absorbed dose to the skin
   (C) the absorbed dose at the tissue level
   (D) the same as the entrance skin dose

70. Which of the following relationships does *not* change when moving from routine to magnification mammography?
   (A) OID
   (B) focal spot size
   (C) SID
   (D) SOD

71. Who performs the compression device check for mammography QC?
   (A) physicist
   (B) any staff technologist
   (C) radiologist
   (D) mammographer

72. A galactocele is
   (A) a lesion associated with trauma to the breast
   (B) a benign milk-filled cyst
   (C) associated with eggshell-like calcification
   (D) associated with a central radiolucent hilus

73. Instead of using a grid, what does magnification mammography use to reduce scatter during normal imaging?

(A) lead shielding
(B) increased OID
(C) a low milliamperes (mAs) technique
(D) increased SID

74. Most of the glandular tissue is arranged in the breast around the

(A) medial and upper-inner quadrants
(B) lateral and lower inner quadrants
(C) central and upper-outer quadrants
(D) medial and upper-outer quadrants

75. A beryllium (Be) window on the x-ray tube enhances contrast by

(A) increasing the output of the x-ray tube
(B) reducing production of scattered radiation
(C) transmitting more low-energy photons
(D) transmitting more high-energy photons

76. Proper compression of the breast is indicated when the

(A) patient is in pain
(B) compression paddle stops
(C) breast is taut
(D) breast feels soft

77. Which factors cause increased skin dose in magnification?

(A) larger OID and smaller focal spot size
(B) increased mA and larger SOD
(C) increased OID and decreased SOD
(D) smaller OID and larger SID

78. In radiology, according to the line-focus principle, the effective focal spot is

(A) larger than the actual focal spot
(B) smaller than the actual focal spot
(C) the same as the actual focal spot
(D) decreased as the target angle increases

79. Figures 6-3A and 6-3B are mammograms of the same patient. Figure 6-3B was taken 6 months after Figure 6-3A. These mammograms have the characteristic appearance of a

(A) resolving oil cyst
(B) galactocele
(C) resolving postsurgical scar
(D) hematoma

80. When using the air-gap technique in magnification mammography what additional step is necessary?

(A) grid use
(B) decrease SID
(C) increase OID
(D) increase SID

81. Which of the following projections would best separate superimposed 12-o'clock and 6-o'clock masses?

(A) MLO
(B) XCCL
(C) CC
(D) AT

82. In positioning terminology, CV means

(A) compressed position
(B) cranial view
(C) cleavage view
(D) compression view

83. Malignant casting-type calcifications can appear on the mammogram as

(A) granulated sugar or crushed stone calcifications
(B) eggshell-like calcifications
(C) elongated, branching, and needle-like calcifications
(D) fragmented, linear branching calcifications

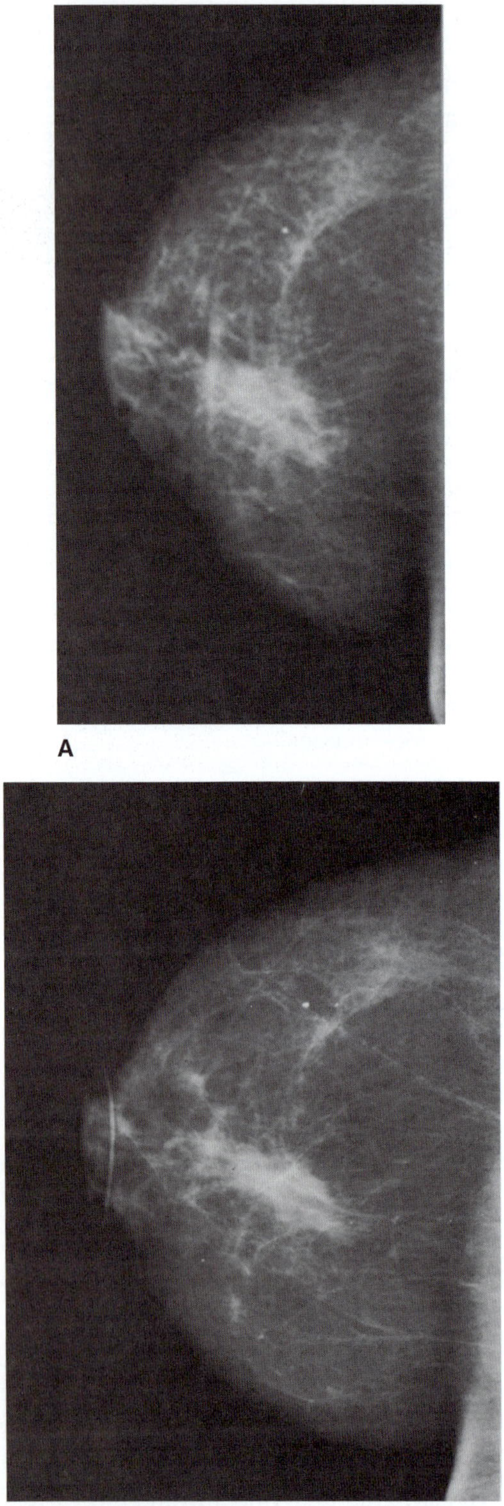

A

B

Figure 6-3. (Reproduced with permission from Peart O: Lange Q&A: Mammography Examination, 2nd ed. New York, NY: McGraw-Hill Education; 2008.)

84. The functional milk-producing units of the breast are contained within the
    (A) lactiferous sinuses
    (B) lobules
    (C) ampulla
    (D) areola

85. What is the grid ratio?
    (A) the height of the lead strips divided by the distance between each strip
    (B) the height of the lead strips multiplied by the distance between each strip
    (C) twice the height of each lead strip
    (D) the distance between each strip divided by the height

86. The AT projection best demonstrates the
    (A) subareolar area
    (B) medial aspect of the breast
    (C) axillary aspect of the breast
    (D) lower-inner quadrant of the breast

87. The lesion seen on Figure 6-4 has the characteristic appearance of a/an
    (A) oil cyst
    (B) stellate lesion
    (C) galactocele, calcified
    (D) fibroadenoma

88. The patient had trauma to the breast 1 month ago and has developed a lump. Such an injury may show mammographically as a
    (A) galactocele
    (B) hematoma
    (C) lymph node
    (D) fibroadenoma

89. A device used to convert light to a digital signal is a/an
    (A) film digitizer
    (B) DICOM
    (C) ADC
    (D) DAC

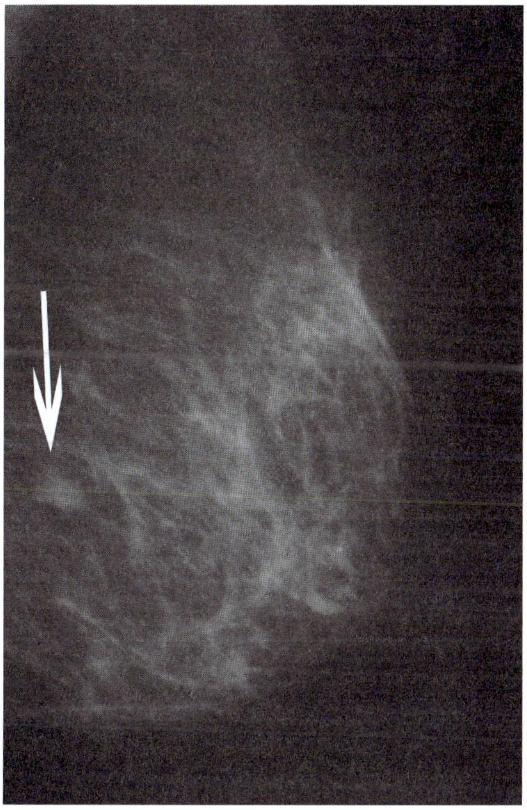

Figure 6-4.

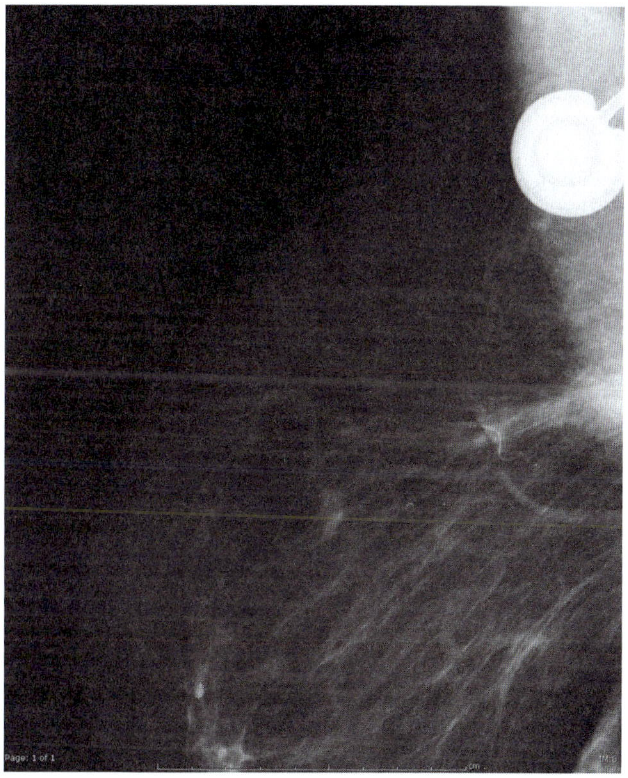

Figure 6-5. (Reproduced with permission from Peart O: Lange Q&A: Mammography Examination, 2nd ed. New York, NY: McGraw-Hill Education; 2008.)

90. If too much upper axilla and shoulder are under the compression paddle when imaging for the MLO, the effect is to

    (A) inhibit proper compression of the upper breast
    (B) inhibit proper compression of the lower breast
    (C) ensure equal compression of the upper and lower breast
    (D) ensure proper compression of the lower breast

91. Which of the following types of breast imaging methods will fall under the category of nuclear imaging?

    (A) PEM
    (B) MRI
    (C) ultrasound
    (D) digital tomosynthesis

92. The area of low optical density in the upper part of Figure 6-5 best represents

    (A) a pacemaker
    (B) the patient's chin
    (C) a hematoma
    (D) port-a-cath

93. A rolled projection can be performed to

    (A) separate superimposed tissues
    (B) identify microcalcifications
    (C) localize a skin lesion
    (D) determine the location of a finding seen only on 1 of the standard projection

94. Ideally, in an open surgical biopsy, when should a breast tissue specimen be imaged?

    (A) immediately after surgery
    (B) within 24 hours of the surgery
    (C) just prior to the surgery
    (D) after the lesion is removed but before the surgical site is closed

95. Which projection gives a mirror image of the MLO?

(A) ML
(B) LM
(C) LMO
(D) AT

96. The nominal focal spot size of the mammography unit is 0.3. This means that the

(A) actual focal spot size is 0.3
(B) effective focal spot size is 0.3
(C) both effective and actual focal spot size is 0.3
(D) actual focal spot is smaller than 0.3

97. Women with postlumpectomy could have magnified images taken of the tumor bed to

(A) confirm the removal of the cancer
(B) check calcium deposits that may result from radiation and surgical changes
(C) all of the above
(D) none of the above

98. Figure 6-6 shows a routine screening mammogram, CC projection. What projection could best image the missed area?

(A) XCCL
(B) CV
(C) ML
(D) AT

99. Where is the grid placed?

(A) above the breast
(B) between the breast and the image plate or detector
(C) below the image plate
(D) between the breast and the x-ray tube

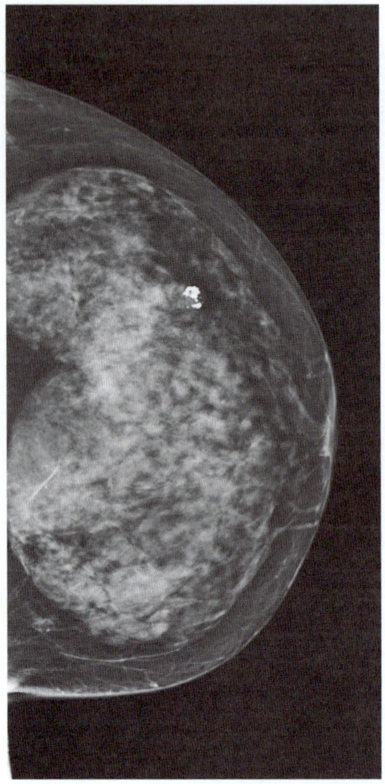

Figure 6-6.

100. All of the following statements are unique to the PSP, CM systems and are not present in flat panel detector FFDM systems *except*

(A) IP can be damaged or dropped during transport
(B) the system has a wide latitude and dynamic range
(C) low exposure can create a noisy image
(D) the imaging system is susceptible to scratches

101. The purpose of the mammography certification and accreditation process is to

(A) provide legal mammography services
(B) enforce minimum national quality standards for mammography
(C) ensure that all women have access to a certified mammography facility
(D) authorize certain states to certify mammography facilities and conduct inspections

102. A facility has a sign posted advising patients to contact a designated person within the organization with comments. This facility is meeting the US Food and Drug Administration (FDA)'s

(A) medical outcome audit program
(B) record-keeping program
(C) patient communication of results program
(D) customer complaint program

103. A hamartoma is

(A) a malignant tumor of the breast
(B) a benign tumor of the breast
(C) associated with trauma of the breast
(D) associated with nursing

104. During lactation the contraction of which cells help to eject milk from the alveoli?

(A) epithelial cells
(B) myoepithelial cells
(C) basement cells
(D) superficial cells

105. A finding of BIRAD 2 on the mammogram means that the mammogram

(A) cannot accurately evaluate the breast
(B) showed benign findings
(C) showed suspicious findings
(D) is suggestive for malignancy

106. Erythema of the breast is an indication

(A) of inflammatory breast cancer
(B) of a breast abscess
(C) of a breast infection
(D) that further testing of the breast is necessary

107. Which of the following is used as a treatment for estrogen-dependent tumors in postmenopausal and premenopausal women?

(A) radiation therapy
(B) chemotherapy
(C) Tamoxifen
(D) antibody therapy

108. In flat-panel detector systems, the spatial resolution of the system is controlled by the

(A) pixel number
(B) DEL size
(C) matrix size
(D) TFT number

109. A thin supportive layer located between the basal surface of the epithelium and the connective tissue layer of the lobule is called

(A) chief cells
(B) myoepithelial
(C) basement membrane
(D) superficial A cells

110. A "camel's nose" breast contour can be prevented in the MLO projection by

(A) including all of the breast under the compression paddle
(B) angling the detector parallel to the pectoralis muscle
(C) properly supporting the anterior breast during compression
(D) ensuring that the nipple remains in profile during compression

111. The superoinferior oblique (SIO) will best demonstrate the

(A) OUQ and the LOQ of the breast
(B) LIQ and the UIQ of the breast
(C) UIQ and LOQ of the breast
(D) LIQ and the OUQ of the breast

112. The basic premise of a medical audit is that

1. all positive mammograms should be followed
2. the pathology results of all biopsies performed should be collected
3. all pathology results should be correlated with the radiologist's findings

(A) 1 and 2 only
(B) 2 and 3 only
(C) 1 and 3 only
(D) 1, 2, and 3

113. Under the MQSA, how long are facilities required to maintain the records of a patient who died shortly after her first mammogram?

(A) 5 years
(B) 10 years
(C) 20 years
(D) permanently

114. Under which of the following circumstances would the triangulation technique be necessary?

(A) to locate an abnormality visualized on 1 projection only
(B) during routine mammography screening
(C) when performing spot magnification
(D) to locate a palpable lesion

115. A dimpled skin condition seen in cases of lymphatic edema of the breast is called

(A) inflammatory carcinoma
(B) ductal ectasia
(C) plasma cell mastitis
(D) peau d'orange

Answer and Explanations

1. **(B)** Many women are choosing conservation therapy that removes the tumor with wide margins (lumpectomy, quadrectomy, or segmental mastectomy) and includes radiation therapy. Treatment starts 3-8 weeks after surgery and includes about 5-6 weeks of daily treatments. Nuclear medicine uses radioactive tracers (also called radioactive isotopes or radiopharmaceuticals). Drugs can be hormonal therapy (estrogen therapy) such as Tamoxifen or chemotherapy.[1,2]

2. **(D)** An annual mammogram is generally recommended for asymptomatic women above age 40 who have not been identified as having significantly higher risk. The mammogram is not an effective screening tool for younger women.[3]

3. **(B)** Studies have suggested that synthetic hormones such as hormone replacement therapy (HRT) or reproductive hormones influence breast cancer risk as well as promote cancer growth. Early menarche (less than 12 years), late menopause (equal to or more than 55 years), oral contraceptive use, and fewer pregnancies will all increase a woman's risk by affecting estrogen levels in the body. Hormones or hormone use, however, are not known to always cause breast cancer and the use of hormones by another family member will not increase a woman's breast cancer risks.[3]

4. **(B)** When imaging implants, the standard projections are used for immobilization purposes only-full compression is not applied. The implant is then displaced and 4 additional compression projections are taken. The result is an 8-projection series (Figure 6-7).[4,5]

5. **(B)** Radiation dose is often the calculation of the entrance skin exposure (ESE) which is the dose received at the skin. However, in mammography the glandular dose, which is a record of the dose to the glandular and more radiosensitive cells and tissues of the breast is considered more significant. The American College of Radiology (ACR) recommends a glandular dose of 3 mGy (0.3 rad) with a grid and 1 mGy (0.1 rad) without a grid.[6,7]

6. **(A)** Screen-film systems have a higher spatial resolution when compared to digital systems. However, digital can manipulate the pixel value after the exposure which compensates for the lower spatial resolution by giving the appearance of a higher contrast resolution. Contrast resolution is the ability to distinguish anatomic structures with similar subject contrast. High-contrast resolution is needed in mammography to distinguish similar soft-tissue densities. All digital systems have high contrast resolution and a wider latitude and dynamic range than screen-film systems. Screen-film systems do not allow manipulation of the image after the exposure. This is a function of digital systems which helps to increase workflow and allows less repeats due to exposure errors.[6,7]

7. **(C)** Digital imaging systems have a linear response to x-ray intensity (Figure 6-8). This means that regardless of the intensity of the x-ray beam, a small change in the intensity is recorded as the same change in the electronic image. In digital imaging, this is possible because there are different devices for acquisition and display, and each can be separately optimized. Digital imaging therefore has a much wider latitude than analog imaging.

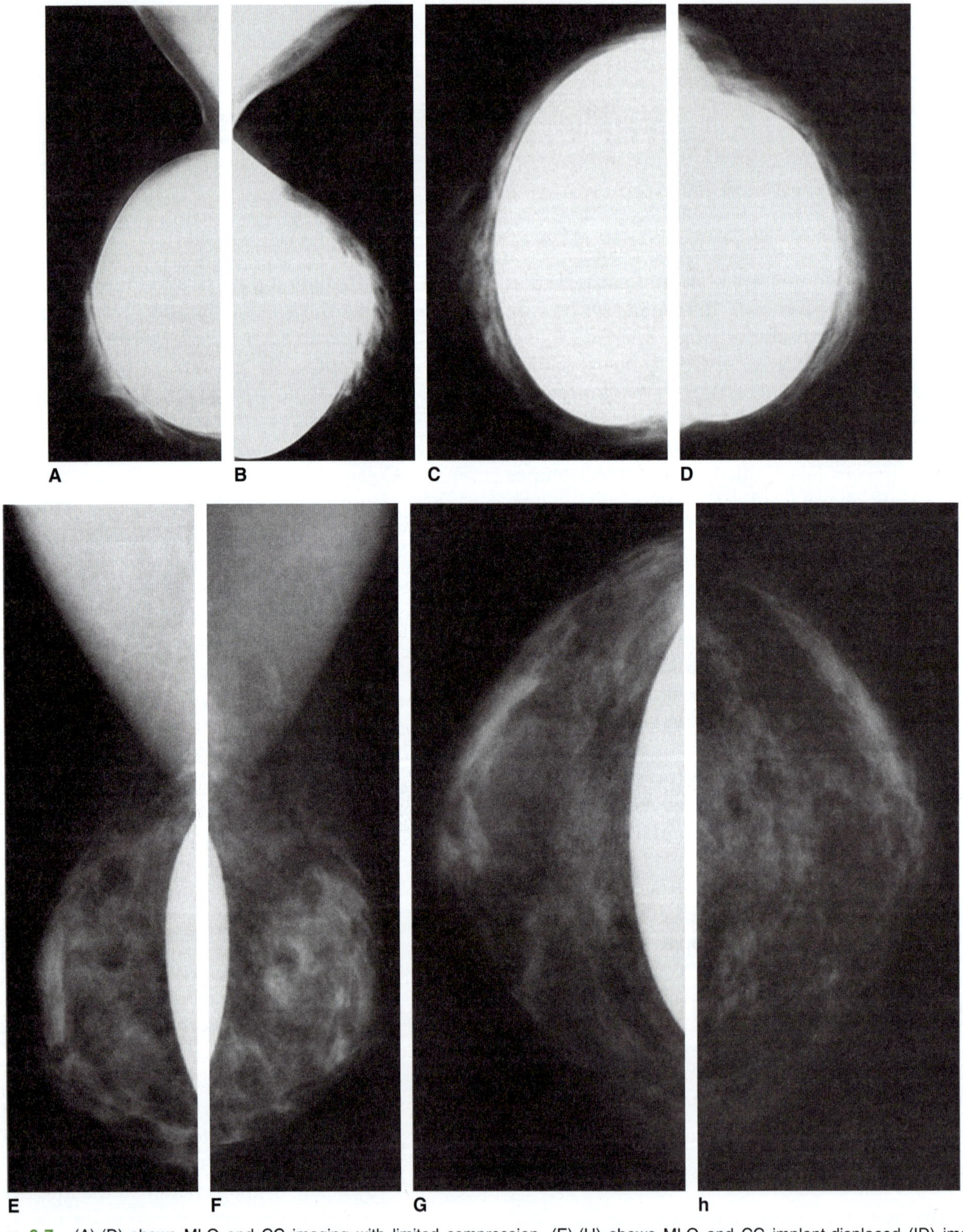

Figure 6-7. (A)-(D) shows MLO and CC imaging with limited compression. (E)-(H) shows MLO and CC implant-displaced (ID) images. (Reproduced with permission from Peart O: Mammography and Breast Imaging PREP: Program Review and Exam Prep. New York, NY: McGraw-Hill Education; 2012.)

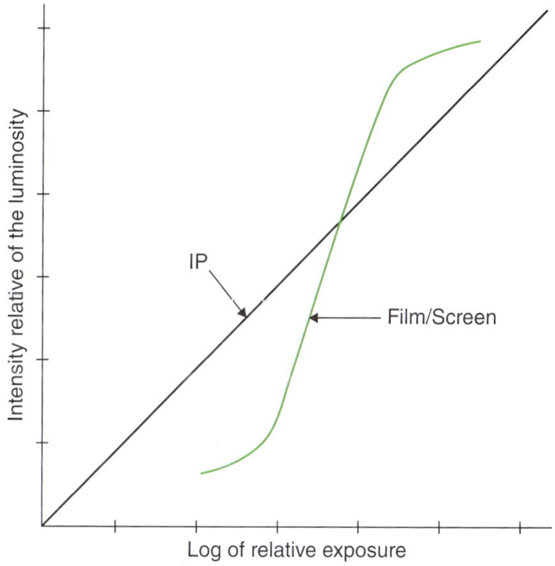

Figure 6-8. Characteristic curve for digital imaging. A graph of the optical density signal and the relative exposure for a digital imaging detector will have a linear response to x-ray. This is unlike the curvilinear response of a screen-film system. (Reproduced with permission from Peart O: Lange Q&A: Mammography Examination, 2nd ed. New York, NY: McGraw-Hill Education; 2008.)

Digital imaging can enhance the contrast resolution of the final image.[8,9]

8. **(C)** Six, five, and five represents the total number of fibers, specks, and masses in each group, but the criteria for the number of objects to meet accreditation requirements are a minimum number of 4 fibers, 3 speck groups, and 3 masses (Figure 6-9). Some digital units require

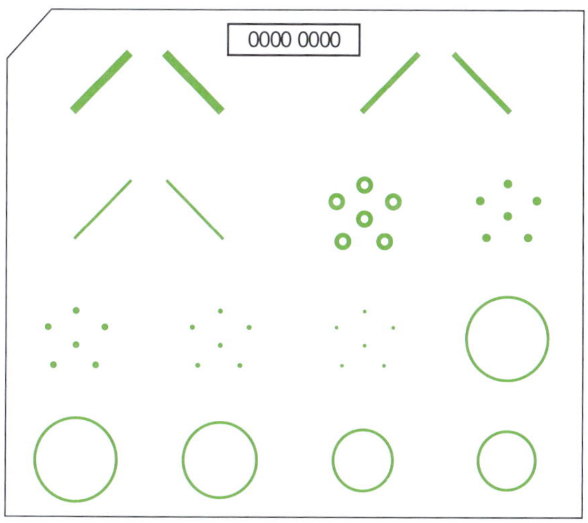

Figure 6-9. Schematic diagram of the phantom showing the relative position of the different objects embedded within the phantom. (Reproduced with permission from Peart O: Lange Q&A: Mammography Examination, 2nd ed. New York, NY: McGraw-Hill Education; 2008.)

5 fibers, 4 speck groups, and 4 masses. When scoring, each fiber, speck group, or mass is counted as 1 point. Partial fibers, speck groups, or masses are counted as 0.5 point or not at all.[9,10]

9. **(B)** The areola is the smooth, darkened area that surrounds the nipple. Skin covers the entire breast tissue, and the Montgomery glands are specialized sebaceous glands on the areola. The ampulla is another name for the lactiferous sinus, a part of the ductal system in the internal breast anatomy.[11,12]

10. **(A)** A keratosis forms on the skin surface of the breast. On the mammogram they are seen as multilobulated lesions with sharply outlined borders. An example of a mixed-density lesion with a radiolucent center is a lymph node. Other mixed-density circular or oval lesions are hematomas, galactoceles, or fibroadenolipomas. Halos are narrow radiolucent rings or ring segments typically seen around the periphery of benign circular or oval lesions. (See Figure 3-22.)[13,14,15]

11. **(A)** Plasma cell mastitis, periductal mastitis, or ductal ectasia is an inflammatory reaction characterized by the presence of plasma cells surrounding a dilated duct. It is a benign condition. Intraductal and/or periductal calcifications are the final results of this condition. The calcifications can be located around or inside the dilated ducts. Most are elongated and sharply outlined with smooth borders; some are needle-like with high density or may have a lucent central area. The fibroadenoma is an oval lesion that may contain calcifications. Keratosis rarely calcifies and mammographically appears as lobulated lesions. Mammographically malignant calcifications often appear in clusters. (See Figure 6-1.)[13,14,15]

12. **(C)** The MQSA is a quality assurance program that involves an overall management of actions needed to ensure the highest quality images and to enhance patient care. It includes regular quality control tests and the collection and evaluation of data. The benefits

of MQSA include: reduction of unnecessary radiation to patient by reducing repeats; improved overall efficiency of service; improved patient satisfaction; consistency of image production; cost-effectiveness. Image manipulation is an advantage of digital imaging systems.[6,7]

13. **(C)** In magnification, the large air gap acts like a grid and reduces scattered radiation, thus improving contrast. Positioning the breast away from the detector takes advantage of the inverse square law: the intensity of the scattered radiation is reduced because the distance between the detector and the object is increased. Mammography imaging uses a fixed source to image-receptor (SID) and it does not change in magnification. With increased object to image-receptor (OID) there is decreased source to object (SOD). However, that will affect the dose to the patient not reduce scatter. With the patient's breast closer to the radiation source there is increased skin dose although the glandular dose remains low. (Figure 6-10)[16,17]

14. **(A)** Magnification uses a large OID with a constant SID. To compensate for the distortion, a small focus spot size is used to allow fine-detail imaging. As the focal spot size decreases the sharpness of detail will increase. Grids are not used in magnification radiography because the large OID serves as an air gap to reduce scatter to the detector. (See Figure 6-10.)[17,18]

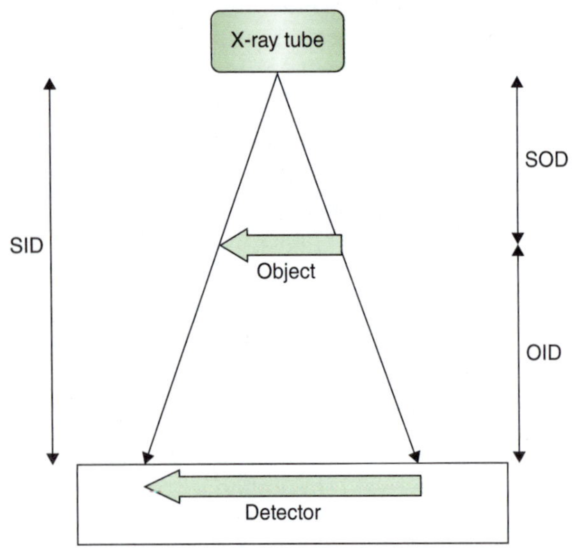

Figure 6-10. Schematic diagram of magnification setup.

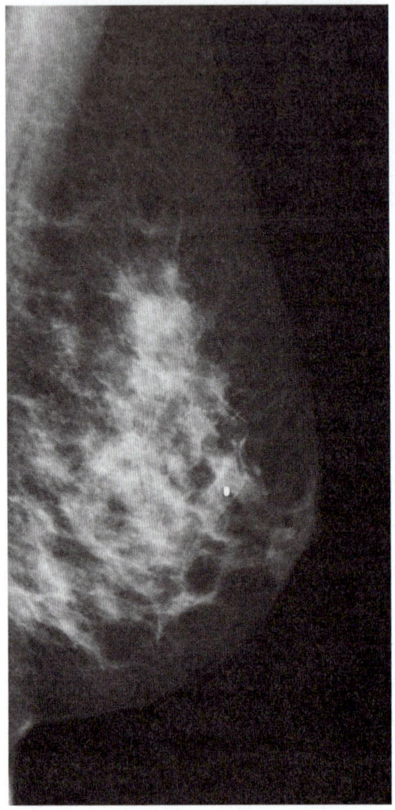

Figure 6-11. After a surgical biopsy, the surgeon may leave a radiopaque clip to indicate the site of the surgery.

15. **(C)** The localization needle wire should be positioned to pass just through the lesion. Most surgeons feel for the tip of the wire before making an incision in the patient's breast. Because the tip is being used as a locator, it should pass through the lesion, not above, below, or beside it (Figure 6-11).[19 20]

16. **(A)** Including the medial breast is very important when imaging the CC projection. The other routine projection, the MLO, will not image the medial breast clearly because it is an oblique projection and the medial tissue will be distorted. A cancer can develop anywhere in the breast but most often in the upper-outer quadrant. Additional projections that can be used to image the medial breast include the CV and the XCCM (Figure 6-12).[4]

17. **(D)** In the TAN projection, the x-ray beam just skims the area of interest. The beam is always

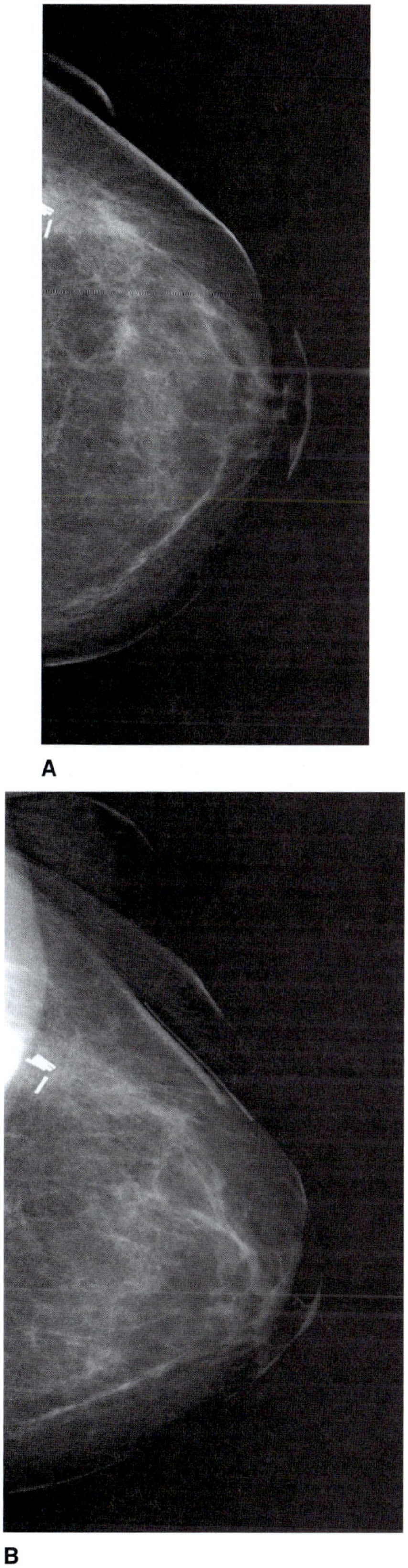

Figure 6-12. (A) Radiograph showing that lateral breast tissue missed on the CC. (B) Missing tissue can be visualized on the XCCL

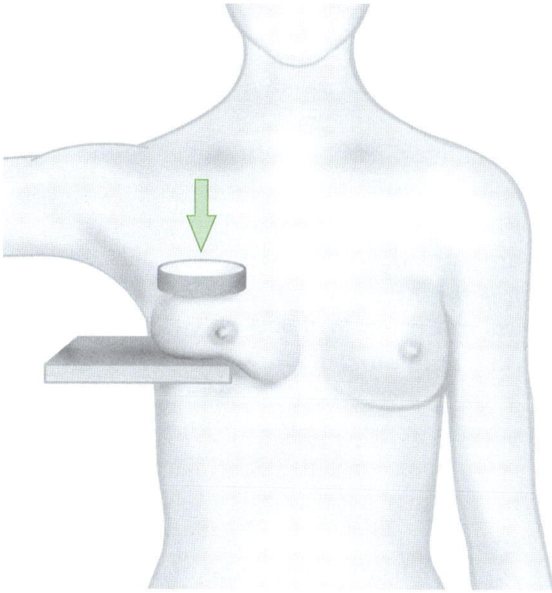

Figure 6-13. Positioning for the TAN projection. (Reproduced with permission from Peart O: Mammography and Breast Imaging PREP: Program Review and Exam Prep. New York, NY: McGraw-Hill Education; 2012.)

tangential or parallel to the skin surface. This projection demonstrates the area of interest free of superimposition. The TAN is possible in any direction or projection (Figure 6-13).[4,5]

18. **(A)** In the RM position, the breast is first positioned for the CC. The top surface of the breast is rolled medially and the bottom surface laterally (Figure 6-14).[4,5]

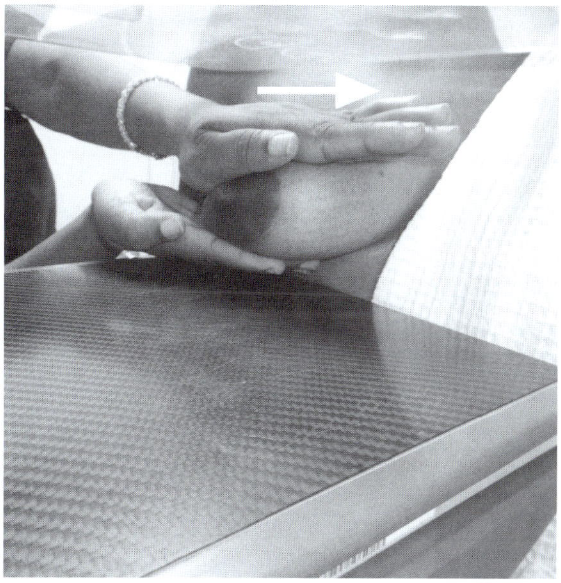

Figure 6-14. Positioning for the RM projection. Arrow shows movement of the superior surface of the breast. The lower surface is rolled laterally.

19. **(D)** The saline implant can be inserted as an expandable sac where the fluid content can be adjusted as needed, during surgery and even after surgery. The saline implants are actually silicone shells filled with a saline solution. Silicone implants are silicone shells filled with silicone gel. The silicone implants are already filled with silicone gel when inserted, therefore the desired size must be known prior to the surgical procedure. The only radiolucent implant available is the autologous myocutaneous flap implant. Flap surgery removes skin and fat from the abdomen, back, or buttock and uses it to form a new breast. Flap techniques can either leave the flap attached to its original blood supply and tunnels the flap under the skin to the breast area, or removes the flap completely, which would involve micro surgery to recreate a blood supply to the flap when it is in position. Mammographically, the flap implant has a fatty or muscular appearance depending on the type of flap technique performed (Figure 6-15).[2]

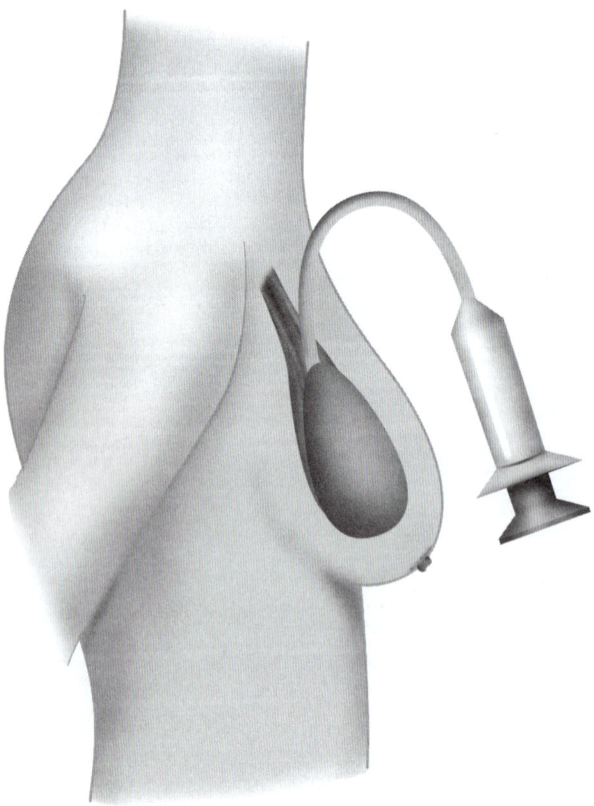

Figure 6-15. Adjusting breast size with tissue expanders.

20. **(B)** After mastectomy, a 3-projection series including the CC, MLO, and ML is often recommended, because without the other breast for comparison, this series gives the radiologist a better opportunity to diagnose any new malignancy. The AT images the axilla and the TAN images skin lesions. The LMO is the true reverse of the MLO.[4,5]

21. **(A)** Even though men generally have a low risk of developing breast cancer, they should be aware of the risk factors, especially family history which could be associated with genetic changes. However, a family history of breast cancer does not mean breast cancer will develop. Slightly over 1% of males in the United States develop breast cancer each year.[1,3,21]

22. **(A)** The CBE is a clinical examination by a trained health-care professional and should be performed every 3 years for women below 40 and every year for women above 40. To be effective, the CBE should be performed in combination with a mammogram (Figure 6-16).[1,21]

23. **(B)** Because of the low x-ray energies used in mammography, the dose to the skin may be high, but dose falls off rapidly as the beam penetrates the breast. The dose to the skin may be as high as 8-12 mGy per projection (800-1200 mR); the dose to the midline of the breast (the average radiation dose to the glandular tissue or glandular dose) will be only about 1.0 mGy (100 mrad). The final rules for mammography, dictated by the MQSA, stated that a single projection mammogram (digital or screen-film) should not give more than 3 mGy (300 mrad) per projection average glandular dose when a grid is used, and should not exceed 1.0 mGy (100 mrad) per projection without a grid.[6,7]

24. **(B)** The actual compression applied to the breast is always under the discretion of the mammographer. However, to ensure that the equipment is working properly the MQSA requires a compression force of a least 111 N (25 lb) and a maximum of 200 N

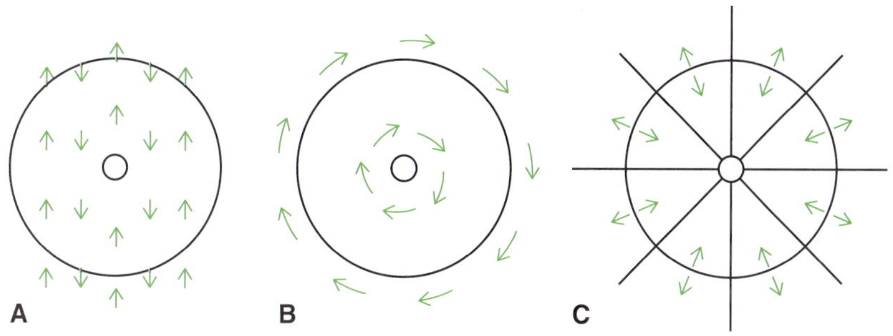

Figure 6-16. CBE and BSE palpation patterns. (Reproduced with permission from Peart O: Mammography and Breast Imaging PREP: Program Review and Exam Prep. New York, NY: McGraw-Hill Education; 2012.)

(20 daN or 45 lb) for the initial power drive. This is an MQSA requirement, necessary to avoid injury to patients.[6,7,22]

25. **(A)** The collimation standard is a MQSA requirement to avoid excess radiation dose to the patient. All units should have a beam-limiting device that allows the entire chest wall edge of the x-ray field to extend to the chest wall edge of the detector and should not extend beyond any of the edges on the detector by more than 1%.[6,7,22]

26. **(C)** The radiation leaving the mammography tube will be filtered by everything in its path. This is the inherent filtration and will include the oil in the tube, the window of the tube, the mirror of the collimation assembly and the compression paddle. In order to reduce the lower energy photons that would only contribute to skin dose added filtration is need. Added filtration can be molybdenum, rhodium, silver, or aluminum.[6,7]

27. **(B)** The Mammography Quality Standards Act (MQSA) was enacted in 1992 with enforcement starting in 1995 to address the need for quality mammograms. Under MQSA all mammography units in the United States must be accredited, certified and inspected regularly. The Act also includes education and continued education requirements for the physicist, radiologist, and radiographer.[6,7,22]

28. **(A)** Grids absorb scatter and increase visibility of image detail and are necessary during normal mammography imaging. The use of a grid typically required increased dose. Grids are placed between the patient's breast and the detector. Grids are not used in magnification radiography or Hologic tomosynthesis imaging. In magnification mammography the large OID serves as an air gap to reduce scatter to the detector. In tomosynthesis, the high contrast is achieved by the tomographic image reconstruction. Grids are also not used in photon counting systems. These systems employ slit scanning with a small detector. They have slot collimation before and after the x-ray passes through the breast tissue, which all serve to provide a high contrast image with lower radiation dose to the patient (Figure 6-17).[6,7,23]

29. **(B)** The breast can reach superiorly to the clavicle (level of the second or third rib), inferiorly to meet the abdominal wall at the level of the sixth or seventh rib (at the inframammary fold or crease), laterally to the edge of the latissimus dorsi muscle and medially to the midsternum.[11]

30. **(B)** The most prominent hormones active in the breast are estrogen and progesterone.

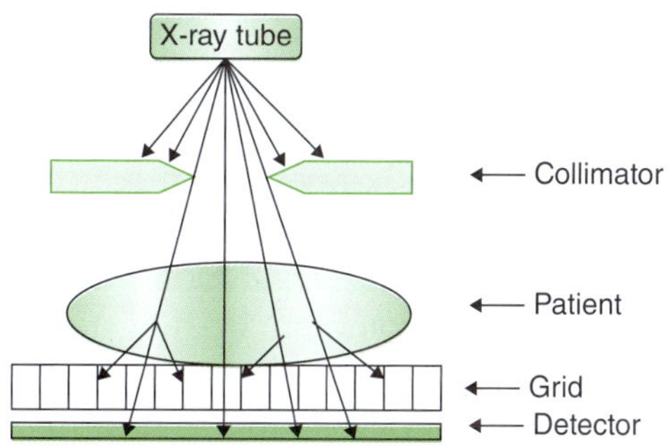

Figure 6-17. Schematic diagram showing the cross-section of a grid. (Reproduced with permission from Peart O: Lange Q&A: Mammography Examination, 2nd ed. New York, NY: McGraw-Hill Education; 2008.)

Estrogen is mostly responsible for ductal proliferation and progesterone is responsible for lobular proliferation and growth. Studies have shown the 2 actually work together to produce full ductal–lobular–alveolar (terminal ductules) development. Prolactin is present in the breast during initial breast growth, pregnancy, and lactation.[11]

31. **(D)** First-degree relatives are immediate relatives such as mother, sister, or daughter.[1,21]

32. **(A)** The BSE involves looking and feeling for changes in the breast. With routine BSE, a woman will become familiar with both the normal appearance and feel of her breasts so that even small changes are noticeable. For this reason BSE should be performed regularly at the same time every month (about 5-10 days after the period begins, or when the breasts are least tender). (See Figure 6-16.)[1,21]

33. **(D)** Unnecessary exposure should be avoided with any mammographic examination. Some studies have shown that the dense cellular breast structure of women younger than 35 is more susceptible to radiation. Dense breast tissue will also need more radiation to penetrate, translating to increased dose.[1,21]

34. **(A)** For mammography tubes made with molybdenum, the most prominent x-rays are characteristic. Characteristic x-rays are produced after a photoelectric interaction. If the target is filtered with molybdenum, the characteristic energy of 19 keV from the K-shell interaction will be prominent. This is within the range of energies that are most effective for mammographic imaging. If the outer shell electron fills the void in the K-shell, the x-ray emissions are termed K-characteristic x-rays. Bremsstrahlung x-rays are produced when an outer projectile electron is slowed by the electric field of the target atom nucleus. This interaction is common in tungsten targets. Coherent or classical scattering describes the interaction between low-energy electrons and atoms. The x-ray loses no energy but changes direction slightly. In Compton scattering, moderate-energy x-rays interact with an outer-shell electron and eject the electron from the atom. The ejected electron is the Compton electron (Figure 6-18).[6,7]

35. **(D)** The QC testing for digital imaging is manufacturer specific. There are tests of the mammographic unit plus additional tests on the display, laser printer if used, and imaging system. Repeat analysis is still needed to monitor repeats due to patient positioning, patient motion, noisy images, or equipment failure. Digital imaging can correct for overexposure, although excessive overexposure increases the patient dose. Digital imaging has a harder time correcting for extreme underexposure, and creates a noisy image (similar to quantum mottle). Digital imaging can enhance the spatial display by enhancing the edges of spiculations or calcifications, making them more visible. Digital imaging cannot correct unsharp images, especially unsharpness caused by motion.[6,7,9]

36. **(A)** Different individuals can perceive different numbers of test objects or may count a different number of objects in the same image. For consistency, the same individual should examine the images each time using the same criteria (same time of day and same viewing conditions). The density calculations are mathematical formulas that do not change. All mammographers should be at least familiar with the basic MQSA guideline.[22]

37. **(A)** The FB (from below) is the reverse CC projection. The beam is directed caudocranially to form an angle of 90 degrees (perpendicular) with the detector (Figure 6-19).[4]

38. **(D)** After radiation therapy the breast may appear red and swollen and may gradually get tighter or harden. The breast may also get smaller and can become distorted after radiation therapy and the surgical procedure. These changes are a result of the radiation and although newer radiation treatment has less effect on the breast, the mammographer should still handle these patients with care because the skin may be delicate and the patient may have tender or painful areas.[2]

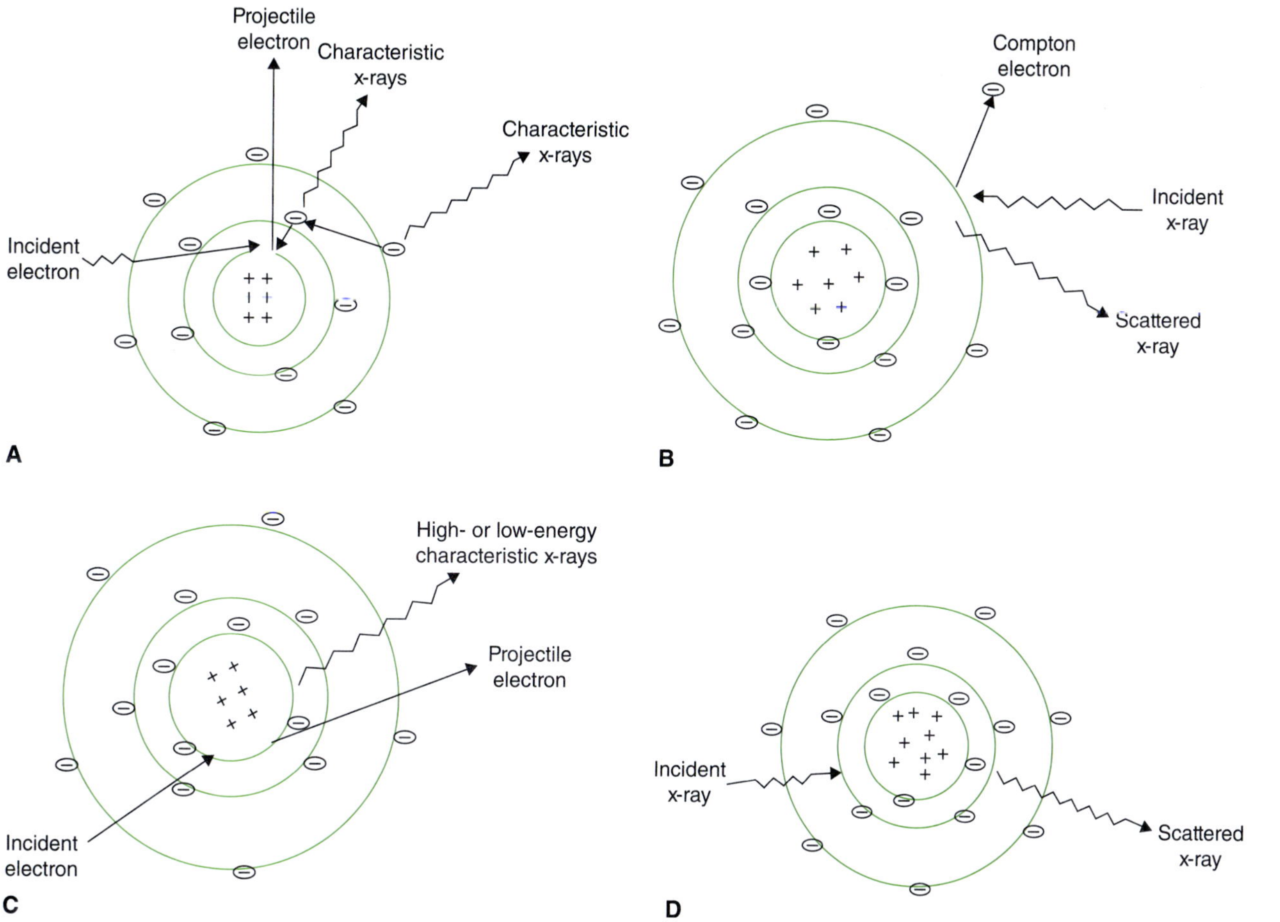

Figure 6-18. Schematic diagram showing (A) characteristic radiation, (B) Compton (C) Bremsstrahlung, and (D) coherent scattering. (Reproduced with permission from Peart O: Mammography and Breast Imaging PREP: Program Review and Exam Prep. New York, NY: McGraw-Hill Education; 2012.)

39. (B) Positron emission mammography (PEM) technology utilizes the fact that cancerous tissue uses vast amounts of sugar. PEM is similar to positron emission tomography (PET) but uses an organ specific high-resolution gamma detector. After the intravenous injection of fluorodeoxyglucose (FDG), the patient sits or relaxes for about 60-90 minutes, giving the body time to absorb the radioactive tracer. Next, each breast is scanned separately using the gamma detector. The pair of detectors is placed above and below the breast to apply mild compression during the scanning process, which takes about 10 minutes. Typically, 2 scans per breasts are taken. The radioactive tracer that is introduced into the body is metabolized in the body like sugar. The tracer will go to the tissues that are most active—normally the cancerous tissue. Before any PEM scan, the patient must fast and no vigorous exercise is allowed 48 hours prior to the PEM scan. Scintigraphy, breast-specific gamma imaging (BSGI) and scintimammography uses the radioactive tracer technetium-99m (Tc-99m) sestamibi. The tracer accumulates in malignant lesions. In lymphoscintigraphy or sentinel node mapping the radiopharmaceutical is injected into the subareolar lymphatic plexus (or lesion). The tracer travels to the sentinel node—identifying that node for dissection and eliminating the need for extensive lymph node dissection (Figure 6-20).[7,19]

40. (B) The LMO provides a mirror image of the MLO. The next best position is the LM projection, which can replace the MLO when imaging patients with difficult body habitus. The LM cannot be used as a routine imaging projection because it does not image the deep

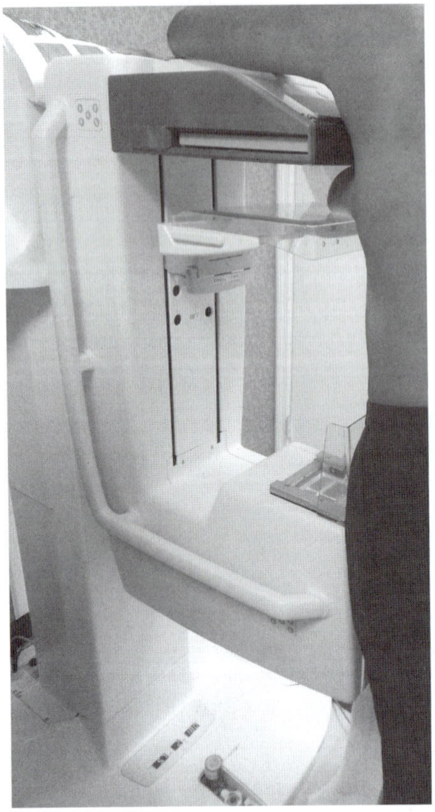

Figure 6-19. Positioning for the FB.

posterior breasts. The LM will also image medially located lesions that are high on the chest wall or in the inferior half of the breast. The ML, although also a true lateral projection, cannot be used because it poorly images the posterior breast. The AT best images the tail of Spence and the RL has the breast positioned for the CC with the upper surface rolled laterally while the lower surface is rolled medially (see Figure 4-9)[4].

41. **(D)** Filtration removes lower energy photons that would only contribute to skin dose. With filtration the average energy of the beam will increase but maximum energy remains the same. With proper filtration the x-ray beam entering the breast will have fewer photons above or below the preferred mammographic energy range. Generally, x-ray tubes use aluminum filtration. Mammography units can use molybdenum, rhodium, silver, or aluminum as the filtration material (Figure 6-21).[6,7]

42. **(C)** The best time to perform the BSE is 5-10 days after the start of the period when

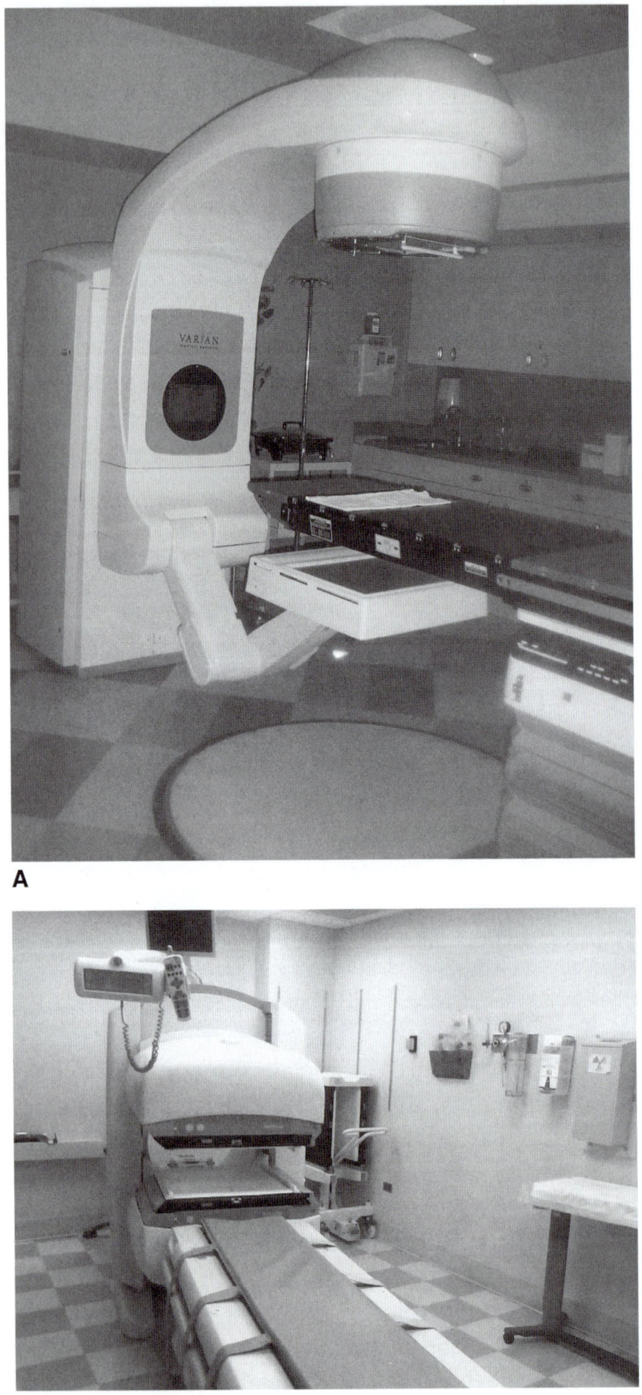

A

B

Figure 6-20. Radiograph showing (A) radiation therapy unit, (B) whole body gamma camera.

the breast is least tender or swollen. If a patient is not having regular periods, the BSE should be done on the same day every month.[1,21]

43. **(C)** The mammography equipment evaluation (MEE) is performed by the physicist. This evaluation is used to determine whether

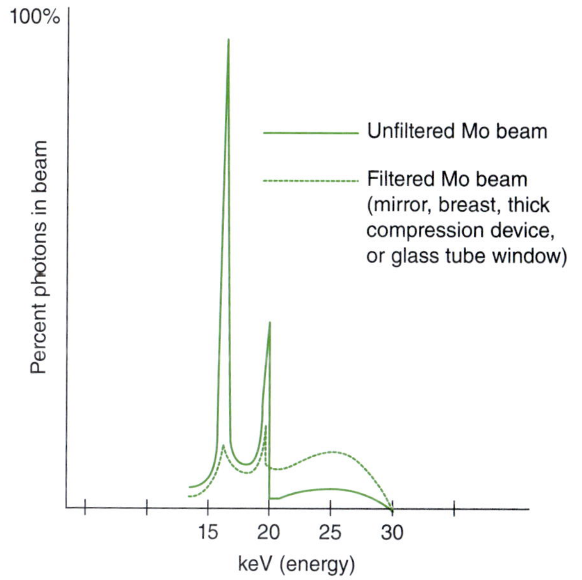

Figure 6-21. Filtration of the x-ray beam. (Reproduced with permission from Peart O: Mammography and Breast Imaging PREP: Program Review and Exam Prep. New York, NY: McGraw-Hill Education; 2012.)

new or changed equipment meets the MQSA requirements. Under the MQSA guidelines there are specific duties for the mammographer, the physicist and the radiologist. The mammographer is responsible for general quality control including daily, weekly, monthly, and semiannual tests. The radiologist is responsible for image interpretation, medical audits, and patient communication. It is the physicists' responsibility to evaluate the mammography unit, review all test, records, and charts plus review policies and procedures and provide a written report of corrective recommendations.[6,7,22]

44. (B) SMPTE (Society of Motion Picture and Television Engineers) is a test pattern used to measure the resolution of a digital system. The pattern can be printed or displayed on a monitor and values calculated. Modulation transfer function (MTF) is a check of the ability of the detector system to produce an image exactly as the object. Contrast measures the minimum density difference between 2 tissues that can be detected in the image as different densities. The contrast-to-noise (CNR) ratio is a check of how well a system will image microcalcifications and distinguish mass or densities from their background density. Signal-to-noise ratio (SNR) is a check of the image noise, the random background information—due to constant flow of current in the circuit—which can obscure the digital image. Noise does not contribute to image quality. On the digital image noise looks like quantum mottle (Figure 6-22).[24,25]

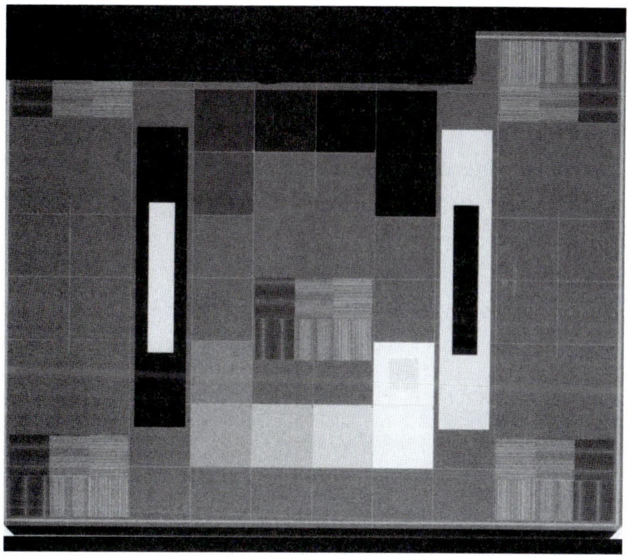

Figure 6-22. SMPTE test pattern.

45. (D) Phantom images are often performed daily or weekly. The repeat/reject analysis is made quarterly. Compression check is tested semiannually, and visual checks are done monthly.

46. (A) Ideally the rate should not exceed 2%, but a rate of 5% is acceptable once a QC program has been established. An analysis of the number of repeated mammograms and rejected images identifies ways to improve efficiency and reduce cost and patient exposure. Because the main purpose of the reject/repeat analysis is to determine problem areas within the department, the one high-rate area should be targeted for improvement.[10,22]

47. (D) The linear-type grids used in mammography typically have a very low ratio because even with the common grid ratio of 4:1, patient exposure doubles (grid ratio = the height of the lead strips/the distance between the strips; ratio = h/d). Most grids are focused to the SID to increase contrast. Grids in mammography typically have a frequency of 30-50 lines per centimeter (Figure 6-23).[6,7]

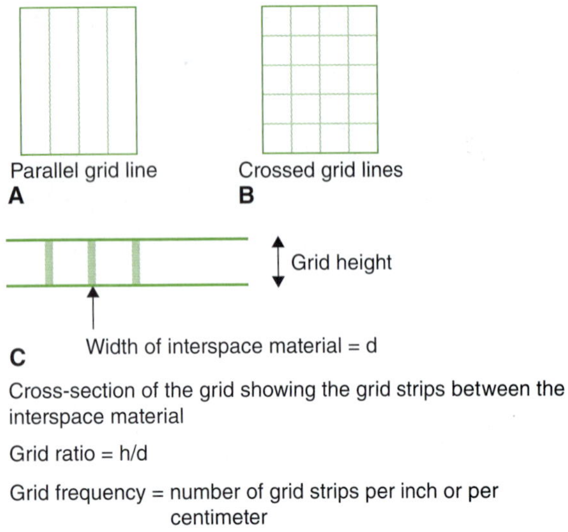

Figure 6-23. Schematic diagrams showing (A) parallel, (B) crossed, and (C) the HTC grid. (Reproduced with permission from Peart O: Lange Q&A: Mammography Examination, 2nd ed. New York, NY: McGraw-Hill Education; 2008.)

48. **(B)** The staging of breast cancer is useful to determine the extent of the spread of the cancer. In general, with the higher stages there is poorer the prognosis. The positron emission tomography or mammography (PET or PEM) technique injects extremely short-lived nuclides into an arm vein. The technology works on the principle that because of the increase in metabolic activity, most cancerous tissue uses vast amounts of sugar (glucose) and at a much higher rate than benign tissue. The radioactive substance used is metabolized in the body like sugar and will therefore go to tissues that are most active. A gamma camera can then be used to measure the emitted radiation signals making the cancer's location visible. The extent of the cancer is then known, which aids the oncologist in determining treatment and monitoring therapy. Currently, PET or PEM imaging is also used to stage lymph node involvement, detect metastases, and in staging and restaging cancerous breast lesions and is becoming a useful tool in molecular imaging.[1,2]

49. **(D)** During the medical history documentation, the physician collects information on the patient's risk factors for benign or malignant breast conditions and any other health problems. Information on past mammograms is also collected because of the importance of comparison. Although the medical history does not prevent breast cancer, it is the first step in evaluating both symptomatic and asymptomatic women and an important step in evaluating treatment options.[3,21]

50. **(D)** The smaller the focal spot size, the greater the resolution. Mammography units use a "half-field" geometry system where the central axis of the x-ray beam will run perpendicular to the plane of the detector at the chest wall. The target of the anode is then angled between 6 and 16 degrees (line-focus principle). The large target angle would force the use of larger focal spot sizes and increase the heel effect (Figure 6-24). However, to reduce the heel effect, an effective anode angle greater than 22 degrees is maintained either by using a 0-dgreee anode angle matched with a 24-degree tube tilt or a 16-degree anode angle matched with a 6-degree tube tile. The result is a 24 and 22 effective anode angle, respectively

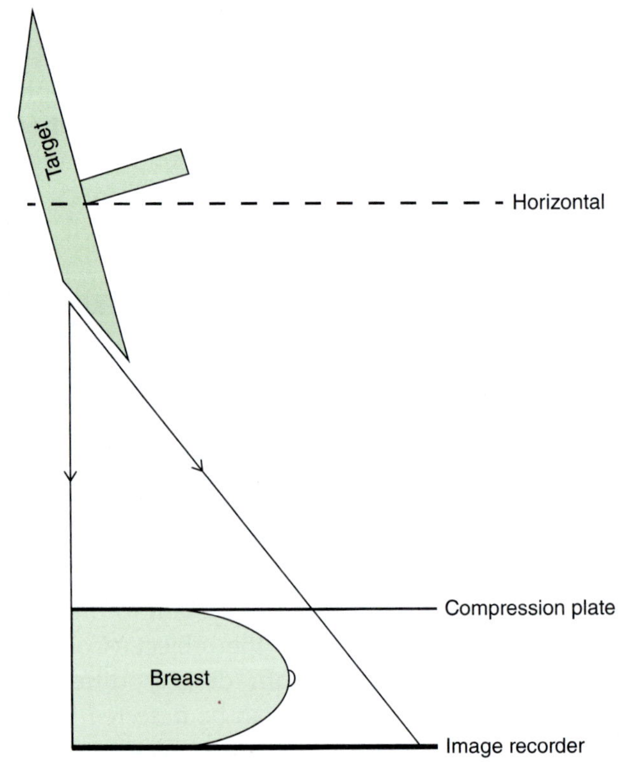

Figure 6-24. Mammography tube tilt. With the x-ray tube tilted about 6 degrees off the horizontal, the central rays run parallel to the chest wall so no breast tissue is missed. 24 × 30 cm FOV requires minimum effective anode angle of 20-24°(therefore = tube tilt + anode angle) Typical 16°anode angle + 6° tube tilt.

(actual anode angle plus the physical tube tilt). As a result, small focal spots are possible, resulting in increased resolution.[6,9]

51. **(A)** The retromammary space separates the breast from the pectoral muscle. This space is filled with a layer of adipose or fatty tissue as opposed to the supporting and connective tissue (stroma), blood vessels, and various ductal structures that make up the glandular and fibrous tissues of the breast.[11,12]

52. **(D)** Cysts occur in the terminal ductal lobular units when the extralobular terminal duct becomes blocked. Fluid accumulates faster than it can be reabsorbed. Cysts vary in size and respond to hormonal fluctuations, but the development of a cyst also depends on a woman's genetic predisposition. Younger women, premenopausal women, and postmenopausal women taking estrogen are likely to have higher hormonal levels and therefore have an increased possibility of having cysts.[13,14]

53. **(C)** By the process of elimination, the best choice is that the lesion is a cyst. Although the fibroadenoma, hematoma, and galactocele are all oval or circular lesions, all are of mixed density (radiolucent and radiopaque) (see Figure 3-19).[13,14]

54. **(B)** As the kVp increases, the relative number of x-rays undergoing Compton interaction also increases. With compression, the part is thinner, less kVp is needed to penetrate the part, and therefore there is less Compton scatter.[26,27]

55. **(B)** The CBE involves both a visual inspection and palpation of the breast. A visual inspection involves looking for changes in the shape and size and appearance of the breast and nipple while noting any skin dimpling, redness, or swelling.[3,21]

56. **(C)** Focused grids have linear lead strips that are slanted to match the divergence of the x-ray beam. A focused grid must be used at the correct SID and correct side of grid must be facing the x-ray tube to prevent grid cutoff. Parallel grids have strips arranged in straight lines in 1 direction (also called linear grids). They can be used with varying SIDs. Crossed grids are in effect 2 linear grids placed on top of each other with the grid lines perpendicular to each other. They offer more efficient scatter cleanup but greater risk of grid cutoff and can result in increased radiation dose to the patient. In mammography the high transmission cellular grid (HTC) is similar to a crossed grid. It uses air as the interspace material and copper instead of lead as the strips to avoid increased patient dose. (See Figure 6-17.)[6,7]

57. **(B)** Fibrous and glandular tissues are together described as fibroglandular densities. X-rays pass more easily through fatty tissue than through fibrous or glandular tissues. Fatty areas are more radiolucent and will appear as black on the mammogram. The fibroglandular tissue is more radiopaque than fatty tissues and results in areas of lower optical density on the mammogram (white areas).[11,12]

58. **(A)** Estrogen and progesterone are 2 of the many hormones responsible for many physiological changes in the breast. Estrogen is responsible for ductal proliferation and progesterone for lobular proliferation. Once a woman starts taking any of these hormones including HRT, the changes to the breast can be spotty, causing lumps, or increased interstitial fluids (cysts) but will generally result in an overall increase in glandular tissue.[11,12]

59. **(C)** By process of elimination, the lesion is likely to be a lymph node. Lymph nodes are lesions with mixed density and generally have a radiolucent center corresponding to the hilus. The fibroadenoma, hematoma, and the galactocele are all mixed-density oval or circular lesions, but none has the lucent center typical of the lymph nodes. (See Figure 3-19.)[13,14]

60. **(D)** In lymphoscintigraphy or sentinel node mapping, the radiopharmaceutical is injected into the subareolar lymphatic plexus (or lesion). The tracer travels to the sentinel node—identifying that node for

dissection and eliminating the need for extensive lymph node dissection. Positron emission mammography (PEM) technology utilizes the fact that cancerous tissue uses vast amounts of sugar. PEM is similar to positron emission tomography (PET) but uses an organ specific high-resolution gamma detector. After the intravenous injection of fluorodeoxyglucose (FDG), the patient sits or relaxes for about 60-90 minutes, giving the body time to absorb the radioactive tracer. Next, each breast is scanned separately using the gamma detector. The pair of detectors is placed above and below the breast to apply mild compression during the scanning process, which takes about 10 minutes. Typically, 2 scans per breasts are taken. The radioactive tracer that is introduced into the body is metabolized in the body like sugar. The tracer will go to the tissues that are most active—normally the cancerous tissue. Before any PEM scan, the patient must fast and no vigorous exercise is allowed 48 hours prior to the PEM scan breast-specific gamma imaging (BSGI) or scintimammography uses the radioactive tracer technetium-99m (Tc-99m) sestamibi. The tracer accumulates in malignant lesions.[1,19]

61. **(C)** As the magnification factor increases, to maintain a sharp image the focal spot must be reduced or the thickness of the part has to decrease. A greater magnification factor will therefore need a smaller focal spot. Small focal spot is therefore used in magnification mammography. Magnification factor equals the SID divided by the SOD. Since the SID is fixed, increasing OID reduces the SOD and therefore increases the magnification factor. (See Figure 6-10.)[6,7]

62. **(A)** The actual focal-spot size is the area on the anode target that is exposed to electrons from the tube current. Because the target is angled, the effective focal spot is made much smaller than the actual area of electron interactions. The effective focal spot is the area projected onto the patient and the detector. The nominal focal-spot size is a measure of

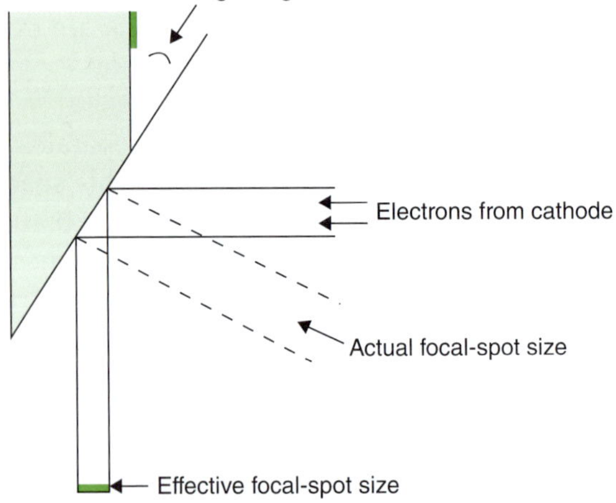

Figure 6-25. Line-focus principle is provides a large actual focal-spot size with a small effective focal-spot size. (Reproduced with permission from Peart O: Mammography and Breast Imaging PREP: Program Review and Exam Prep. New York, NY: McGraw-Hill Education; 2012.)

the effective focal-spot size and is the value used by manufacturers when identifying large or small focal spots (Figure 6-25).[6,7,16]

63. **(C)** The MQSA governs final assessment findings in the evaluation of mammographic images. In an effort to guide referring physicians and radiologists in the breast cancer decision making process, the ACR came up with the BIRAD, which is a standardized mammographic reporting system that can be used as a coding and assessment system. To ensure recognition of the system the ACR collaborated with the National Cancer Institute (NCI), the Center for Disease Control and Prevention (CDC), the FDA, the American Medical Association (AMA), the American College of Surgeons and the American College of Pathologists. The BIRAD system is now well recognized and used by radiologists, physicians, and surgeons across the United States, Canada, and much of Europe and Asia. The MQSA also has a category assessment; however, the ACR assessment categories were already in existence prior to the publication of the final regulations of MQSA. Because the assessment categories developed by the ACR are so widely recognized, the FDA accepts the ACRs BIRAD categories; however, to avoid confusion in addition to the category name (e.g., BIRAD 1) the report must include the word identifier, for example, BIRAD 1: negative.

BREAST IMAGING REPORTING AND DATA SYSTEM (BIRAD)	
BIRAD 0:	Need additional imaging information and/or prior mammograms for comparison
BIRAD 1:	Negative
BIRAD 2:	Benign finding
BIRAD 3:	Probably benign finding—short-interval follow-up suggested
BIRAD 4:	Suspicious abnormality—biopsy should be considered
BIRAD 5:	Highly suggestive of malignancy—appropriate action should be taken
BIRAD 6:	Known biopsy proven malignancy—appropriate action should be taken[10, 22]

64. **(B)** Rejects are all discarded images. Repeats are images that resulted in a dose to the patient. The causal repeat rate is the percentage of repeats from a specific cause. It is equal to the number of repeats of a specific cause divided by the total number of repeats, times 100. The total repeat rate is the number of repeated images divided by the total number of images taken, times 100. In mammography the department repeat rates should not exceed 2%.[10,22]

65. **(C)** Epithelial hyperplasia is also known as proliferative breast disease and is an overgrowth of cells that line either the ducts or the lobules. When hyperplasia involves the duct, it is called ductal hyperplasia or duct epithelial hyperplasia. When it affects the lobules, it is referred to as lobular hyperplasia. Depending on how it looks under the microscope, it may be classified as usual or atypical. An epidermoid cyst, often incorrectly referred to a sebaceous cyst, is a pimple-like cyst that occurs in the oil glands of the skin, and the hematoma is a pooling of blood as a result of trauma or surgery. Over time a hematoma may slowly calcify, resulting in the formation of an oil cyst, and later a calcified hematoma.[13,14]

66. **(A)** This is a ruptured implant. In an implant rupture the silicone may leak into the fibrous capsule or may escape from the capsule leaking into the surrounding breast tissues and muscle causing pain or discomfort. In the encapsulated implant, the implant hardens or calcifies but does not rupture. A herniated implant shows the implant pushing out of the fibrous capsule, but does not indicate a silicone leak. Patients with implant removal may have traces of residual silicone in the breast. (See Figure 6-2.)[13]

67. **(C)** The first step is to determine the location of the lesion by applying the rules for lesion movement. When comparing the MLO projection to the ML, a lateral abnormality will move down from its position on the MLO. A medial abnormality will move up from its position on the MLO. A centrally located lesion and lesions at the areola will show little or no movement. Once the location of the lesion is determined, an XCCL for a lateral lesion or the CV or the XCCM for medial lesions will locate the lesion in the craniocaudal position. The AT images the axilla of the breast only and is not needed.[4]

68. **(A)** During ductography, a collecting duct that ends at the nipple is cannulated and a small amount of contrast agent is injected. Generally, approximately 1 cc is enough to fill the duct.[19]

69. **(C)** The glandular dose is used in mammography because the biological effects of radiation are most likely to be related to the total energy absorbed by glandular tissue. The glandular dose is the average radiation dose to the glandular tissue in the middle of the breast. The other measure of dose is the ESE. The ESE is most often referred to as the patient dose. It is the exposure at the skin's surface. In mammography the ESE may be very high because of low-energy x-rays, but the dose falls quickly as the x-rays penetrate the breast.[6,10]

70. **(C)** The SID of mammography units do not change. Obtaining a magnified image requires increasing the OID while maintaining a constant SID. Any change in OID will result in a corresponding change in SOD. To maintain a sharp image, a smaller focal spot must be used in magnification. (See Figure 6-10.)[6,16]

71. **(D)** QC testing should always be performed by the dedicated QC personnel or the same individual. Here the mammographer would be the most obvious person.[10,22]

72. **(B)** Galactoceles are small, milk-filled cysts with a high fat content. These are associated with lactation, may be mixed density, and are circular/oval with sharply defined contours. A hematoma is associated with breast trauma or surgery and the oil cyst appears mammographically as eggshell-like calcifications. Lymph nodes typically have a central radiolucent area corresponding to the hilus.[13,14]

73. **(B)** Using increased OID or the air gap technique is effective in reducing scatter to the detector. The air gap technique provides a large OID s increase which allows the scatter to be dissipated in the air before reaching the detector. An OID of at least 6 in (10-15 cm) is required to be effective. (See Figure 6-10.)[6,7]

74. **(C)** With the 4 quadrants terminology, the breast can be described as: the upper-outer quadrant (UOQ), upper-inner quadrant (UIQ), lower outer quadrant (LOQ), and lower inner quadrant (LIQ). The exact locations within the quadrant are represented by viewing each breast separately as a clock face. The upper-outer quadrant, which extends toward the axilla, is known as the axillary tail, tail of the breast or tail of Spence. Most glandular tissue is found centrally and extends laterally toward the axilla in the UOQ. This distribution increases or decreases with hormonal fluctuations, but generally mirrors the opposite breast (Figure 6-26).[21]

75. **(C)** Mammography uses very low-energy kVp and it is very important that the x-ray tube window not attenuate the low-energy photons. Most mammography units use beryllium window as the port window. With a low atomic number of 4 it is ideal and provides an inherent filtration of approximately 0.1 mm Al (aluminum). The material of the glass window has no effect on scattered radiation, nor can it increase or decrease the output of the x-ray tube.[6,7,16]

76. **(C)** Compression is important in mammography to reduce breast thickness, radiation dose, and motion unsharpness. Compression also separates superimposed areas of the breast tissue and brings abnormalities closer to the detector. Unfortunately, compression is painful for some women. In general, the breast should be compressed until taut to ensure adequate compression. Compression, however, should not be applied to cause the patient severe pain.[4]

77. **(C)** In magnification mammography, the object to image-receptor distance (OID) is increased, the source to object distance (SOD) is decreased but the source to image-receptor (SID) remains fixed. Magnification factor = SID/SOD or image size/object size. The greater the magnification factor, the greater OID and the smaller the SOD therefore the greater the skin dose to the patient.

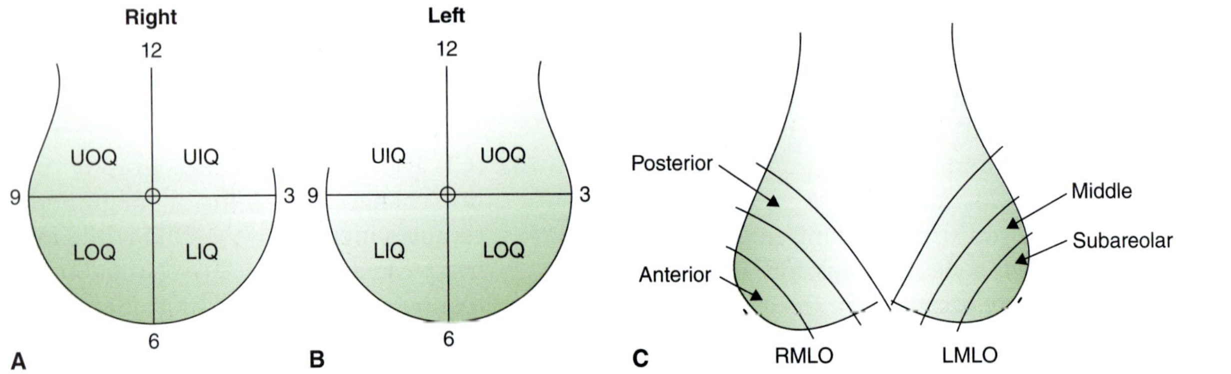

Figure 6-26. Schematic diagram showing the (A) clock-face, (B) region, and (C) quadrant locations of the breast. (Reproduced with permission from Peart O: Mammography and Breast Imaging PREP: Program Review and Exam Prep. New York, NY: McGraw-Hill Education; 2012.)

In magnification the patient's skin dose increases because the breast is closer to the source. The small focal-spot size used to maintain a sharp image requires that the mA be reduced with a corresponding increase in exposure time. (See Figure 6-10.)[4,6,7]

78. **(B)** The actual focal-spot size is the area on the anode target that is exposed to electrons from the tube current. As the size of the focal spot decreases, the heating of the target is concentrated into a smaller area. In the design known as the line-focus principle, the target is angled allowing a larger area for heating while maintaining a small effective focal spot. Because the target is angled, the effective focal spot is made much smaller than the actual area of electron interactions. The effective focal spot is the area projected onto the patient and the detector. As the target angle is made smaller, the effective focal spot decreases. (See Figure 24)[6,7]

79. **(C)** Postsurgical scarring is a benign process that can mimic a radial scar. It follows a surgical intervention and can appear as an area of architectural distortion or an irregular shaped lesion with spiculated margins. It may or may not be associated with calcifications. Typically, the surgical scar will resolve over time. A benign surgical scar has no central tumor, although there may be long spicules radiating from the center of the lesion. Regardless of the size of the spicules in the surgical scarring, there is no associated skin thickening, dimpling, or nipple reaction. As shown on the radiograph (see Figure 6-3) the lesion is resolving. A galactocele is a benign, milk-filled cyst with a high fat content. These lesions are generally associated with lactation. They are usually circular, with sharply defined borders, and have densities that are a combination of radiolucent and radiopaque. They are often left alone, but if painful they can be drained using needle puncture. Often they yield a yellow fluid. Oil cysts are generally seen mammographically as eggshell-like calcifications. Hematomas are generally associated with trauma. They are mixed-density oval or circular lesions and can calcify to become high-density calcifications. (See Figure 3-18.)[13,14]

80. **(C)** When the air gap technique is used, the OID must increase to allow the scatter to be dissipated in the air before reaching the detector. An OID of at least 6 in (10-15 cm) is required to be effective. (See Figure 6-10.)[6,7]

81. **(A)** Using clock-face terminology there are 4 main clock positions (12-o'clock, 3-o'clock, 6-o'clock, and 9-o'clock). In the XCCL and the CC, the central rays are directed superiorly to inferiorly; therefore, 12-o'clock and 6-o'clock lesions will be superimposed. The AT images the axilla and would miss any 6-o'clock lesion. In the MLO, the beam is directed medially to laterally separating the upper aspect of the breast (12-o'clock position) from the lower aspect (6-o'clock position). (See Figure 6-26.)[4]

82. **(C)** The cleavage view (CV) is the standard terminology adopted by the ACR. All projections in mammography are compression or compressed projections. (See Figure 4-9.)[4]

83. **(D)** Malignant casting calcifications are produced when carcinoma in situ fills the ducts and their branches. The shape of the cast is determined by the uneven production of calcification and the irregular necrosis of the cellular debris. The contours of the cast are always irregular in density, width, and length and the cast is always fragmented. A calcification is seen as branching when it extends into adjacent ducts. Additionally, the width of the ducts determines the width of the castings. Eggshell-like and needle-like, sharply outlined, or elongated branching calcifications are typically benign mammographically. Granulated sugar or crushed stone calcifications are termed pleomorphic or granular-type calcifications and are often malignant. (See Figure 3-19.)[13,28]

84. **(B)** Starting at the TDLU or terminal ductal lobular unit, the collecting ductal system gradually widens in tree-like branches forming segmental ducts. Immediately behind the nipple it further distends to form an ampulla, also called the lactiferous sinus. This is a pouch-like structure immediately behind

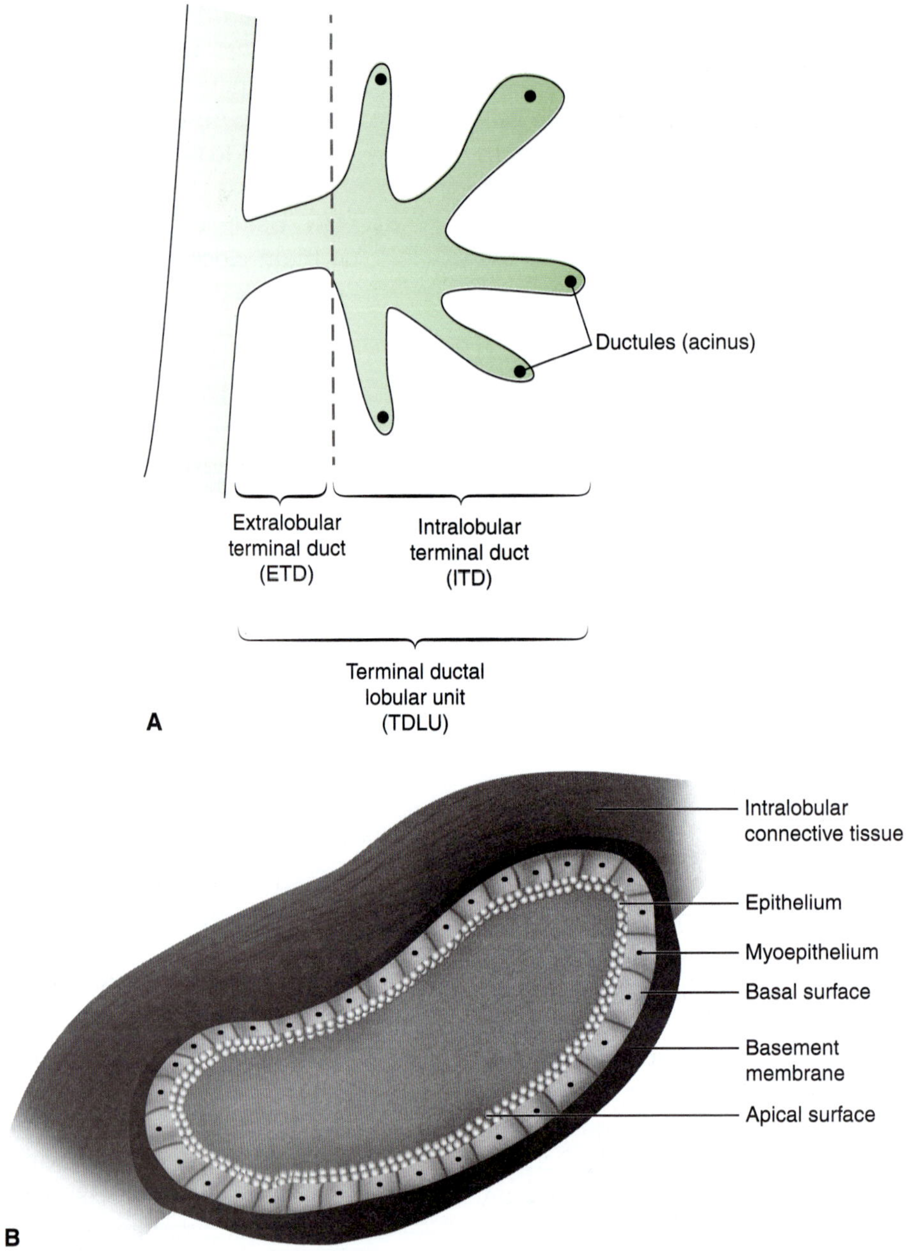

Figure 6-27. Schematic diagram of the (A) TDLU, (B) epithelium layers of TDLU. (Reproduced with permission from Peart O: Mammography and Breast Imaging PREP: Program Review and Exam Prep. New York, NY: McGraw-Hill Education; 2012.)

the nipple. The ducts again narrow to end at the nipple (Figure 6-27).[11]

85. **(A)** The grid ratio is equal to the height of the lead strips divided by the distance between each lead strip (or width of interspace material). (See Figure 6-23)[17]

86. **(C)** The AT projection best demonstrates the axillary tail of the breast. The medial and subareolar areas are not visualized on the AT projection. The upper-outer quadrant, which extends toward the axilla, is known as the axillary tail, tail of the breast, or tail of Spence. (See Figure 4-9.)[4]

87. **(D)** The fibroadenoma is generally a mixed density lesion (radiolucent and radiopaque). Galactoceles are small, milk-filled cysts with a high fat content associated with lactation. Over time the galactocele can calcify to form a high density lesion. If the hematoma

calcifies, it slowly becomes a mixed-density oil cyst with the typical eggshell-like calcifications and then eventually a high-density radiopaque lesion. Stellate lesions are high-density lesions with spiculated margins. (See Figure 3-19.)[13]

88. **(B)** A hematoma is associated with breast trauma or surgery. Generally, the result is a pooling of blood, which can show mammographically as a low-density radiopaque lesion. If the hematoma calcifies, it slowly becomes a mixed-density oil cyst with the typical eggshell-like calcifications and then eventually a high-density radiopaque lesion. Galactoceles are small, milk-filled cysts with a high fat content associated with lactation. Fibroadenomas are benign tumors common in women at any age and the intramammary lymph nodes can be found in any quadrant of the breast and are not related to injury. (See Figure 3-19)[13,14]

89. **(C)** The analog-to-digital converter (ADC) converts analog signal (light or electronic) from the image receptor or detector to a digital signal for computers to manipulate for processing, display, and storage. The ADC assigns each picture element or pixel a value which corresponds to a level of brightness. The entire image is divided into a matrix of pixels based on the brightness of each pixel. The digital-to-analog converter (DAC) converts digitally manipulated data back to an analog (electronic) signal and the film digitizers converts an analog produced radiograph (film) to a digital version via a scanning device. DICOM is a set of computer software standards that permit a wide range of digital imaging programs to communicate with each other.[17,18]

90. **(B)** Generally, when the shoulders are not relaxed or if the height of the detector is too high, most of the axilla and shoulders will fall into the compression area. The thick area of the axilla and shoulder can stop the compression paddle before adequate compression is applied to the lower or anterior breast.[4]

91. **(A)** Digital breast imaging including digital tomosynthesis, ultrasound, and MRI will all image the structure and anatomy of the breasts. Molecular imaging looks at the biological activity and shows what the cells are doing or how they are functioning. Nuclear imaging studies all use radioactive tracers or radiopharmaceuticals. These include position emission tomography or mammography (PET or PEM) imaging, breast-specific gamma imaging (BSGI) or scintimammography and lymphoscintigraphy.[1,19]

92. **(D)** In this case the circular lucency in the center suggests a port-a-cath. A pacemaker generally presents as a low optical density object with wirings. A hematoma is generally associated with trauma or surgery. They are mixed-density oval or circular lesions possible with calcifications. The patient's chin would present as a uniform area of low optical density. (See Figure 3-19.)[13]

93. **(A)** The rolled positions are helpful when dense breast tissue is superimposed on a lesion. The dense tissue is rolled off the lesion.[4]

94. **(D)** The specimen must be imaged after biopsy to ensure that the lesion was completely removed. In imaging the specimen, it should be compressed and magnified to prevent the appearance of pseudomasses and to assess calcifications. The specimen should also be compared to the initial mammograms. Imaging the specimen before the open surgical biopsy is completed will allow the surgeon to take an additional biopsy specimen if indicated.[19]

95. **(C)** The LMO is useful for patients with prior chest surgery or patients with pacemakers, which prevent compression to the medial breast. The LMO is an inferolateral to superomedial projection. The x-ray tube is angled approximately 125 degrees. The detector is positioned at the medial aspect of the breast and compression is applied from the lateral aspect. AT images the tail of the breast (tail of Spence); LM and ML are both 90-degree lateral projections. (See Figure 4-9.)[4]

96. **(B)** The actual focal-spot size is the area on the anode target that is exposed to electrons from the tube current. Because the target is angled, the effective focal spot is made much smaller than the actual area of electron interactions. The effective focal spot is the area projected onto the patient and the detector. The nominal focal-spot size is a measure of the effective focal-spot size and is the value used when identifying large or small focal spots. (See Figure 6-25.)[6,7]

97. **(C)** Radiation and surgical treatment can cause changes in the breast and can cause calcium formation. After any breast surgery, including lumpectomy, magnification can be useful as a preassessment and postassessment of any calcifications. Magnification imaging can also be used to confirm complete removal of malignant calcifications.[19]

98. **(A)** The posterior lateral breast tissue is missing on this CC and the XCCL is the best option to image the missed area. The CV shows the medial breast. The AT images the axillary tail and the ML is a 90-degree lateral that will best image the medial breast. (See Figure 4-9.)[4]

99. **(B)** Grids absorb scatter and increase visibility of image detail. They are a thin, rectangular device made of alternating strips of radiopaque materials (usually lead) and radiolucent materials. The radiolucent material allows x-ray photons traveling in a straight line to pass through to the detector while the lead strips absorb scatter radiation photons before they reach the detector. Grids are placed between the patient and the detector. Grids are not used in magnification radiography. The large OID serves as an air gap to reduce scatter to the detector. (See Figure 6-23.)[17,18]

100. **(B)** Mammography imaging systems using photostimulable phosphor (PSP), sometime called computed mammography (CM), and systems using flat panel technology, sometime called digital mammography(DM) or full-field digital mammography (FFDM), both have a wide latitude and dynamic range. Advantages of CM include: A wide latitude and dynamic range; CM is a faster imaging system when compared to screen-film; there is reduced repeats and no lost films; there is increased workflow. Disadvantages of CM include: lower spatial resolution. (All digital imaging can manipulate the pixel value after the exposure which compensates for the lower spatial resolution is digital imaging system but CM is not as effective as DM in compensating for the lower resolution of the imaging system); CM uses IPs which can be damaged during transport; The IPs used in CM are susceptible to scratches in computer reader; low exposure can create a noisy image; the photostimulable phosphor (PSP) is very sensitive to radiation which can contribute to a noise image. Advantages of DM include: no plates to drop or damage; no plates to be transferred; DM has increased DQE over CM (DQE describes how efficient the system is in converting x-ray input signals into a useful image). Disadvantages of DM include: image lag or memory effect because the charge is trapped in the metastable band and is released slowly over time. Image lag time varies and is shorter for flat-panel digital detectors based on indirect conversion. Low exposure can create a noisy image.[6,7]

101. **(B)** The MQSA was established in the US on October 27, 1992, to enforce minimum national standards for mammography. Under the MQSA requirements, the FDA can authorize individual states to certify mammography facilities, conduct inspections, and enforce the MQSA quality standards. After October 1994, the MQSA required all legal providers of mammography services to be accredited by an approved accreditation body and certified by the FDA. The FDA cannot ensure that all women have access to a certified mammography facility.[10,22,30]

102. **(D)** The MQSA final regulations require facilities to have a written and documented policy of resolving consumer complaints. The facility may select its own format. Medical outcome audit is required by MQSA to follow up positive mammographic assessments and to correlate pathology results with the radiologist's findings. Record keeping refers to the section of MQSA standards dealing with the maintenance of mammograms and reports in a permanent file (for not less than 5 years, or not less than 10 years if no additional mammograms of the patient are performed at the facility, or longer if required by state or local laws). To satisfy the communication-of-results section of the standards, all mammographic facilities must send each patient a summary of the report, written in lay terms, within 30 days of the mammographic examination. If assessments are suspicious or highly suspicious for malignancy, the facility should contact the patient as soon as possible with the results.[10,22,30]

103. **(B)** A harmartoma is a benign tumor. It is considered self-limiting because the tumor consists of an overgrowth of normal tissue and the tumor cells do not reproduce. Breast lesions associated with trauma and nursing are hematomas and galactoceles, respectively. (See Figure 3-19.)[13,14]

104. **(B)** Parturition is the process of giving birth. In the immature breast, a 2-layer epithelium of cells lines the ducts and alveoli. After puberty this epithelium proliferates, forming 3 alveolar cell types—superficial (luminal) A cells, basal B cells (chief cells), and myoepithelial cells forming the innermost layer or basal surface of the epithelium. The myoepithelial cells are arranged in a branching, starlike fashion located around the alveoli and excretory milk ducts. Contraction of the myoepithelial cells helps to propel milk toward the nipples. Beneath the epithelium is connective tissue that helps to keep the epithelium in place. Between the epithelium and the connective tissue is a layer called the basement membrane. The basement membrane provides support and acts as a semipermeable filter under the epithelium (Figure 6-27).[11,12]

105. **(B)** A benign finding means that although something was seen it is considered totally benign. When using the BIRAD, the verbal identifier must be used to avoid confusion with the MQSA assessment. The MQSA categories numbers 1-7 and places all mammographic findings in categories similar to the BIRAD system but it is rarely used today. (See Table question 63)

BREAST IMAGING REPORTING AND DATA SYSTEM (BIRAD)

BIRAD 0:	Need additional imaging information and/or prior mammograms for comparison
BIRAD 1:	Negative
BIRAD 2:	Benign finding
BIRAD 3:	Probably benign finding—short-interval-follow-up suggested
BIRAD 4:	Suspicious abnormality—biopsy should be considered
BIRAD 5:	Highly suggestive of malignancy—appropriate action should be taken
BIRAD 6:	Known biopsy proven malignancy—appropriate action should be taken[10,22,30]

106. **(D)** Erythema is a redness or inflammation of the skin. Although it can indicate inflammatory breast cancer, it can also be an indication of breast abscess or other infectious changes. Further evaluation and testing, including mammography, would be necessary to determine the cause.[13,14]

107. **(C)** Tamoxifen is a nonsteroidal antiestrogen drug given to patients with breast cancer. It is considered an antiestrogen drug because it prevents estrogen from latching onto tumor cell receptors and will shrink or stop the recurrence of breast cancer. Tamoxifen will also lower the risks of breast cancer recurrence in postmenopausal women. Tamoxifen is considered a palliative treatment because it will not cure the disease. The drug can cause serious side effects including an increased risk for endometrial cancer, uterine cancer, pulmonary embolism, stroke, deep vein thrombosis, blood clots, and increased menopausal symptoms. Because of these risks, Tamoxifen is often not given for more than 5 years. However, other studies suggest the benefits of Tamoxifen outweigh the risks and the drug can be taken and will be effective for longer periods. There are now a number of similar drugs on the market with less dangerous side effects. Radiation therapy may be used to destroy cancer cells remaining after surgery or to reduce the size of a tumor before surgery. Chemotherapy uses a combination of drugs to kill undetected tumor cells that may have migrated to other parts of the body. Antibody therapy works by blocking the effect of the protein HER-2—important in regulating the growth of breast cancer cells.[1,2]

108. **(B)** The detector elements (DELs or dexels) are located within the thin-film transistor (TFT). DEL size controls the recorded detail, or spatial resolution, for the flat-panel device. DEL size also contributes to the image blur present in a flat-panel detector receptor. The larger DELs in a flat-panel detector cause more image blur.The DEL is a part of the complex circuit device of the TFT and is the sensitive component of the TFT which collects electrons emitted from either amorphous selenium or amorphous silicon that represent individual components of a digital image. Each square in the TFT matrix can have sensitive and nonsensitive areas. The *fill factor* is the ratio of the sensitive area to the entire detector area and is usually expressed as a percentage. Fill factor will affect the spatial resolution and signal-to-noise ratio. A typical fill factor is 80%. The technologist can't change the size of the DEL, which is fixed for that piece of equipment. Once the DELs are read, the flat-panel detector automatically erases and is ready for another exposure. The actual digital image produced is a matrix of picture elements (*pixels*). Each cell corresponds to a specific location in the image. The matrix is therefore a box of cells with numeric values arranged in rows and columns. The *image resolution* is controlled by the number of pixels with the greater the number of pixels; the greater the image resolution.[6,7]

109. **(C)** After puberty, the epithelium of the lobules proliferates, becoming multilayered and forming 3 alveolar cell types, superficial (luminal) A cells, basal B cells (chief cells), and myoepithelial cells. The innermost layer or basal surface of the epithelium consists of myoepithelial cells. Beneath the epithelium is connective tissue that helps to keep the epithelium in place. Between the epithelium and the connective tissue is a layer called the basement membrane. The basement membrane provides support and acts as a semipermeable filter under the epithelium.[12,13]

110. **(C)** The "camel's nose" contour refers to the sloping of the anterior breast in the MLO projection, caused by insufficient compression. The result is poor separation of the breast tissues. Preventing "camel's nose" involves pulling the anterior breast up and out and supporting it during the initial stage of compression. The mammographer should use one hand to maintain support of the breast until enough compression is in place to keep the breast in position (Figure 6-28).[4]

111. **(C)** With the 4 quadrants terminology, the breast can be described as UOQ, UIQ, LOQ, and LIQ. The exact locations within the

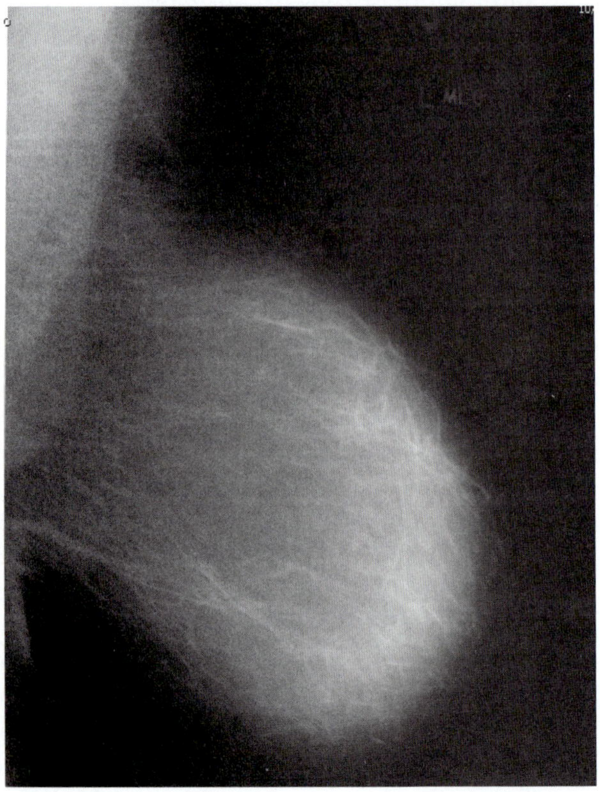

Figure 6-28. Poor compression of the anterior breast in the MLO projection results in drooping of the anterior breast "camel nose." (Reproduced with permission from Peart O: Lange Q&A: Mammography Examination, 2nd ed. New York, NY: McGraw-Hill Education; 2008.)

quadrant are represented by viewing each breast separately as a clock face. The SIO best demonstrates the UIQ and the LOQ of the breast, free of superimposition. This projection can be used to demonstrate these quadrants free of the implant especially when using the implant-displaced ID or Eklund compression techniques. (See Figure 6-26.)[4]

112. (D) The medical audit is used to check the reliability of the mammographic image. As per the MQSA each facility must establish and maintain a system to track positive mammographic findings and to correlate such findings with the biopsy results the facility obtains on an annual basis. This is the medical audit. At a minimum, the system must track all positive mammographic findings which can include "suspicious" or "highly suggestive of malignancy." Each facility can set up and maintain a tracking system that works best for it but the system must include a set of procedures to track mammograms, determine whether biopsies were done on the patient, determine whether the biopsy specimen was benign or malignant, and report this information back to the interpreting physician. The system must also include patients whose cancers not initially detected by the mammogram. The audit analysis must be initiated within 12 months after the date the facility becomes certified and must be conducted and reviewed by the interpreting physician at least once every 12 months.[30]

113. (B) The MQSA requires facilities to maintain records of the original mammograms and reports for a period of not less than 5 years and not less than 10 years if no additional mammograms of the patient are performed at the facility. Some state and local laws may require longer storage times. Facilities are also allowed to permanently or temporarily transfer a patient's records to another medical institution, physician, or healthcare provider if requested by the patient.[30]

114. (C) Triangulation is used to determine the location of a nonpalpable lesion seen mammographically. After triangulation the lesion can be spot compressed or magnified. Triangulation could also be used to determine the shortest skin-to-abnormality distance for the purpose of stereotactic biopsy. To determine the location of the lesion relative to the nipple, the mammographer should measure (1) the distance from the nipple to the level of the lesion posteriorly on the CC or MLO projection, (2) from that level to the lesion in the superior-to-inferior (as on the MLO) or medial-to-lateral direction (as on the CC), and (3) from the lesion to the skin surface (Figure 6-29).[4]

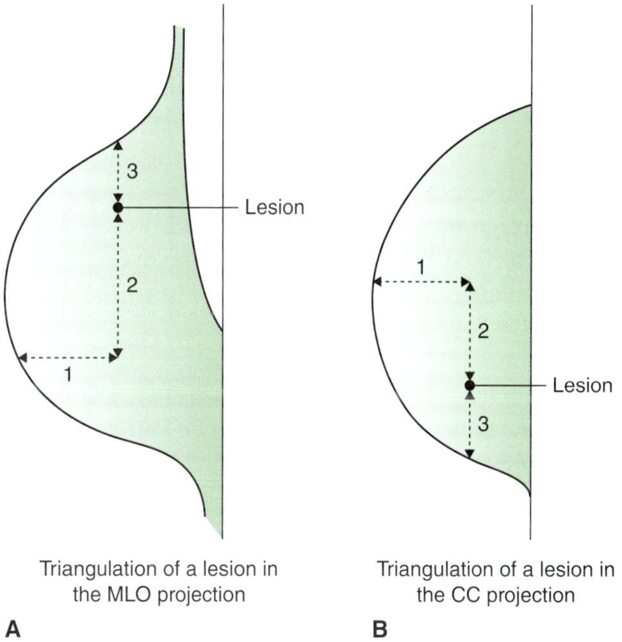

Figure 6-29. The triangulation technique is used to determine the shortest skin-to-abnormality distance in the (A) MLO and (B) CC projections. 1 = distance from nipple to the level of the lesion posteriorly, 2 = distance from level to lesion, 3 = distance from lesion to skin surface.

115. (D) Peau d'orange describes the skin of the breast wherein the breast skin thickens and resembles an orange. The condition occurs secondary to obstruction of the axillary lymphatics and may be a result of either benign or malignant conditions such as inflammatory carcinoma. Plasma cell mastitis or ductal ectasia are both inflammatory conditions. Plasma cell mastitis calcifications follow the course of the ducts. Some may be elongated and branching, some needle-like, and some ring-like or oval, but all are sharply outlined, high density, and have smooth borders. If they are periductal, they have central lucencies. Ductal ectasia involves the lactiferous ducts and may or may not cause nipple discharge or inversion. Both conditions are characterized by the presence of plasma cells surrounding a dilated duct. (See Figure 3-19.)[13,14]

References

1. American Cancer Society: Early Detection, Diagnosis, and Staging. Can breast cancer be found early? http://www.cancer.org/cancer/breastcancer/detailedguide/breast-cancer-detection. Last Review 01/31/2014. Accessed March 14, 2014.
2. Peart O. Treatment options. In: *Mammography and Breast Imaging: Prep*. New York, NY: McGraw-Hill; 2012:397-432.
3. American Cancer Society: Causes, Risk Factors and Prevention. What are the risk factors for breast cancer? http://www.cancer.org/cancer/breastcancer/detailedguide/breast-cancer-risk-factors. Last Medical Review: 01/14/2014. Accessed March 14, 2014.
4. Peart O. Breast imaging mammography. In: *Mammography and Breast Imaging: Prep*. New York, NY: McGraw-Hill; 2012:213-262.
5. Andolina VF, Lille SL, Willison KM. The mammogram. In: *Mammographic Imaging: A Practical Guide*. 3rd ed. Philadelphia, PA: Lippincott Williams & Wilkins; 2010:119-274.
6. Bushong SC. Advanced x-ray imaging. In: *Radiologic Science for Technologists—Physics, Biology and Protection*. 10th ed. St. Louis, MO: Mosby; 2004: 371-384.
7. Fostbinder R, Orth D. Special imaging techniques. In: *Essentials of Radiologic Science*. Philadelphia, PA: Lippincott Williams & Wilkins; 2012: 204-252.
8. Peart O. Breast imaging digital mammography, ultrasound and MRI. In: *Mammography and Breast Imaging: Prep*. New York, NY: McGraw-Hill; 2012:263-332.
9. Bushberg JT, Seibert JA, Meidholdt EM, Boone JM. Mammography. In: *The essential physics of medical imaging*. 3rd ed. Philadelphia, PA: Lippincott Williams & Wilkins; 2012:238-281.
10. Papp J. Mammography quality standards. In: *Quality Management in the Imaging Sciences*. 3rd ed. St. Louis, MO: Mosby; 2006:195-229.
11. Peart O. Breast anatomy, physiology and pathology of the breast. In: *Mammography and Breast Imaging: Prep*. New York, NY: McGraw-Hill; 2012:263-332.
12. Tortora GJ, Derrickson B. The reproductive systems. In: *Principles of Anatomy and Physiology*. 12th ed. New York, NY: John Wiley & Sons; 2009:1110-1112.
13. Peart O. Breast benign and malignant diseases of the breast. In: *Mammography and Breast Imaging: Prep*. New York, NY: McGraw-Hill; 2012:263-332.
14. Venes D, Biderman A, Adler E. *Taber's Cyclopedic Medical Dictionary*. 21st ed. Philadelphia, PA: F.A. Davis; 2005:1-2518.
15. Tabár L, Dean PB. Circular/oval lesion. In: *Teaching Atlas of Mammography*. 4th ed. New York, NY: Thieme; 2011:17-92.
16. Peart O. Mammography equipment. In: *Mammography and Breast Imaging: Prep*. New York, NY: McGraw-Hill; 2012:117-156.
17. Bushong SC. The radiographic image. In: *Radiologic Science for Technologists—Physics, Biology and Protection*. 10th ed. St. Louis, MO: Mosby; 2004: 161-264.
18. Fostbinder R, Orth D. Special imaging techniques. In: *Essentials of Radiologic Science*. Philadelphia, PA: Lippincott Williams & Wilkins; 2012:92-183.
19. Peart O. Interventional procedures. In: *Mammography and Breast Imaging: Prep*. New York, NY: McGraw-Hill; 2012:363-396.
20. Andolina VF, Lille SL, Willison KM. Special procedures. In: *Mammographic Imaging: A Practical Guide*. 3rd ed. Philadelphia, PA: Lippincott Williams & Wilkins; 2010:275-284.
21. Peart O. Patient education and assessment. In: *Mammography and Breast Imaging: Prep*. New York, NY: McGraw-Hill; 2012:23-64.
22. Peart O. The US Mammography Quality Standard Act (MQSA). In: *Mammography and Breast Imaging: Prep*. New York, NY: McGraw-Hill; 2012:437-500.
23. Hologic Inc. Selenia Dimensions with acquisition workstation 8000. Product and Clinical Education Training manuals. Courtesy of Hologic Inc. www.hologic.com. Acquired December 2013.
24. Bushberg JT, Seibert JA, Meidholdt EM, Boone JM. Image quality. In: *The Essential Physics of Medical Imaging*. 3rd ed. Philadelphia, PA: Lippincott Williams & Wilkins; 2012:60-100.
25. Bushong SC. The digital radiographic image. In: *Radiologic Science for Technologists—Physics, Biology and Protection*. 10th ed. St. Louis, MO: Mosby; 2004:265-332.
26. Bushong SC. X-radiation. In: *Radiologic Science for Technologists—Physics, Biology and Protection*. 10th ed. St. Louis, MO: Mosby; 2004:83-160.
27. Fostbinder R, Orth D. Circuits and x-ray production. In: *Essentials of Radiologic Science*. Philadelphia, PA: Lippincott Williams & Wilkins; 2012:45-91.

28. Tabár L, Dean PB. Calcifications on mammogram. In: *Teaching Atlas of Mammography*. 4th ed. New York, NY: Thieme; 2011:149-238.
29. Peart O. Breast imaging emerging modalities. In: *Mammography and Breast Imaging: Prep*. New York, NY: McGraw-Hill; 2012:333-362.
30. FDA U.S. Food And Drug Administration. Policy Guidance Help System. http://www.fda.gov/Radiation-EmittingProducts/MammographyQualityStandardsActandProgram/Guidance/PolicyGuidanceHelpSystem/default.htm#Quality. Last Update March 20, 2013. Accessed March 22, 2014.

CHAPTER 7

Practice Test 2

Questions

1. A clinical breast examination (CBE) and breast self-examination (BSE) are similar in that both

   (A) involve looking and feeling for changes in the breast
   (B) are done by a trained medical professional
   (C) are done monthly
   (D) are done yearly

2. The most common cause of undercompression is

   (A) a faulty compression paddle
   (B) inadequate compression by the mammographer
   (C) patient pain tolerance level
   (D) broken automatic compression device

3. The Health Insurance Portability and Accountability Act (HIPAA) of 1996 affects radiology and other hospital departments by its focus on

   (A) patient record confidentiality
   (B) facility reimbursement
   (C) quality management
   (D) risk management

4. Ductal papilloma is

   (A) a benign proliferation of tissue in the male breast
   (B) a malignant tumor involving the ducts
   (C) a collection of blood in the breast, which can occur after surgery
   (D) benign growths involving the milk ducts

5. The right craniocaudal (RCC) of the routine imaging series showed a small, irregular-shaped lesion at posterior margin of the image plus scattered calcifications including calcification clusters (Figure 7-1). Typically, the radiologist will recommend _______ as the next immediate step.

   (A) ultrasound to assess the content of the lesion and provide an analysis of the calcifications
   (B) spot compression including magnification to assess calcifications and the margins of the lesion
   (C) magnetic resonance imaging (MRI) to assess for malignancy and to assess any calcifications
   (D) a breast biopsy to check for malignancy

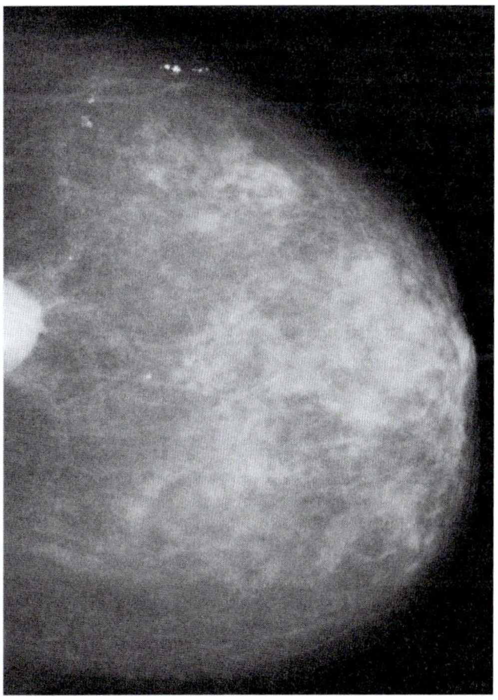

Figure 7-1.

6. A bunch of 8 bits equals 1
   (A) pixel
   (B) byte
   (C) matrix
   (D) bit depth

7. Which of the following could be used when imaging extremely small breasts in the craniocaudal (CC) position?
   (A) spatula
   (B) mediolateral (ML)
   (C) cleavage view (CV)
   (D) exaggerated craniocaudal (XCCL)

8. In the tangential (TAN) projection, any tube angulation will depend on
   (A) the size of the patient's breast
   (B) the location of the abnormality
   (C) the position of the midaxillary line in relation to the detector
   (D) whether the abnormality is palpable or nonpalpable

9. A small but growing cancer may not be obvious to the individual because it often presents as
   (A) skin irritation
   (B) inverted nipples
   (C) a painless mass
   (D) a painful mass

10. Mammography is more accurate in
    (A) premenopausal women
    (B) postmenopausal women
    (C) women with fibrocystic breast
    (D) women with dense breast tissue

11. In taking medical history, hormone use (both natural and artificial) are taken into account because
    (A) hormones cause breast cancer
    (B) early menarche can increase breast cancer risks
    (C) late menarche can increase breast cancer risks
    (D) contraceptive use lower the risks for breast cancer

12. One major difference between collimation in mammography and collimation in general radiography is that
    (A) in mammography the entire detector area is exposed
    (B) decreasing collimation increases exposure in mammography
    (C) mammography uses a variety of beam-limiting devices
    (D) in radiography the entire detector area is always exposed

13. Line pair per millimeter is the unit of
    (A) matrix size
    (B) spatial resolution
    (C) field-of-view (FOV)
    (D) bit depth

14. Image brightness is adjusted changing by changing the
    (A) milliamperes (mAs)
    (B) peak kilovoltage (kVp)
    (C) window level
    (D) window width

15. The retromammary space is filled with
    (A) supportive and connecting tissue
    (B) adipose tissue
    (C) fibroglandular tissue
    (D) blood vessels

16. The fatty versus fibroglandular nature of breast tissue is affected by which of the following?

    (A) age
    (B) hormone use
    (C) number of pregnancies
    (D) all of the above

17. In positioning for the exaggerated craniocaudal (XCCL) projection, if the shoulder of the affected side is in the way of the compression device

    (A) push the shoulder down
    (B) a 5-degree lateral tube angulation can be utilized
    (C) use 5-degree medial tube angulation to avoid superposing the shoulder on breast tissue
    (D) reduce the patient's lateral rotation

18. In the craniocaudal (CC) position the pectoral muscle is seen

    (A) all the time
    (B) rarely if ever
    (C) about 30%-40% of the time
    (D) about 50% of the time

19. Between ages 20 and 39, a woman should have a clinical breast examination (CBE) every

    (A) year
    (B) 2 years
    (C) 3 years
    (D) 4 years

20. The lesion seen in Figure 7-2 is not palpable and is not associated with nipple or skin changes. It has the characteristics of a/an

    (A) invasive ductal breast carcinoma
    (B) mammographically malignant tumor
    (C) mammographically benign tumor
    (D) nonspecific lesion; further testing is indicated

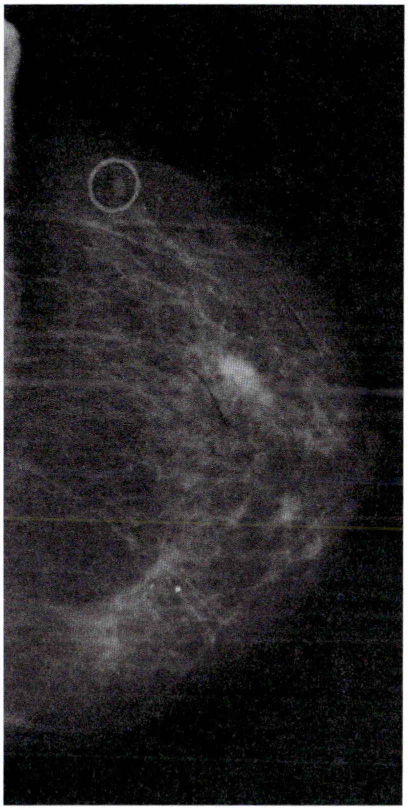

Figure 7-2.

21. Regardless of the reason, if the proper amount of compression cannot be applied which of the following *must* apply?

    (A) The patient must be told.
    (B) The patient's doctor must be told.
    (C) The radiologist must be told.
    (D) It must be noted on the patient's history form.

22. On the craniocaudal (CC) image the posterior nipple line (PNL) line should extend to the

    (A) level of the nipple
    (B) posterior breast or edge of the image
    (C) level of the inframammary crease
    (D) most anterior breast

23. The interspace material of the mammography linear grid is generally made of
    (A) carbon or wood
    (B) aluminum
    (C) any high radiopaque material
    (D) lead

24. Which section of the breast is poorly visualized on the craniocaudal (CC) projection?
    (A) medial
    (B) axial
    (C) lateral
    (D) superior

25. Figure 7-3 shows a radiograph of the left mediolateral oblique (LMLO). Why should this radiograph be repeated? The patient and mammographer's identification plus the projection has been removed to avoid Health Insurance Portability and Accountability Act (HIPAA) violations.
    (A) The pectoral muscle should be concave anteriorly.
    (B) The pectoral muscle should be convex anteriorly.
    (C) The inframammary fold is closed.
    (D) The posterior breast tissue is missing.

26. Increasing the image contrast is achieved by
    (A) increasing window level
    (B) decreasing window level
    (C) increasing window width
    (D) decreasing window width

27. Which projection could be used to demonstrate a deep medial lesion not seen on the craniocaudal (CC)?
    (A) axillary tail (AT)
    (B) exaggerated craniocaudal (XCCL)
    (C) cleavage view (CV)
    (D) mediolateral oblique (MLO)

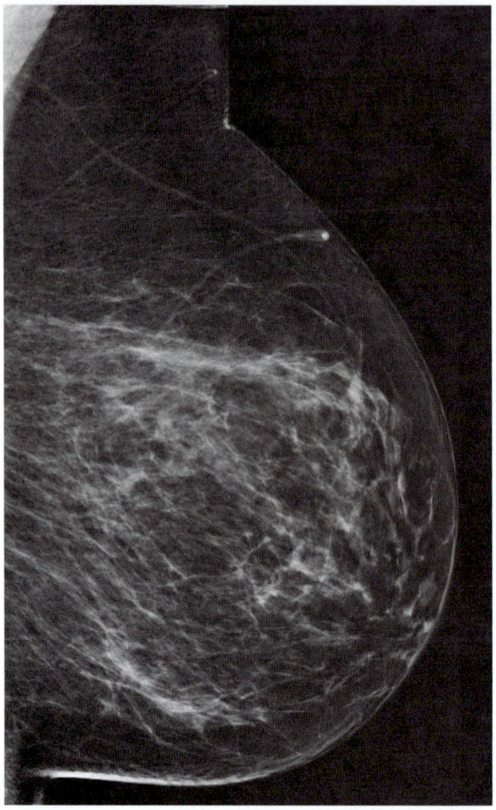

Figure 7-3.

28. After a routine 4-projection mammographic series, the nipple is not seen in profile on any of the images. Additional projections are done if
    1. the nipple is indistinguishable from a mass
    2. a subareolar abnormality is suspected
    3. the nipple is not marked with a BB (lead shot)
    (A) 1 and 2 only
    (B) 2 and 3 only
    (C) 1 and 3 only
    (D) 1, 2, and 3

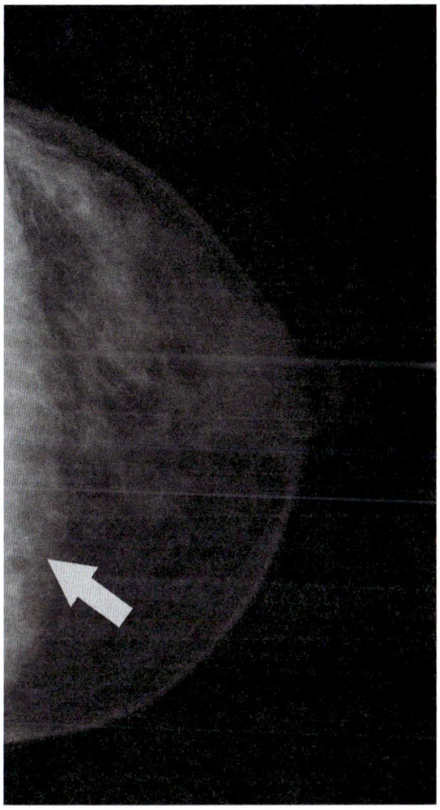

Figure 7-4.

29. On the radiograph, Figure 7-4, the arrow indicates

    (A) a malignant lesion
    (B) glandular tissue
    (C) muscle
    (D) fatty tissue

30. Your patient's sister was diagnosed with breast cancer at age 35. Your patient is considered to have

    (A) a greater risk for breast cancer
    (B) a lower risk for breast cancer
    (C) no significantly increased risk for breast cancer
    (D) a personal history of breast cancer

31. The Mammography Quality Standards Act (MQSA) mandates that the average glandular dose received per projection/position during routine mammography screening should not exceed

    (A) 1 mGy (100 mrad)
    (B) 2 mGy (200 mrad)
    (C) 3 mGy (300 mrad)
    (D) 4 mGy (400 mrad)

32. The device used to convert films in an analog imaging system to a digital version is called

    (A) film digitizer
    (B) Digital Imaging and Communications in Medicine (DICOM)
    (C) analog-to-digital converter (ADC)
    (D) digital-to-analog converter (DAC)

33. The computer network that allows images to be viewed at various monitors or transmitted or stored is termed

    (A) local area network (LAN)
    (B) picture archiving and communications system (PACS)
    (C) Digital Imaging and Communications in Medicine (DICOM)
    (D) wide area network (WAN)

34. Which of the following statement on heath-care records is *false?*

    (A) Health records must include all signed informed consent forms.
    (B) Patients have a right to amend their health-care records.
    (C) Patients can access their health records.
    (D) Health-care records cannot be used in a court of law.

35. Montgomery glands are specialized

    (A) sweat glands
    (B) sebaceous gland
    (C) Cooper ligaments
    (D) hair follicles

36. A woman taking estrogen replacement therapy may notice changes in the breast such as
    (A) breast enlargement
    (B) increase in fibroadenomas
    (C) increase in breast cysts
    (D) all of the above

37. Paget disease of the breast is a (an)
    (A) infiltrating carcinoma generally limited to the breast
    (B) form of carcinoma associated with changes of the nipple
    (C) benign breast condition that is relatively common
    (D) malignant form of breast carcinoma involving the lobules

38. In a digital image what determines the matrix size?
    (A) the number of bit in each pixel
    (B) the number of pixels in the rows and columns
    (C) the picture element in the matrix
    (D) the number of gray shades that a pixel can produce

39. A set of computer software standards that permits a wide range of digital imaging programs to understand each other
    (A) DIGCOM
    (B) PACS
    (C) DICOM
    (D) PCAS

40. Picture archiving and communications system (PACS) network typically would include
    (A) digital images from multiple modalities
    (B) images from a single modality only
    (C) all patients' records
    (D) surgical and radiography patient records

41. Women who were exposed to diethylstilbestrol (DES) in utero may have
    (A) a lower risk for breast cancer
    (B) a higher breast cancer risk if they also take HRT
    (C) a lower risk for breast cancer if they also take HRT
    (D) breast tissue that is extra sensitive to radiation

42. In which of the following modified projections is the superior surface of the breast rolled medially?
    (A) medial roll (RM)
    (B) lateral roll (RL)
    (C) medial (M)
    (D) lateromedial (LM)

43. Factors that lower breast cancer risk include
    1. having your first child after age 30
    2. breast-feeding your child
    3. late menarche
        (A) 1 and 2 only
        (B) 2 and 3 only
        (C) 1 and 3 only
        (D) 1, 2, and 3

44. PACS stands for
    (A) picture access to communication system
    (B) picture archiving and computer systems
    (C) picture archiving and communication system
    (D) pixel access and computer systems

45. The computer processing or photostimulable phosphor (PSP) reader functions to
    (A) focus a beam of infrared light on the PSP
    (B) trap excited electrons at a higher energy level
    (C) scan, read, and erase the exposed PSP
    (D) provide energy to the trapped electrons

46. Gynecomastia defines

(A) a localized abscess
(B) increased breast tissue in the male breast
(C) decreased breast tissue in the female breast
(D) a risk of carcinoma for the male patient

47. Photostimulable luminescence (PSL) is

(A) emission of bluish-purple light from electrons as they transition from higher energy to a lower energy state
(B) conversion of light energy to an electrical signal by the photomultiplier tube (PMT)
(C) conversion the analog signal to a digital signal by the analog-to-digital converter (ADC)
(D) conversion light into an analog signal by the charge-coupled device (CCD)

48. According to Mammography Quality Standards Act (MQSA) regulations, which of the following is not required on the final mammographic image?

(A) date of the examination
(B) technical factors used
(C) mammographer/technologist identification
(D) projection identification

49. The inframammary crease is located at approximately the level of the

(A) second to third rib
(B) third to fourth rib
(C) fourth to fifth rib
(D) sixth to seventh rib

50. Identify Cooper ligament in Figure 7-5.

(A) site A
(B) site B
(C) site C
(D) site D

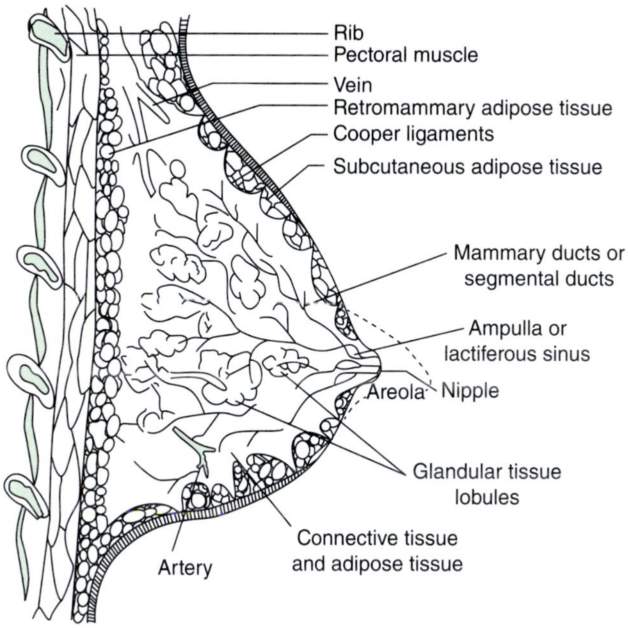

Figure 7-5. (Reproduced with permission from Peart O: Lange Q&A: Mammography Examination, 2nd ed. New York, NY: McGraw-Hill Education; 2008.)

51. Identify the lactiferous sinus in Figure 7-5.

(A) site A
(B) site B
(C) site C
(D) site D

52. Scattered radiation is reduced during magnification mammography by

(A) using a small focal spot size
(B) using a grid
(C) using the air-gap technique
(D) increasing the source-to-image receptor distance (SID)

53. Ductography can be used to determine

(A) the location of the lesions in the ducts
(B) if a lesion is benign or malignant
(C) changes or abnormalities associated with the ducts
(D) more than 1 of the above

54. When imaging small breasts a useful option is
    (A) replacing the craniocaudal (CC) with the exaggerated craniocaudal (XCCL)
    (B) using the mediolateral (ML) instead of the mediolateral oblique (MLO)
    (C) using a spatula to avoid compressing fingers
    (D) reducing the angulation to avoid compressing too much pectoral muscle

55. During magnification, positioning the breast away from the detector utilizes which law/principle in scatter reduction?
    (A) inverse-square law
    (B) reciprocity law
    (C) heel effect
    (D) line-focus principle

56. A woman who is nulliparous has a lower risk for breast cancer than a woman with
    (A) late menopause
    (B) late menarche
    (C) a personal history of breast cancer
    (D) early menarche

57. The primary purpose of the grid in mammography is to
    (A) improve image sharpness
    (B) reduce the production of scatter
    (C) reduce patient dose
    (D) increase the subject contrast

58. The implant-displaced (ID) projection is possible on all of the following cases *except*
    (A) implants placed posterior to the pectoral muscle
    (B) implants placed anterior to the pectoral muscle
    (C) soft implants
    (D) encapsulated implants

59. A palpable mass that is not seen on a diagnostic mammogram generally means
    (A) breast cancer is ruled out; the mass is probably benign
    (B) other diagnostic testing must be considered
    (C) the mass is likely breast cancer
    (D) the mass is likely caused by fluctuating hormones

60. Which of the following patients has the greatest risk for breast cancer?
    (A) a nulliparous woman at age 40
    (B) a never married woman
    (C) a woman, age 70
    (D) a woman, age 30

61. A mammographer using a 0.1-mm focal spot size is most likely performing
    (A) routine mammography work
    (B) magnification imaging
    (C) spot compression imaging
    (D) stereotactic work

62. Which of the following patients cannot give consent?
    (A) minor who is married
    (B) minor serving in the military
    (C) competent adult
    (D) mentally challenged adult

63. In the photostimulable phosphor (PSP) computer reader the photomultiplier tube
    (A) collects the blue/purple light given off by the trapped electrons
    (B) scans the PSP with a red laser light
    (C) provides energy to the trapped electrons in the phosphor layer
    (D) erases the PSP by releasing electrons

64. Which of the following statements is true when imaging the breast?
    (A) Fold and or wrinkles should be eliminated by pushing the fold or wrinkle posteriorly.
    (B) Skin folds or wrinkles may be impossible to avoid in the elderly.
    (C) When imaging the elderly the study will always be compromised by a fold or wrinkle.
    (D) Fold and or wrinkles can be eliminated by pulling the fold or wrinkle anteriorly.

65. The base of the breast refers to the
    (A) the nipple area of the areola
    (B) areas adjacent to the chest wall
    (C) axilla area of the breast
    (D) lower outer quadrant of the breast

66. Fibrous tissues are presented radiographically as
    (A) black or radiolucent areas
    (B) gray and less dense areas
    (C) white or denser areas
    (D) black and less dense areas

67. The calcifications in Figure 7-6 are characteristic of
    (A) invasive ductal carcinoma
    (B) mammographically malignant calcifications
    (C) calcifications due to plasma cell mastitis
    (D) numerous oil cysts

68. The mediolateral oblique (MLO) projection demonstrates a large encapsulated lesion occupying almost the entire breast. The contour is sharp and the lesion is radiolucent. This lesion is most likely to be a (an)
    (A) oil cyst
    (B) hematoma
    (C) fibroadenoma
    (D) lipoma

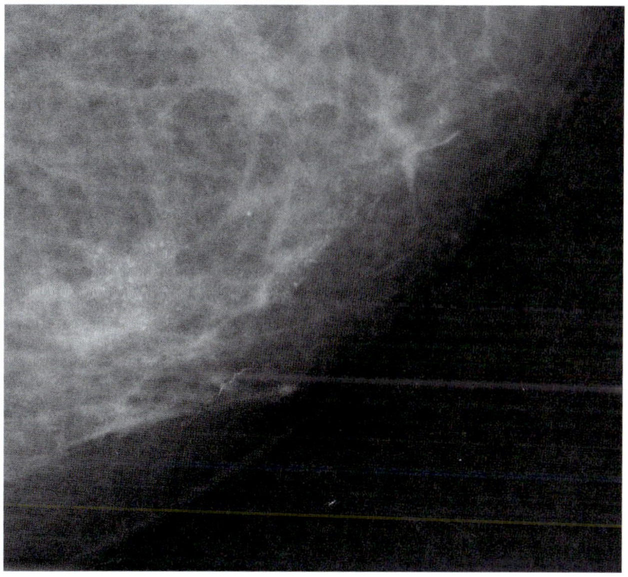

Figure 7-6.

69. The latent image on the photostimulable phosphor (PSP) can last several hours but will lose
    (A) 50% of its energy in 4 hours
    (B) 50% of its energy in 8 hours
    (C) 25% of its energy in 4 hours
    (D) 25% of its energy in 8 hours

70. Disadvantages of photostimulable phosphor (PSP) or computed mammography (CM) technology includes
    (A) reduced repeats
    (B) wide latitude and dynamic range of the system
    (C) the PSPs sensitively to radiation
    (D) speed of the imaging system

71. In the nonscintillator direct based flat-panel digital mammography (DM) system, the x-ray beam strikes a/an
    (A) scintillator
    (B) photoconductor
    (C) thin-film transistor
    (D) photomultiplier

72. Spot compression
    1. applies more compression to a localized area
    2. can be performed with magnification
    3. employs a coned collimated field to limit the area of interest
    (B) 1 only
    (C) 1 and 2 only
    (D) 2 and 3 only
    (E) 1, 2, and 3

73. Identify the minus density structure shown in the middle of the breast on Figure 7-7.
    (A) closed inframammary fold
    (B) skin fold
    (C) pectoralis muscle
    (D) vein

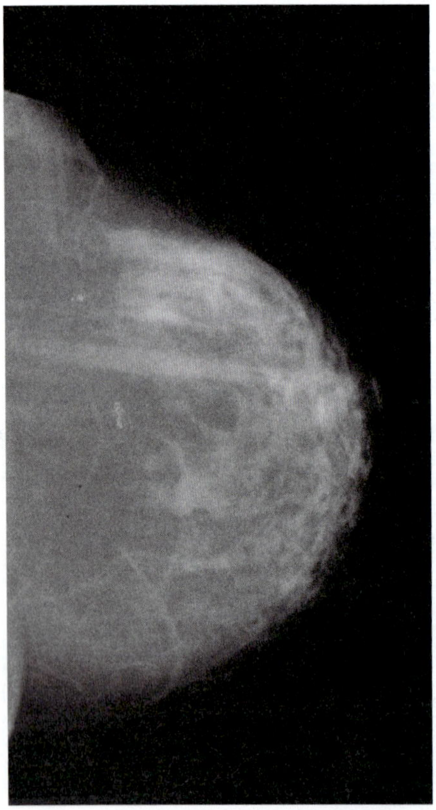

Figure 7-7.

74. To reduce the possibility of projecting the abdomen on the mediolateral oblique (MLO) image, the mammographer could
    (A) have the patient stand just at the detector and bend back
    (B) have the patient stand away from the detector and bend forward
    (C) have the patient turn medially to image the lateral breast on the craniocaudal (CC)
    (D) discard the MLO and image the breast in the lateral position instead

75. A 4-projection mammography series shows a solitary tumor, with the halo sign, in the upper-outer quadrant (UOQ) of the left breast. The lesion is partially obscured. The next recommended step is
    (A) biopsy
    (B) ultrasound
    (C) stereotactic localization
    (D) aspiration

76. Why is the specimen magnified?
    (A) to ensure that the lesion has been completely removed
    (B) to visualize the calcifications within the specimen
    (C) to compare the magnified and nonmagnified images
    (D) to check the number and placement of calcifications

77. In digital mammography, a grossly underexposed image
    (A) appears excessively noisy
    (B) is too light
    (C) is too dark
    (D) appears correctly exposed

78. Which of the following patients is likely to be diagnosed with pathological gynecomastia?

(A) lactating woman
(B) elderly man
(C) premenopausal woman
(D) young man

79. Montgomery glands are located on the breast's

(A) skin
(B) nipple
(C) areola
(D) muscle

80. Aluminum can be used as the filtration material in

(A) digital units when imaging dense breast
(B) digital tomosynthesis units
(C) digital units when imaging fatty breast
(D) analog units with tungsten targets

81. Digital mammography units often use _____ as the target material.

(A) molybdenum
(B) rhodium
(C) aluminum
(D) tungsten

82. Over age 40, it is recommended that women have a clinical breast examination (CBE) every

(A) year
(B) 2 years
(C) 3 years
(D) 4 years

83. When imaging the breast using the craniocaudal (CC) projection, if the detector is too high or too low the inframammary fold (IMF) will be over or under elevated. Over elevation of the IMF will result in

(A) loss of posterior and superior breast tissue
(B) loss of anterior and posterior breast tissue
(C) loss of superior and posterior breast tissue
(D) loss of inferior and posterior breast tissue

84. Capture elements in the flat-panel detector system can include all of the following *except*

(A) photomultiplier
(B) cesium iodide
(C) gadolinium oxysulfide
(D) amorphous selenium

85. Which of the following involves the use of a small-gauge needle to remove cell samples from a suspected cancerous lesion in the breast for cytological analysis?

(A) core biopsy
(B) excisional biopsy
(C) needle localization
(D) fine-needle biopsy (FNB)

86. A lesion is superimposed by breast tissue in the craniocaudal (CC) projection. A projection/position used to demonstrate the lesion in the same orientation but free of superimposition is the

(A) mediolateral oblique (MLO)
(B) implant-displaced (ID)
(C) exaggerated craniocaudal (XCCL)
(D) medial roll (RM)

87. In imaging the breast in the mediolateral oblique (MLO) projection, compression to the lower, anterior portion of the breast is compromised if

(A) the detector is too high
(B) the pectoral muscle extends to the nipple line
(C) too much axilla and shoulder are under compression
(D) the inframammary fold is not horizontal

88. Involution of the breast describes a process by which

(A) milk is removed from the breast by suckling
(B) breast epithelium proliferates during menstruation
(C) the glandular tissue in the breast is replaced by fat
(D) estrogen use causes an overall density decrease in the breast

89. In imaging the breast for the craniocaudal (CC) projection, what technique is used to minimize skin folds in the lateral aspect of the breast?

(A) Lift the posterior lateral aspect of the breast onto the detector.
(B) Drape the contralateral breast over the corners of the detector.
(C) Have the patient's head turned facing the ipsilateral breast.
(D) On the side being imaged, the patient's arm hangs relaxed with humerus externally rotated.

90. Phosphor crystals in the flat-panel detector system are classified as _______ phosphors when they are scattered through the phosphor level.

(A) needle
(B) turbid
(C) amorphous
(D) selenium

91. Grid use in magnification mammography is contraindicated because

(A) the use of a grid will increase subject contrast
(B) scatter is already minimized
(C) grid use increase scatter
(D) grids would result in decrease subject contrast

92. The breast can be imaged in the from below (FB) projection

(A) to improve visualization of lesions in uppermost aspect of breast by reducing object-to-image receptor distance (OID)
(B) during needle localization to provide a shorter route to inferior lesions
(C) to maximize the amount of tissue visualized in patients with kyphosis
(D) all of the above

93. Figure 7-8 shows a radiograph of the right mediolateral oblique (RMLO). What major problem makes this radiograph suboptimal? The patient and mammographer's identification plus the projection has been removed to avoid Health Insurance Portability and Accountability Act (HIPAA) violations.

(A) The skin marker does not fully cover the skin lesion.
(B) The posterior breast is not imaged.
(C) There is a skin fold in the posterior area of the breast.
(D) The inframammary fold is missing.

94. Which statement *best* describes a parallel or linear grid?

(A) Lead strips are aligned adjacent to one another and placed lengthwise in the same direction within the structure of the grid.
(B) Lead strips are aligned at right angles to each other.
(C) Lead strips are designed to take advantage of the divergence of the x-ray beam as it leaves the x-ray tube.
(D) Lead strips are designed to move during the exposure.

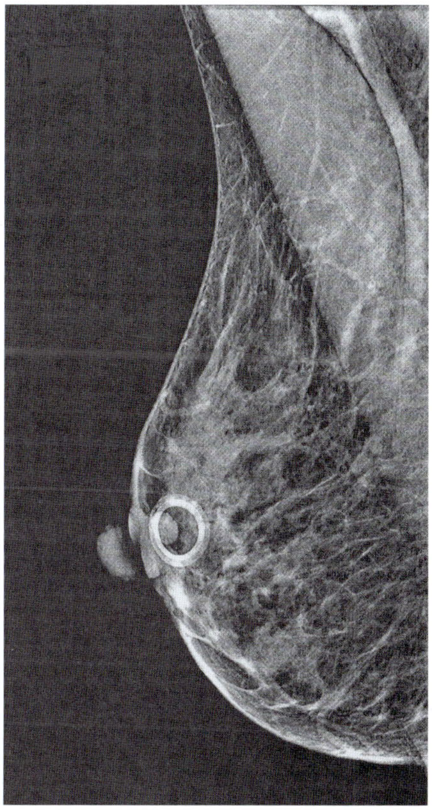

Figure 7-8.

95. The charge-coupled device (CCD) serves to convert
    - (A) x-rays to light
    - (B) x-rays to electrons
    - (C) light to electrons
    - (D) electrons to light

96. The scintillators are used to convert
    - (A) x-rays to light
    - (B) x-rays to electrons
    - (C) light to electrons
    - (D) electrons to light

97. The photoconductor in the direct digital radiography system is used to convert
    - (A) x-rays to light
    - (B) x-rays to electrons
    - (C) light to electrons
    - (D) electrons to light

98. The repeat rate should be analyzed if the rate changes from the previous measure rate by more than
    - (A) ±2% points
    - (B) ±3% points
    - (C) ±4% points
    - (D) ±5% points

99. A magnification image of a breast shows several oval-shaped radiolucent lesions with eggshell-like calcifications. These are most likely to be
    - (A) ductal papilloma
    - (B) fibroadenomas
    - (C) oil cysts
    - (D) hematomas

100. The thin-film transistor (TFT) in the flat-panel detector systems collects
    - (A) light
    - (B) pixels
    - (C) electrons
    - (D) x-rays

101. In general, the implant-displaced (ID) series are taken using the
    - (A) axillary tail (AT) and mediolateral oblique (MLO) projections
    - (B) craniocaudal (CC) and ML projections
    - (C) CC and MLO projections
    - (D) CC and lateromedial (LM) projections

102. Today all mammographers (technologists or radiographers performing mammograms independently) must have
    - (A) satisfied the final requirements of the Food and Drug Administration (FDA)
    - (B) completed at least 20 hours of documented training in mammography
    - (C) performed at least 75 examinations under direct supervision of a qualified mammographer
    - (D) none of the above

103. The criteria for a properly positioned mediolateral oblique (MLO) includes
   1. a concave pectoral muscle on the anterior border
   2. fat visualized posterior to the fibroglandular tissues
   3. an open inframammary fold (IMF)
      (A) 1 and 2 only
      (B) 2 and 3 only
      (C) 1 and 3 only
      (D) 1, 2, and 3

104. A benign inflammatory condition of the lactiferous ducts leading to nipple discharge, nipple inversion, or periareolar sepsis is called
   (A) ductal ectasia
   (B) Paget disease of the breast
   (C) peau d'orange
   (D) ductal papilloma

105. The cells lining the alveoli in the lobules are called
   (A) epithelial cells
   (B) myoepithelial cells
   (C) basement cells
   (D) superficial cells

106. Informed consent implies that the patient
   1. has already signed the authorization for treatment
   2. was informed of the procedure or operation, its risks, possible consequences and any alternative options
   3. the patient was given information about the procedure in their language
      (A) 1 and 2 only
      (B) 2 and 3 only
      (C) 1 and 3 only
      (D) 1, 2, and 3

107. A technique describing reshaping of the breast is called
   (A) reduction mammoplasty
   (B) mammoplasty
   (C) breast augmentation
   (D) breast biopsy

108. Smaller pixels will result in
   (A) lower spatial resolution
   (B) lower image resolution
   (C) greater spatial resolution
   (D) greater image resolution

109. The detector elements (DELs) are located within the
   (A) scintillator
   (B) thin-film transistor (TFT)
   (C) charge-coupled device (CCD)
   (D) complementary metal-oxide silicon (CMOS)

110. In positioning for the superoinferior oblique (SIO), the ________ of the breast will rest on the detector.
   (A) lateral surface
   (B) superior surface
   (C) medial surface
   (D) inferior aspect

111. Imaging the craniocaudal (CC) projection in males will present the same difficulty as imaging small, firm-breasted females. An added problem may be that
   (A) males have more problems with the compression
   (B) the male breast is smaller than the smallest female breast
   (C) males have more muscular breast tissue
   (D) hair on the chest of males makes compression difficult

112. For the superoinferior oblique (SIO) projection, the central ray is directed

(A) inferolateral to superomedial
(B) superomedial to inferolateral
(C) inferomedial to superolateral
(D) superolateral to inferomedial

113. Which of the following are considered agencies granting accreditation under the Food and Drug Administration (FDA) regulation?

(A) State of California
(B) American College of Radiology (ACR)
(C) NY State Department of Health
(D) State of Florida

114. Which alternative projection could be used, in addition to the craniocaudal (CC), in imaging a patient with a prominent pacemaker?

(A) mediolateral (ML)
(B) lateromedial oblique (LMO)
(C) exaggerated craniocaudal (XCCL)
(D) mediolateral oblique (MLO)

115. The 2 main classifications of breast cancer are

(A) tubular and lobular
(B) lobular and medullary
(C) lobular and ductal
(D) inflammatory and ductal

116. In addition to the patient's name, all mammographic reports should have the

(A) final assessment of findings
(B) hospital number or additional patient identifier
(C) name of the radiologist
(D) all of the above

Answers and Explanations

1. **(A)** Both the clinical breast examination (CBE) and the breast self-examination (BSE) are examinations of the breast where changes in the shape, contour, and texture of the breast are assessed and the breast is checked for lumps. The CBE is performed by a health professional, whereas the BSE is performed by the woman on herself. The BSE should always be done monthly after age 20. The CBE is recommended every 3 years for those below 40 and every year for those older than 40.[1,2]

2. **(B)** Studies have shown that although there are many reasons for undercompression, the main reason is a lack of communication between the mammographer and the patient. The mammographer undercompresses the breast either because the patient refuses further compression, is unable to tolerate more compression, or the mammographer wants to "protect" the patient from further pain. Patients generally tolerate more compression if they fully understand the reason for the compression. Faulty or broken compression devices are generally easily repaired.[1,2]

3. **(A)** The Health Insurance Portability and Accountability Act of 1996 (HIPAA) are privacy rules that provide all patients with federal protections of their health information. It gives patients an array of rights with respect to their health records and monitors the disclosure of health information needed for patient care.[3]

4. **(D)** An intraductal papilloma generally occurs near the nipple within the larger ducts, but can also occur deep within the breast. The papilloma may produce spontaneous discharge from the nipple or if deep within the breast may appear radiographically as a mass. Ductal papillomas are benign and can be visualized with ductography or galactography. However, ultrasound is becoming the modality of choice when evaluating the ducts.[4,5]

5. **(B)** Further imaging depends on the preference of the radiologist. However, whenever possible, imaging should demonstrate a lesion in its entirety. Before moving to another modality, such as magnetic resonance imaging (MRI) or ultrasound, the radiologist is likely to recommend further mammography imaging such as spot compression to demonstrate the margins of the lesion and/or magnification to assess the calcifications. Also, MRI and ultrasound do not image calcifications well.[6,7]

6. **(B)** A digital image consists of a box of cells or picture elements (pixels) corresponding to numeric values arranged in rows and columns. Each pixel contains bits of information. The rows and columns form a matrix and each cell corresponds to a specific location in the image. The matrix size is determined by the number of pixels in the rows and columns. The bit depth is the number of gray shades that a pixel can produce. A bunch of 8 bits is a byte (Figure 7-9).[7,8]

7. **(A)** The spatula can be used instead of the mammographer's fingers to pull extremely small breasts into position for compression. The mediolateral (ML) is a lateral projection. Cleavage view (CV) images the extreme medial breast from the craniocaudal position and exaggerated craniocaudal (XCCL)

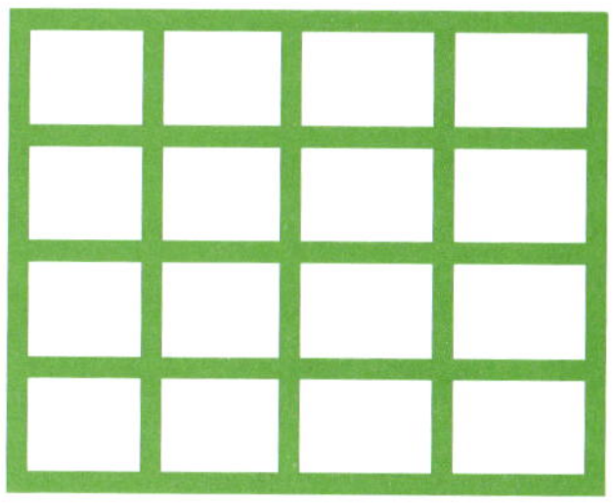

Figure 7-9. Schematic diagram of the matrix.

images the extreme lateral breast from the craniocaudal position.[9,10]

8. **(B)** In the tangential (TAN) projection, the technique is to take a skimming projection of the area of interest. Because the TAN can be taken in any projection, the degree of obliquity and the projection depends on the location of the abnormality. A BB marker can be used to establish the area of interest (Figure 7-10).[9,10]

9. **(C)** Although pain can be associated with breast cancer, a painless mass is the more common symptom of breast cancer. Painful masses are associated with cysts. Less common symptoms of advanced breast cancer include skin thickening, skin irritation or distortion, and sudden nipple inversion, discharge, erosion, or tenderness.[1,11]

10. **(B)** On average, a mammogram can detect up to 90% of breast cancers in women without symptoms and is more accurate in postmenopausal compared to premenopausal women. Some cancers are not visualized mammographically. The reasons are varied. The patient may have extremely dense breast or the mammogram may not be the best method of detection for a particular type of cancer. Poor imaging techniques by the mammographer and the interpretation skills of the radiologist can also be contributing factors.[1,11]

11. **(B)** Hormone use influences breast cancer risk, but does not actually cause breast cancer. All factors that increase the number of menstrual cycles in a woman's lifetime can increase the breast cancer risks.[1,11]

12. **(A)** In general, the use of any beam-limiting device in radiography or mammography requires increased exposure. Both imaging methods use varying sized beam-limiting devices. However, unlike general radiography where the beam should be limited to the size of the part, in mammography the entire field (not just the breast) is exposed. This was necessary to reduce extraneous light when viewing the analog image on the view box and the technique was not changed with digital.[6,7]

13. **(B)** The spatial resolution of a digital system is the minimum separation between 2 objects

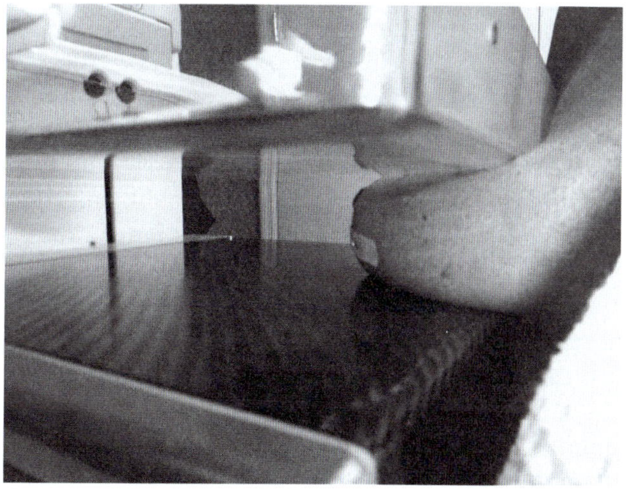

Figure 7-10. TAN.

at which they can be distinguished as 2 separate objects in the image. In digital imaging spatial resolution is determined by the pixel size. Smaller pixels have better spatial resolution. Spatial resolution is measured as line pairs per millimeter (lp/mm). The matrix size is determined by the number of pixels in the rows and columns. The bit depth is the number of gray shades that a pixel can produce. The field-of-view (FOV) sets the collimation for breast size and describes how much of the patient breast is imaged in the matrix.[7,8]

14. **(C)** In a digital imaging the term brightness replaces density. Brightness can be altered after the exposure. The controlling factors are milliamperes (mAs), processing software and predetermined digital algorithms. Increasing window level will increase brightness. Window width controls the black-and-white display therefore the contrast. Increasing window width will decrease contrast. The peak kilovoltage (kVp) plus processing software and digital algorithms will also be factors in controlling contrast.[7,8]

15. **(B)** The retromammary space separates the breast from the pectoral muscle. It is filled with a layer of adipose or fatty tissue as opposed to the supporting and connective tissue (stroma), blood vessels, and various ductal structures that make up the glandular and fibrous tissues of the breast.[12,13]

16. **(D)** Generally, glandular tissues predominate in younger women and adipose or fatty tissues in older patients. This ratio is not fixed, and depends on the woman's age and genetic predisposition. It fluctuates with hormone levels, whether the hormonal changes are caused by medication use, pregnancy, lactation, or menopause.[12,13]

17. **(B)** The purpose of the exaggerated craniocaudal (XCCL) projection is to image the lateral aspect of the breast. After positioning the patient for the craniocaudal (CC) projection, the patient is rotated to bring the outer lateral aspect of the breast on the detector. If the ipsilateral shoulder is in the way a 5-degree lateral tube angulation can be used to avoid superimposing of the humeral head on the breast. The ipsilateral arm should hang down and both shoulders should be at the same level. The patient can hold the support bars with the contralateral hand. Pushing the shoulders down will distort the lateral aspect of the breast (Figure 7-11).[9,10]

18. **(C)** Depending on patient body habitus, the pectoral muscle is imaged on the posterior aspect of the breast on about 30%-40% of all craniocaudal (CC) projections. It may be visualized unilaterally or bilaterally. Routine CC imaging that includes the pectoral muscle all the time can indicate faulty positioning with loss of medial or lateral breast tissue.[9,10]

19. **(C)** The American Cancer Society (ACS) guidelines for early detection of breast cancer include having a clinical breast examination (CBE) every 3 years between ages 20 and 39 and every year after age 40.[1,2]

20. **(D)** Whenever a large radiating structure or area of architectural distortion (even when superficial) is not associated with skin changes or nipple retraction, the mammogram is considered nonspecific. Further testing is indicated and a malignancy cannot be ruled out. Also, a definitive diagnosis such as benign lesion, invasive ductal carcinoma, or malignant tumor, can only be made after a biopsy. This lesion is a radial scar. Radial scars are complex sclerosing lesions. They are not truly scars and are often unrelated to prior surgery or trauma. Some possible causes of the radial scar are localized inflammatory reaction or chronic ischemia with a slow infection. The radial scar can be a benign condition, but can be associated with premalignant—atypical ductal hyperplasia—and malignant conditions. A benign radial scar has no central tumor, although there may be long spicules radiating from the center of the lesion. Regardless of the size of the spicules in the benign radial scar, there is no associated skin thickening, dimpling, or nipple reaction. Because of the possible

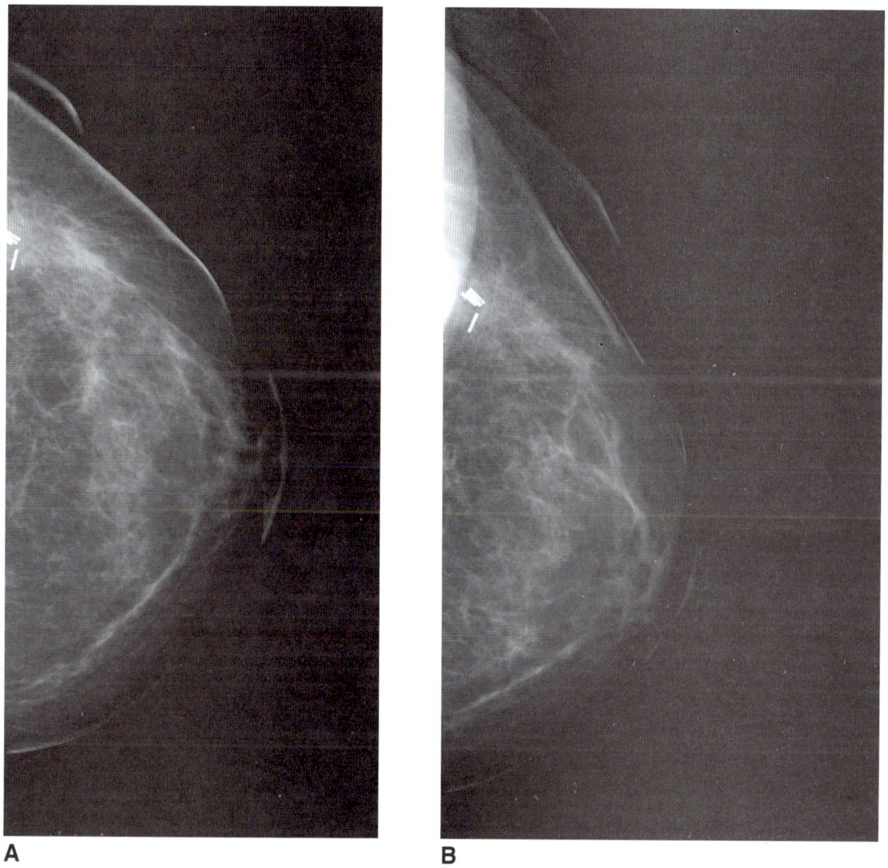

Figure 7-11. (A) Normal CC can miss tissue in the lateral breast. (B) XCCL demonstrates the missed tissue clearly.

association with malignancy it is recommended that all stellate lesions, including radial scars, should be biopsied.[4]

21. **(D)** Although the mammographer should inform the radiologist and can also inform the patient, anything unusual must be documented in the the patient's medical records or on the patient's medical history form. The patient's records are a means of communication between the mammographer and the radiologist and can be important legal documents used to define what was or was not done to a patient. Records can also be used as evidence in court cases.[1,2]

22. **(B)** On the craniocaudal (CC) projection, the posterior nipple line (PNL) measures the distance from the nipple to the edge of the image. On the mediolateral oblique (MLO) the PNL is drawn from the nipple extending posteriorly to meet the pectoral muscle at a right angle (perpendicularly). The length of the PNL on the CC view should be within 1 cm of its length on the MLO when the MLO is properly positioned. This means that the PNL is usually longer on the MLO when compared to the CC. However, in approximately 10% of the cases, the PNL is greater on the CC (Figure 7-12).[9]

23. **(A)** Grids absorb scatter and increase visibility of image detail. Mammography grids usually use carbon or wood as the interspace material. Some mammography units have a high transmission cellular grid (HTC) which uses air as the interspace material and copper instead of lead as the strips (Figure 7-13).[14,15]

24. **(C)** All effort should be made to image the medial breast tissue on the craniocaudal (CC) mammogram; eliminating it could eliminate

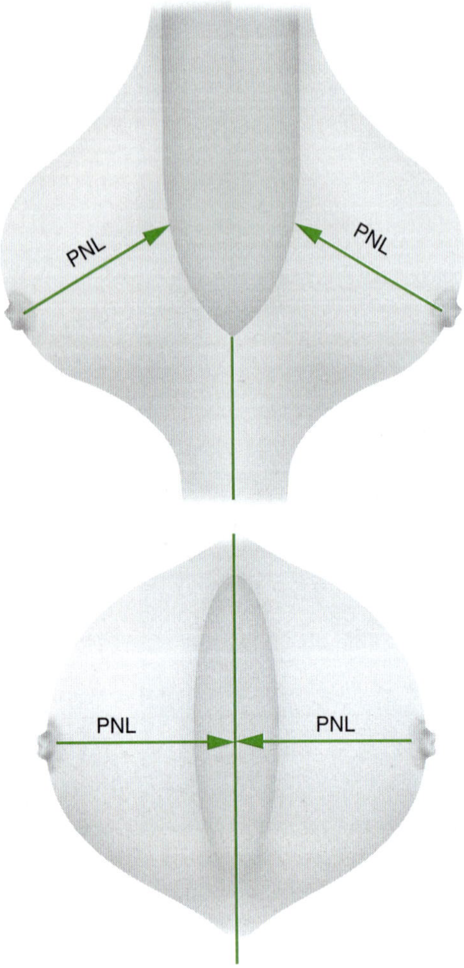

Figure 7-12. PNL schematic diagram showing the PNL on CC and MLO.

this area of the breast from the study. The CC best demonstrates the anterior, central, medial, and posteromedial portions of the breast but is poor at visualizing the lateral breast tissue. When imaging the CC, if the breast is too wide to fit on the detector, additional images must be taken to ensure coverage of the medial breast. Although the medial breast is imaged on the mediolateral oblique (MLO), superimposition of glandular structures and increased object-to-image receptor distance (OID) and the oblique nature of the projection often cause distortion of that area (Figure 7-14).[9,10]

25. **(D)** The image does not have enough pectoralis muscle and is therefore missing the posterior breast. The mediolateral oblique (MLO) projection best demonstrates the posterior and upper-outer quadrant (UOQ) of the breast. Considerations when evaluating the MLO projection includes: the pectoral muscle should be wide superiorly with a convex anterior border and should extend to or below the level of the posterior nipple line; the inframammary fold should be open; dense areas of the breast should be adequately penetrated; there should be no drooping of the anterior breast and distortion

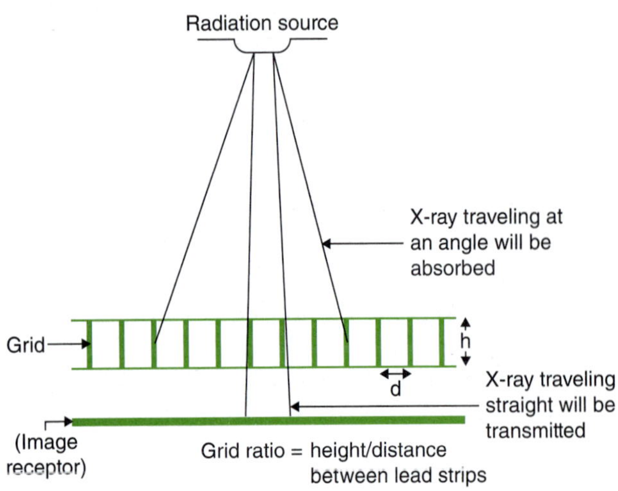

Figure 7-13. The cross-section of a grid. (Reproduced with permission from Peart O: Lange Q&A: Mammography Examination, 2nd ed. New York, NY: McGraw-Hill Education; 2008.)

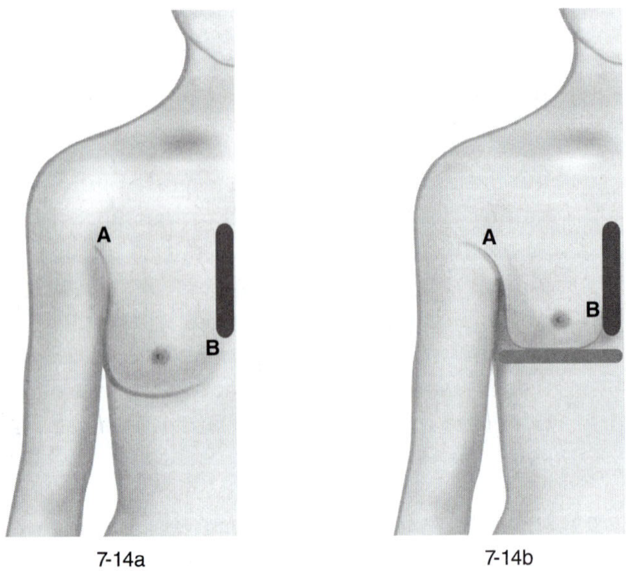

Figure 7-14. The CC and MLO are complimentary projections. A lesion in the lateral breast (lesion A) could be missed on the CC yet imaged on the MLO. A lesion in the medial breast (lesion B) could be missed on the MLO yet imaged on the CC.

of the architectural structures; the skin fold must be open and abdominal tissue should not overlap the breast tissue.[9,10]

26. **(D)** In a digital imaging the term brightness replaces density. Brightness can be altered after the exposure. The controlling factors are milliamperes (mAs), processing software and predetermined digital algorithms. Increasing window level will increase brightness. Window width controls the black-and-white display, therefore the contrast. Increasing window width will decrease contrast. The peak kilovoltage (kVp), plus processing software and digital algorithms will also be factors in controlling contrast.[7,8]

27. **(C)** The cleavage view (CV) best images the medial breast. The mediolateral oblique (MLO) will best demonstrate the posterior and upper-outer quadrant (UOQ) of the breast. The exaggerated craniocaudal (XCCL) and axillary tail (AT) will demonstrate the lateral and axilla portion of the breast, respectively.[9,10]

28. **(D)** Putting the nipple in profile is sometimes counterproductive. Breast tissue is lost either superiorly, inferiorly, laterally, or medially, depending on the projection and the location of the nipple on the breast. Missed tissue can then lead to undetected breast cancer. If the nipple is not in profile, additional images are needed for the above reasons, but should not be done solely to place the nipple in profile, especially if the nipple is marked with a BB marker (small radiopaque marker) (Figure 7-15).[9,10]

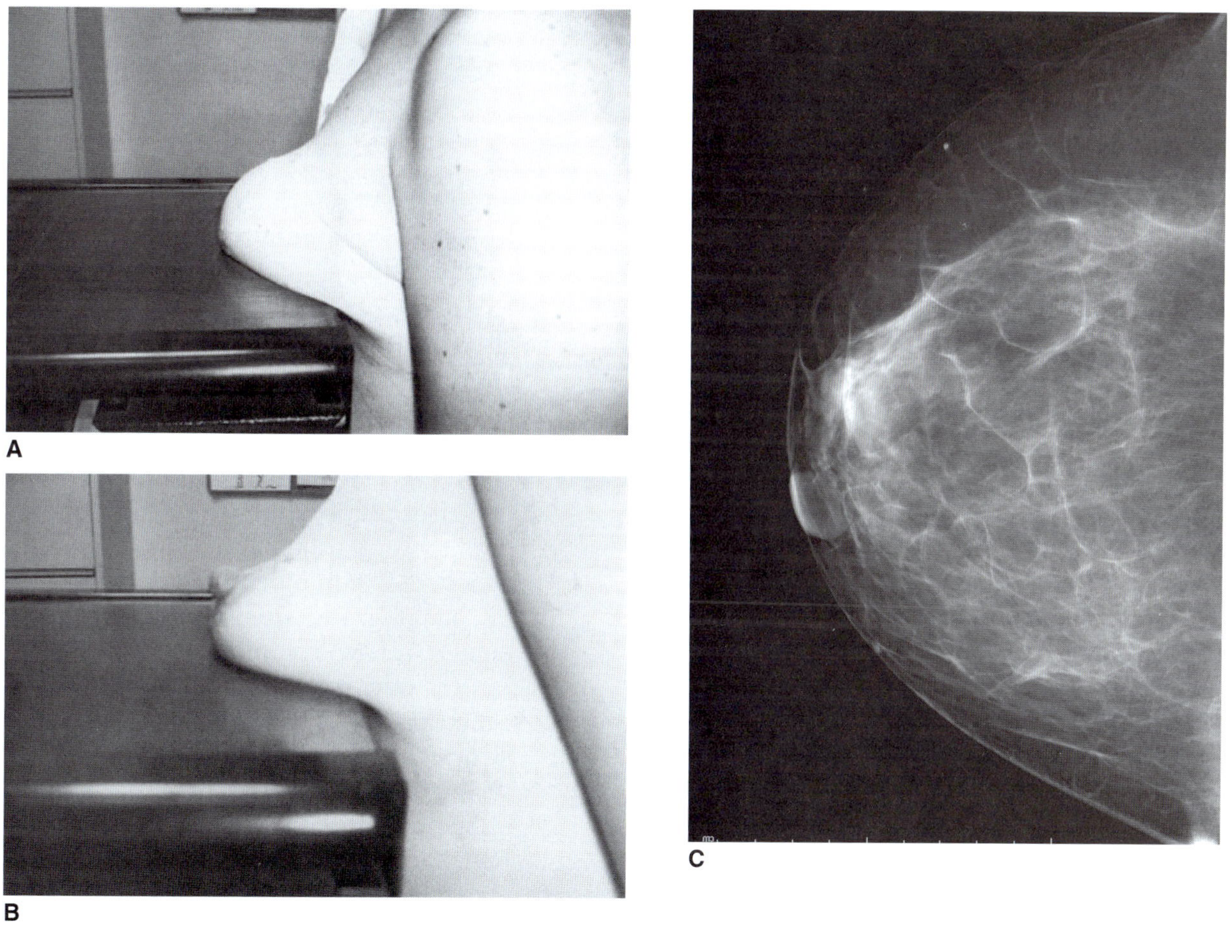

Figure 7-15. Nipple not in profile (A & B) patient positioning. (C) Radiograph showing the nipple not in profile. (Reproduced with permission from Peart O: Mammography and Breast Imaging PREP: Program Review and Exam Prep. New York, NY: McGraw-Hill Education; 2012.)

29. **(C)** The low-density structure indicated by the arrow is the pectoralis muscle. On the craniocaudal (CC) the pectoralis muscle is seen in approximately 30%-40% of cases. If the pectoral muscle is seen on all cases, imaging may be losing medial breast tissue. In any CC projection the nipple should be centered on the radiograph. However, do not eliminate breast tissue to center the nipple. Also the medial and lateral aspects of the breast must be included in the collimated area. The length of the posterior nipple line (PNL) on the CC view should be within 1 cm of its length on the mediolateral oblique (MLO) when the MLO is properly positioned.[9,10]

30. **(A)** Although the biggest risk factor of breast cancer is gender (female), having a sister with breast cancer can significantly increase a person's risks for the disease. A personal history applies only if the patient has had breast cancer.[1,2]

31. **(C)** The final rule of mammography, dictated by the Mammography Quality Standards Act (MQSA), states that a single projection/position mammogram should not give more than 3 mGy (300 mrad) average glandular dose when a grid is used and should not exceed 1 mGy (100 mrad) per projection/position without a grid.[16,17]

32. **(A)** The analog-to-digital converter (ADC) converts analog signal (light or electronic) from the image receptor or detector to a digital signal that the computer can manipulate for processing, display, and storage. The ADC assigns each picture element or pixel a value which corresponds to a level of brightness. The entire image is divided into a matrix of pixels based on the brightness of each pixel. The digital-to-analog converter (DAC) converts digitally manipulated data back to an analog (light or electronic) signal and the film digitizer converts analog produced radiographs (films) to a digital version via a scanning device. Digital Imaging and Communications in Medicine (DICOM) is a set of computer software standards that permit a wide range of digital imaging programs to communicate with each other (Figure 7-16).[7,8,18]

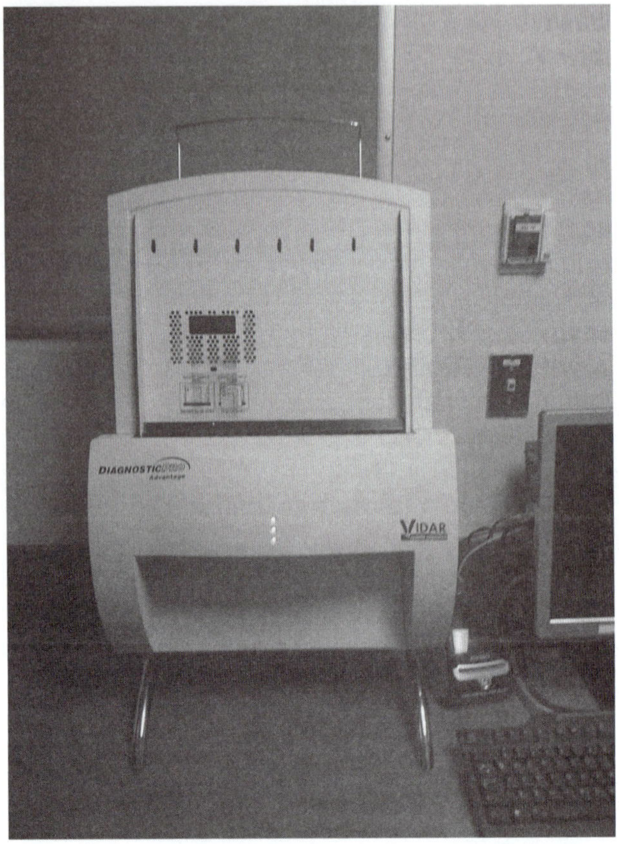

Figure 7-16. A film digitizer.

33. **(B)** The picture archiving and communications system (PACS) is a computer network that allows digital images from multiple modalities, e.g., general computed tomography (CT), magnetic resonance imaging (MRI), or ultrasound, to be viewed at a single monitor, at various monitors, transmitted or stored. All equipment used must be Digital Imaging and Communications in Medicine (DICOM)-compliant. A PACS system can include: reading station with processing capabilities (e.g., radiologists view reconstructed tomosynthesis images); physician review stations; web access; technologist quality control station; administrative stations; archive system; and interface to various hospital and radiology systems. DICOM is a set of computer software standards that permit a wide range of digital imaging programs to communicate with each other. A local area network, or LAN, is a computer network serving a limited or small geographical area. Typically, LAN devices will share a server loaded with appropriate applications and data for the LAN user group. An example of a LAN network could be the computer network serving a group of CT scanners, monitors and a single storage device or a hospital network. A wide area network, or WAN, is a computer network serving a large geographical area. Typically, WAN networks can be transmitted by major carriers, such as a telephone or cable co[7,8]

34. **(D)** Patients health records can contain: the patient demographic information (name, date of birth, health record number plus other identifying information); clinical observations and complete medical and surgical history; reports of relevant physical examinations; signed informed consents if relevant; diagnostic or therapeutic orders; the physician ordering the procedures, documentation of the amount, date and time of any medication administered; reports of all diagnostic tests; and documentation of evaluations or treatments. Patients have a right to access and amend their health records. When amending the health records, the original entry is not altered and the amendment becomes a part of the record. Health records are legal documents and can be admissible as evidence in a court of law.[1,2]

35. **(B)** The Montgomery glands (glands of Montgomery) are seen as protrusions on the surface of the areola and are actually specialized sebaceous glands. (The openings to the protrusions are called Morgagni tubercles.) They usually become more prominent during pregnancy and lactation and secrete a fluid which helps lubricate the nipple and areola.[12,13]

36. **(D)** Estrogen and progesterone are 2 of the many hormones responsible for many physiological changes in the breast. Estrogen is responsible for ductal proliferation and progesterone for lobular proliferation. Once a woman starts estrogen, the changes can be spotty, causing lumps or increased interstitial fluids (cysts), but will generally result in an overall increase in glandular tissue.[1,2]

37. **(B)** Paget disease of the breast (first described by Jean Paget in 1874) is a special form of ductal carcinoma associated with eczematous changes of the nipple. Generally it presents as a malignant nipple lesion. Infiltrating carcinoma implies that the cancer has left the point of origin and is spreading into the surrounding tissues.[5,12]

38. **(B)** A digital image consists of a box of cells or picture elements (*pixels*) corresponding to numeric values arranged in rows and columns. Each pixel contains *bits* of information. The number of bits per pixel determines the shade of gray demonstrated. The rows and columns form a *matrix* and each cell corresponds to a specific location in the image. The matrix size is determined by the number of pixels in the rows and columns. The *bit depth* is the number of gray shades that a pixel can produce. With a greater bit depth there will be more shades of gray and therefore the image will provide more information (a more accurate visualization of the object).[7,8]

39. **(C)** The picture archiving and communications system (PACS) is a computer network that allows digital images from multiple modalities, e.g., general computed tomography (CT), magnetic resonance imaging (MRI), or ultrasound, to be viewed at various monitors, or transmitted or stored. Digital Imaging and Communications in Medicine (DICOM) is a set of computer software standards that permits a wide range of digital imaging programs to communicate with each other. DIGCOM & PCAS are detractors.[7,8]

40. **(A)** The picture archiving and communications system (PACS) is a computer network that allows digital images from multiple modalities, e.g., general computed tomography (CT), magnetic resonance imaging (MRI), or ultrasound, to be viewed at a single monitor, at various monitors, or transmitted

or stored. All equipment used must be Digital Imaging and Communications in Medicine (DICOM)-compliant. A PACS system can include: reading station with processing capabilities (e.g., radiologists view reconstructed tomosynthesis images); physician review stations; web access; technologist quality control station; administrative stations; archive system; and interface to various hospital and radiology systems.[7,8]

41. **(B)** Diethylstilbestrol (DES) was used by pregnant women in the United States during 1940-1971. It was used to prevent miscarriage and studies show that women who took DES during pregnancy have a slightly increased risk of breast cancer. Also, women who were exposed to DES in utero, or whose mothers took DES while they were pregnant, may also have a slightly increased risk of breast cancer after age 40. Hormone replacement therapy (HRT) will also cause and increased breast cancer risks. A woman with took DES and is also taking HRT will therefore have a higher risk for developing breast cancer than a woman who took DES but did not use HRT.[1]

42. **(A)** In the rolled positions, the superior surface of the breast is rolled in 1 direction and the lower (inferior) surface in the other direction. With the medial roll (RM) the patient is positioned for the craniocaudal (CC). From the CC position the superior portion of the breast is rolled medially and the inferior portion is rolled laterally. For the lateral roll (RL) the patient is positioned for the CC. From the CC position the superior portion of the breast is rolled laterally and the inferior portion is rolled medially. The medial and lateral roll (RM and RL) are both useful in separating glandular structures of the breast to resolve questions of superimposed structures. The lateromedial (LM) is a 90-degree lateral projection, with the x-rays traveling from lateral to medial and magnification (M) produces a magnified image of an area (Figure 7-17)[9,10]

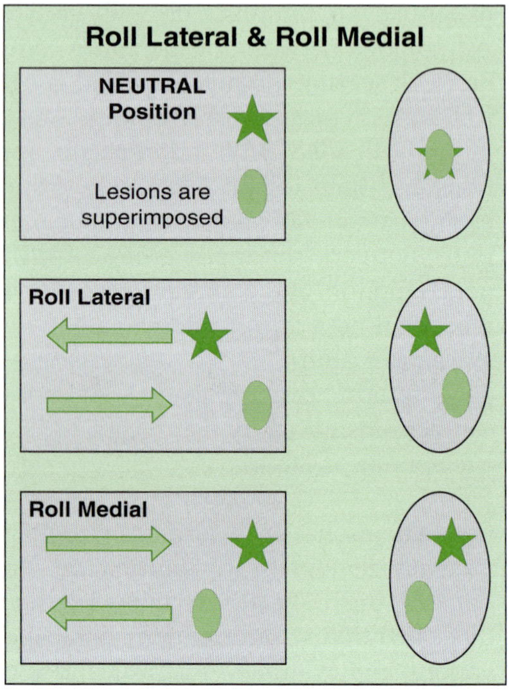

Figure 7-17. The roll positions (RM and RL) can be used to remove superimposed lesions.

43. **(B)** Breast cancer risk decreases among women who have a first child before age 30, who breast-feed, or who experience late menarche or early menopause. Studies have suggested that reproductive hormones influence breast cancer; and can increase breast cancer risk. Factors affecting the risk for breast cancer could include any factor that affects the reproductive hormones, such as early menarche (before 12); late menopause (after 55); late age at first full-term pregnancy (after 30); the use of oral contraceptives; or the use of estrogen replacement therapy.[1,2]

44. **(C)** The picture archiving and communications system (PACS) is a computer network that allows digital images from multiple modalities, e.g., general computed tomography (CT), magnetic resonance imaging (MRI), or ultrasound, to be viewed at various monitors, a single monitor, transmitted or stored.[7,8]

45. **(C)** In the computed mammography (CM) imaging system the image is captured on a photostimulable phosphor (PSP). In the process of PSP image capture, the x-ray photon strikes the phosphor crystals in the PSP. This action causes electrons in the crystals to move from normal orbital location to a

higher level. This is the latent image formation. The number of electrons affected is directly proportional to the amount of energy absorbed by the PSP. Some but not all of the electrons raised to a higher energy level will spontaneously return to their resting state. The image plate (IP) containing the PSP is placed in a computer PSP reader. The computer reader functions to open the IP and remove the PSP, then to scan, read, and erase the exposed PSP. A red laser light source scans the PSP to extract the image data. The laser light causes electrons at high-energy (latent image) to release energy absorbed from the x-ray beam as blue-purple light and to return to a lower energy resting state. The blue-purple light released is collected by the light guide and used to record the image. The entire process takes about 60 seconds. After scanning the PSP, it is returned to the IP and the IP is ejected from the computer reader (Figure 7-18).[7,8,18]

46. **(B)** Gynecomastia is a benign increase of tissue in the male breast. It can occur bilaterally or unilaterally. Gynecomastia does not increase the risk of breast cancer for male patients (Figure 7-19).[4,5]

47. **(B)** When the image plate (IP) is placed in a computer reader, the *photostimulable phosphor* (PSP) is extracted and an infrared laser light scans the PSP plate. The red laser light provides energy to the trapped electrons in the phosphor of the PSP plate. The laser causes the metastable electrons to return to the ground state. The electrons emit a blue-purple visible light as they relax to the lower energy levels. *Photostimulable luminescence* (PSL) is the emission of bluish-purple light from electrons as they transition from higher energy to a lower energy state (Figure 7-20).[7,8]

48. **(B)** Although the Mammography Quality Standards Act (MQSA) recommends that technical factors appear on the image, this is not an MQSA requirement. Other recommendations for analog imaging includes, a flash card implant-displaced (ID) versus stick-on labels because the flash ID is more permanent along with separate date stickers because

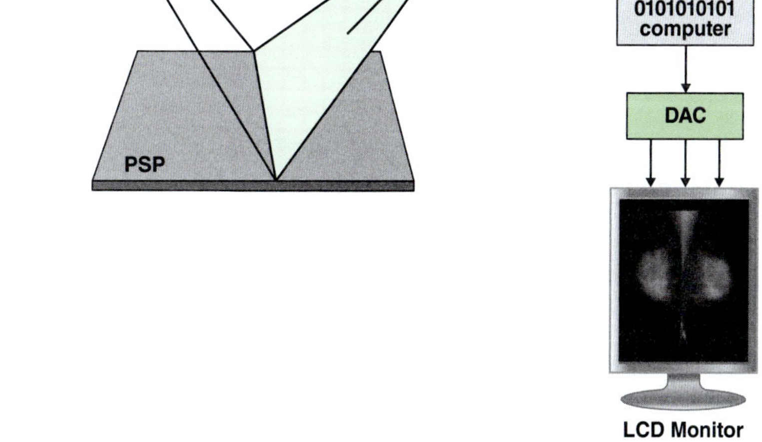

Figure 7-18. Schematic diagram showing PSP scanning.

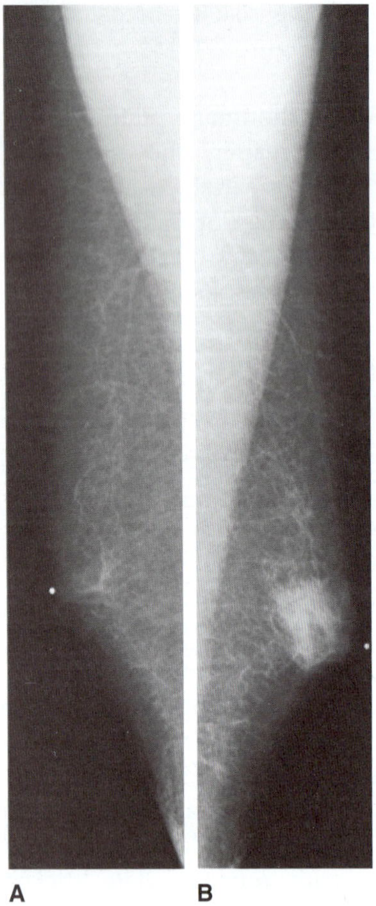

Figure 7-19. Radiograph showing gynecomastia. (Reproduced with permission from Peart O: Mammography and Breast Imaging PREP: Program Review and Exam Prep. New York, NY: McGraw-Hill Education; 2012.)

they are easy to read and can be color coded by year.

General requirements are

- name of patient and additional patient identifier
- date of examination
- projection and right or left marker—placed near the axilla using the standardized codes
- facility name and location (must include city, state, and zip code)
- mammographer identification
- mammography unit identification (if more than 1 unit per site)
- cassette/screen identification (analog imaging systems)[16,17]

49. **(D)** The breast can reach superiorly from the clavicle (second or third rib), and inferiorly to meet the abdominal wall at the level of the sixth or seventh rib. This lowest point of the breast is called the inframammary crease or fold.[12]

50. **(A)** The Cooper ligaments are fibrous membranes that support the lobes providing shape and form to the breast. The ligaments attach to the base of the breast and extend outward attaching to the anterior superficial fascia of the skin.[12]

51. **(C)** Starting at the TDLU or terminal ductal lobular unit, the collecting ductal system gradually widens in tree-like branches forming segmental ducts. Immediately behind the nipple it further distends to form an ampulla, also called the lactiferous sinus. This is a pouch-like structure immediately behind the nipple. The ducts again narrow to end at the nipple (Figure 7-21).[12]

52. **(C)** Scattered radiation is produced whenever the useful beam intercepts any object causing it to diverge. There are 2 methods of reducing

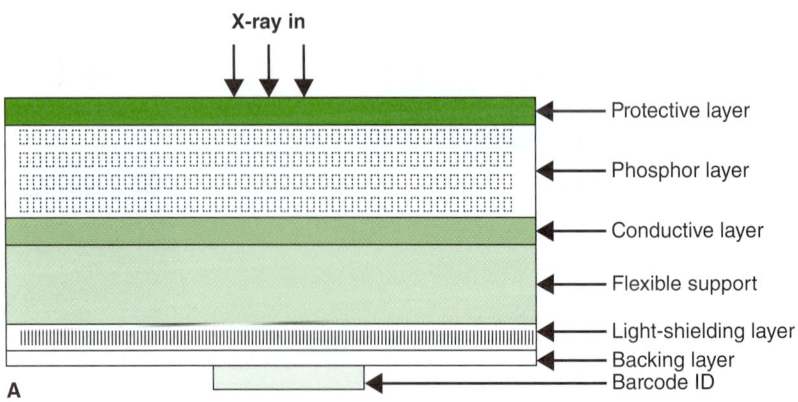

Figure 7-20. The photostimulable phosphor (PSP) layers.

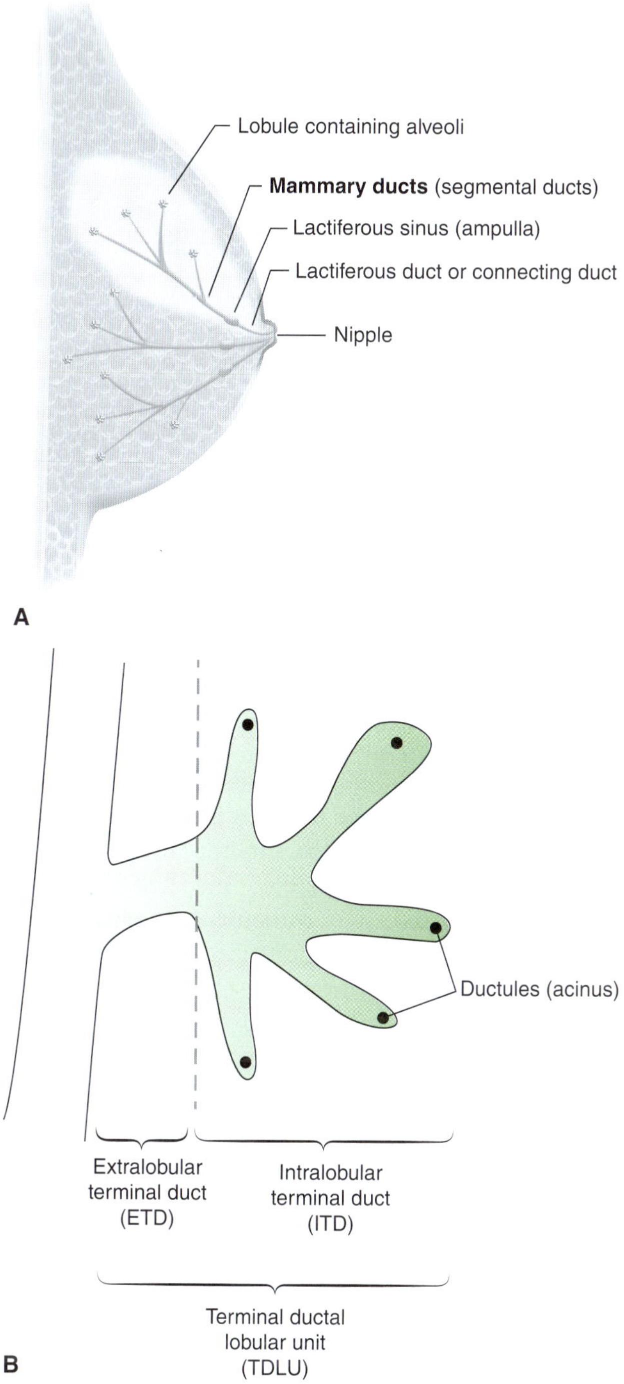

Figure 7-21. (A) Schematic diagram of the ductal tree. (B) TDLU. (Reproduced with permission from Peart O: Mammography and Breast Imaging PREP: Program Review and Exam Prep. New York, NY: McGraw-Hill Education; 2012.)

the amount of scattered radiation reaching the detector: limiting the x-ray field size (not an option in mammography) and the use of grids or air-gaps. In magnification mammography, the large air gap acts as a grid in reducing scattered radiation. Grid use in magnification is therefore not necessary and would unnecessarily increase the exposure dose to the patient. Increasing the source-to-image receptor distance (SID) reduces magnification but does not reduce the amount of scatter production. Also it is not an option in magnification mammography where the SID is fixed. The small focal spot is necessary to increase resolution, but this does not affect the amount of scattered radiation reaching the detector.[14]

53. **(D)** Ductography will not determine if a lesion is malignant or benign, but it can determine the location and number of lesions or changes associated with the ducts. Only a cytological or histological analysis can accurately determine the true nature of the lesion.[19]

54. **(C)** Sometimes the breast is very thin and the mammographer's fingers are compressed before compression is complete. A rubber spatula can be used to hold the breast in place before compression takes over. The ML does not image the posterior breast and cannot replace the mediolateral oblique (MLO) and too much pectoral muscle is not normally an issue with small breasts. The exaggerated craniocaudal (XCCL) images the lateral aspect of the breast with the x-ray beam directed craniocaudally.[9]

55. **(A)** Positioning the breast away from the detector takes advantage of the inverse-square law: the intensity of the scattered radiation is reduced because the distance between the detector and the object is increased. The heel effect describes the process that causes the radiation intensity at the cathode side of the x-ray field to be higher than that on the anode side. The line-focus principle is used in an angled design of the tube target, that allows a large area for heating while maintaining a small focal spot. The reciprocity law states that the density produced on a radiograph is equal for any combination of mA and exposure times as long as the product of mA and the ms is equal (Figures 7-22 and 7-23).[6,7]

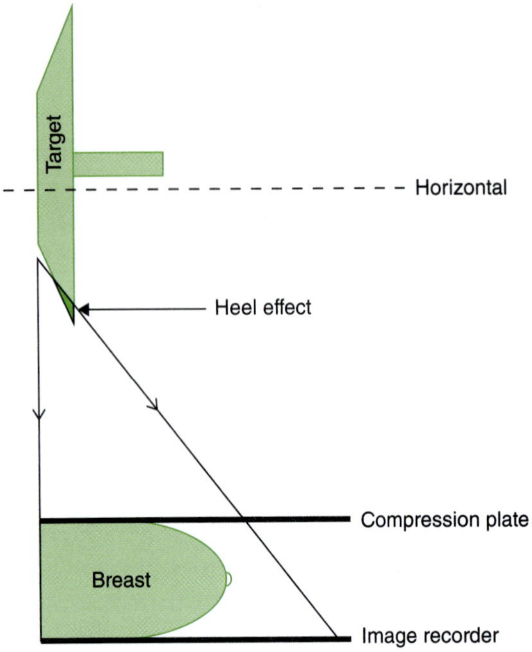

Figure 7-22. Heel effect. (Reproduced with permission from Peart O: Mammography and Breast Imaging PREP: Program Review and Exam Prep. New York, NY: McGraw-Hill Education; 2012.)

56. (C) Risk factors increases a woman's risk for breast cancer. Risks factors can be relatively high risk, moderate risks, and minor risks. High-risks factors include gender (female), age, genetic factors, and family or personal history of breast cancer. Moderate risk factors include having 1 first-degree relative with breast cancer, having atypical hyperplasia confirmed on biopsy, high radiation dose to the chest area and high bone density after menopause. Minor risk factors are associated with hormonal use or changes in the body and include not having children or having the first child after age 30, not breast-feeding, early menarche (before age 12) or late menopause (after age 55), postmenopausal obesity, recent and long-term use of hormone replacement therapy (HRT) or oral contraceptive, alcohol consumption, and obesity.[1,20]

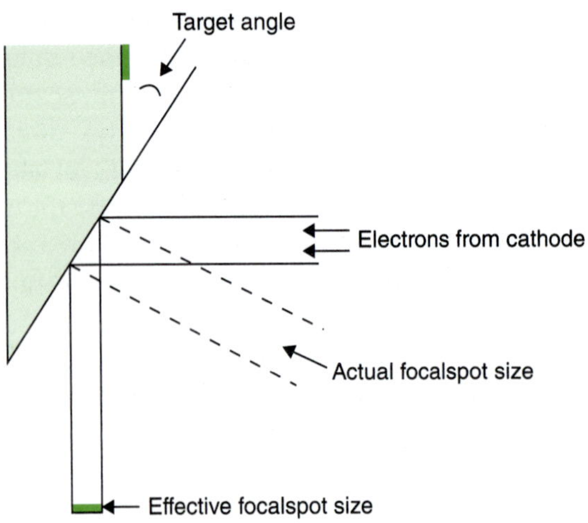

Figure 7-23. Line-focus principle. The nominal focal spot size is larger than the actual focal spot. (Reproduced with permission from Peart O: Mammography and Breast Imaging PREP: Program Review and Exam Prep. New York, NY: McGraw-Hill Education; 2012.)

57. (D) Grids do not improve image sharpness; the sharpness of an image is affected by the focal-spot size, source-to-image receptor distance (SID), object-to-image receptor distance (OID), type of intensifying screens (in analog imaging only), and motion. Grids increase patient dose and reduce the amount of scattered radiation striking the detector, but do not affect the production of scatter radiation. Grid use will, however, result in increased subject contrast. (See Figure 7-13.)[14,15]

58. (D) As long as the implant is soft and remains free of encapsulation, the implant-placed (ID) projections are possible. Once the implant is encapsulated, it is difficult if not impossible to displace. Most modern implants are placed behind the pectoral muscle (subpectoral or retropectoral placement) versus the placement in front of the pectoral muscle (subglandular or retromammary placement) that was done in the past. The placement of the implant behind the pectoral muscle allows better imaging and better displacement of the implants for the ID projections. Implants placed behind the pectoral muscle are also less likely to become encapsulated.[4]

59. (B) On average, a mammogram can detect up to 90% of breast cancers in women without symptoms, and is more accurate in postmenopausal than premenopausal women. Some cancers are not visualized mammographically. The reasons are varied. The patient may have extremely dense breast or the mammogram may not be the best method of detection for a particular type of cancer. Poor imaging techniques by the mammographer and the interpretation skills of the radiologist can also

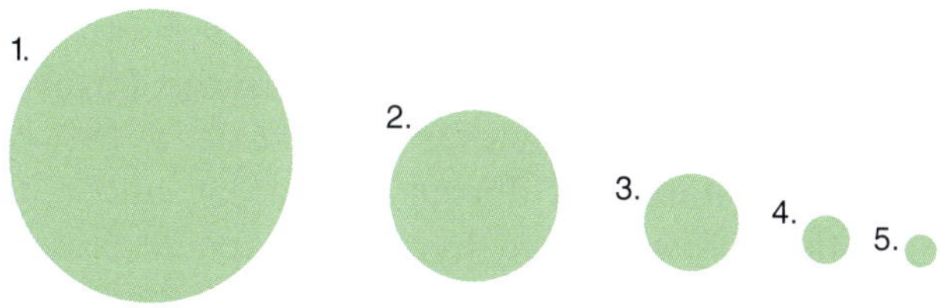

Figure 7-24. A size of the lesion at detection can depend on a variety of factors.
1. size found by chance (3.6-4.2cm)
2. size with occasional BSE
3. size found with regular BSE (approximately 2 cm)
4. size found by 1st or regular mammograms (1 cm)
5. size found by regular mammograms on fatty breast (5 mm)

be contributing factors. If the mammogram is normal and the patient feels a palpable mass, the mass could be normal or abnormal. The patient must contact her doctor immediately for further testing (Figure 7-24).[1,2]

60. **(C)** Risk factors increase a woman's risk for breast cancer. Risks factors can be relatively high risk, moderate risks, and minor risks. High-risk factors include gender (female), age, genetic factors, and family or personal history of breast cancer. Moderate risk factors include having 1 first-degree relative with breast cancer, having atypical hyperplasia confirmed on biopsy, high radiation dose to the chest area or, high bone density after menopause. Minor risk factors are associated with hormonal use or changes in the body and include not having children or having the first child after age 30, not breast-feeding, early menarche (before age 12) or late menopause (after age 55), postmenopausal obesity, recent and long-term use of hormone replacement therapy (HRT) or oral contraceptive, alcohol consumption, and obesity.[1,2]

61. **(B)** The focal spot size is important in mammography and many x-ray tubes have 2 focal spot sizes—1 for routine and 1 for magnification work. In routine work, the focal spot size can be 0.4 or smaller. In magnification work, the focal spot may be 0.15 or smaller. Any work done with a 0.1-mm focal spot size would be for magnification.[6,7,21]

62. **(D)** Consent can only be give if the person possesses substantial understanding and is mentally and physically able to give consent. The following can give informed consent: a competent adult; legal guardian or representative of an incompetent adult; individuals obligated by court order; an emancipated minor (14-18 years) or a minor who is married, serving in the military, self-supporting—living on own, pregnant, (a pregnant minor can give consent for child but not for self), suffering from conditions, e.g., sexually transmitted disease (STD).[22]

63. **(A)** When the image plate (IP) is placed in a computer reader, the photostimulable phosphor (PSP) is extracted and an infrared laser light scans the PSP. The red laser light provides energy to the trapped electrons in the phosphor of the PSP plate. The laser causes the metastable electrons to return to the ground state. The electrons emit a blue-purple visible light as they relax to the lower energy levels. Photostimulable luminescence (PSL) is the emission of bluish-purple light from electrons as they transition from higher energy to a lower energy state. A *Photomultiplier tube* (PMT), *photodetector* (PD), or *charge-coupled device* (CCD) will collect the blue-purple light given off by the trapped electrons as they return to their normal neutral state. The PMT will convert the light energy to an electrical or electronic signal that is transmitted to an analog to digital converter (ADC). The digital signal is sent to a computer for processing. After processing the signal is sent as an image to the liquid crystal display (LCD). Instead of the CCD some systems use a complementary metal-oxide silicon (CMOS) to convert light into an analog signal that is sent to the ADC. The CMOS is a semiconductor transistor similar to the CCD in that it has either a fiber optic coupling or a lens system. Each array of metal-oxide-semiconductor capacitors (MOS capacitors) represents a pixel. The CMOS is smaller than the CCD and will therefore take up less space (see Figure 7-18).[7,8]

64. **(B)** Skin folds or wrinkling will not always be present but when present may be impossible to avoid in the elderly. The best method is

to smooth folds or wrinkles using the index finger during compression. However, avoid pushing breast tissue outside of the compression field, posteriorly to eliminate a fold or wrinkle. Pulling breast tissue anterior will increase the number of folds or wrinkles in the compressed breast. Added projections will be needed if any breast tissue is eliminated when removing wrinkling or folds.[12]

65. **(B)** The breast includes the nipple, inframammary fold, and tail of Spence. The tail of Spence (tail, axilla, or axillary tail are other names used) describes the area of the breast stretching up into the axilla. The base describes the region where the inframammary fold is located, and the area of breast that is closest to the chest wall. The apex is the nipple region, and the most anterior part of the breast.[12]

66. **(C)** Fibrous tissue is usually described with glandular tissue together as fibroglandular densities. X-rays pass more easily through fatty tissue than through fibrous or glandular tissue. Fatty areas appear radiolucent (black on the mammogram). The fibroglandular or fibrous tissue is more radiopaque than fatty tissue, and shows as areas of lower optical density (white) on the mammogram (Figure 7-25).[12]

67. **(B)** Figure 7-6 shows casting-type calcifications which are often malignant. The shape of the cast is determined by the uneven production of calcifications and the irregular necrosis of the cellular debris. The contours of the cast are always irregular in density, width, and length, and the cast is always fragmented. A calcification is seen as branching when it extends into adjacent ducts. Also, the width of the ducts will determine the width of the castings. A diagnosis of invasive ductal carcinoma is only made on cytological or histological analysis. Oil cysts are eggshell-like calcifications and plasma cell mastitis is composed of large linear periductal or intraductal calcifications.[23]

68. **(D)** Of the choices, the only huge radiolucent breast lesion is a lipoma, which is a common benign tumor composed of fatty tissue. Another large lesion is the fibroadenolipoma or hamartoma. It is a benign proliferation of fibrous, glandular, and fatty tissue surrounded by a thin capsule of connective tissue. The oil cyst is benign and appears mammographically as eggshell-like calcifications and plasma cell mastitis are large linear periductal or intraductal calcifications Both the fibroadenoma and the hematoma are seen as circular-oval lesions with mixed densities and generally will not occupy the entire breast. (See Figure 3-19.)[4,5]

69. **(D)** The latent image formed on the photostimulable phosphor (PSP) can last for several hours but loses 25% of its energy in 8 hours. *Fading* is the term used to describe the time it takes for the latent image to disappear.[7,8]

70. **(C)** Advantages of photostimulable phosphor (PSP) technology or computed mammography (CM) include: the wide latitude and dynamic range, CM is a faster imaging system when compared to screen-film, there is reduced repeats, less change of lost films, and there is increased workflow. Disadvantages of CM include: lower spatial resolution (the digital imaging system can manipulate the pixel values after the exposure which compensates for the lower spatial resolution, but CM is not as effective as flat-panel technology or digital mammography (DM) in compensating for the lower resolution of the imaging system); CM imaging plates (IPs) can be easily damaged during transport; CM use PSPs which are susceptible to scratches in the computer reader; low exposure can create a noisy image; and the PSP, which is located in the IP, is very sensitive to radiation which can contribute to a noisy image (Figure 7-26).[7,8]

71. **(B)** Nonscintillator-based imaging systems have a direct 2-step process: x-ray beam strikes the photoconductor, e.g., amorphous selenium (a-Se). The a-Se converts x-ray to electrons. The electrons migrate to the thin-film transistor (TFT) after which the signal is sent to the workstation monitor (Figure 7-27).[7,8]

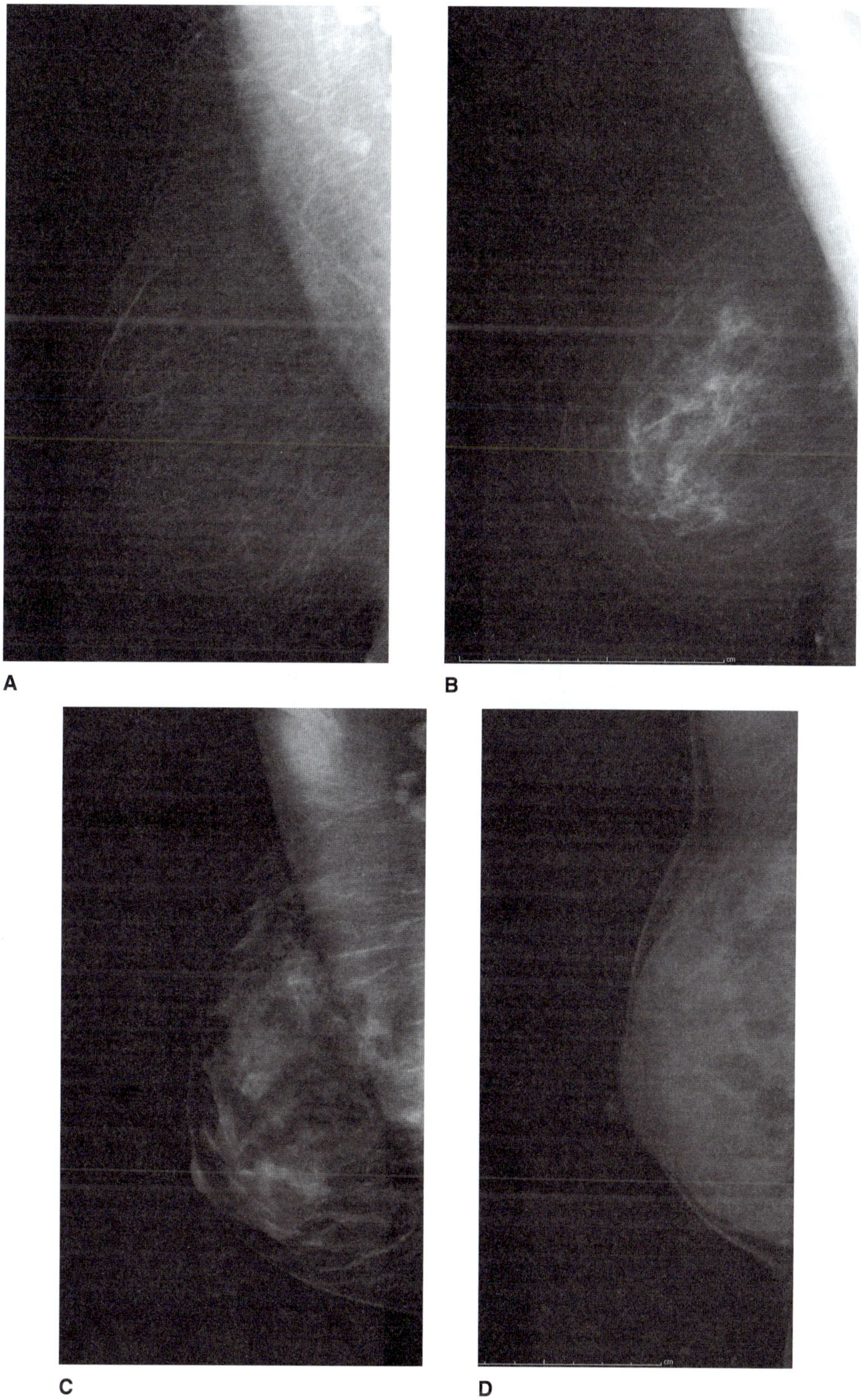

Figure 7-25. Different density breast tissue. (A) All fatty. (B) Scattered fibroglandular tissue. (C) Heterogeneously dense. (D) Extremely dense.

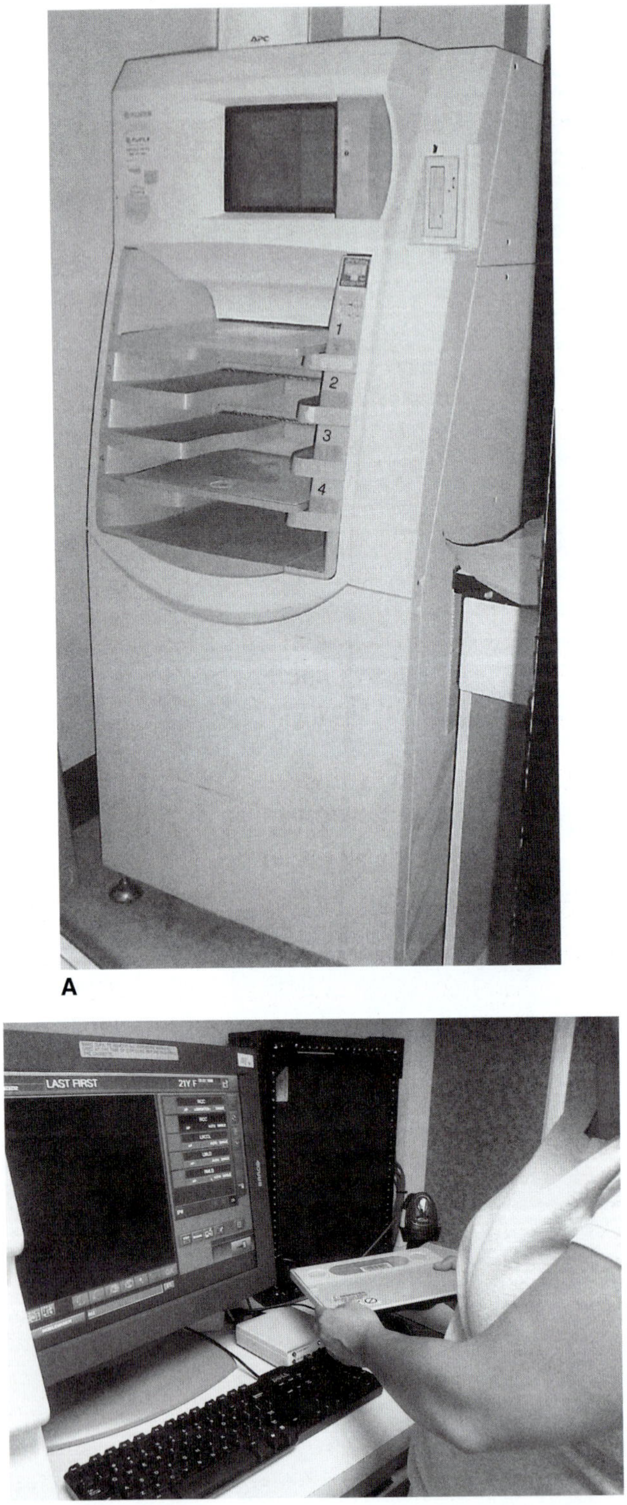

Figure 7-26. (A) CM reader and (B) scanning the IP. The patient identification and projection information is input by scanning it to the barcode reader.

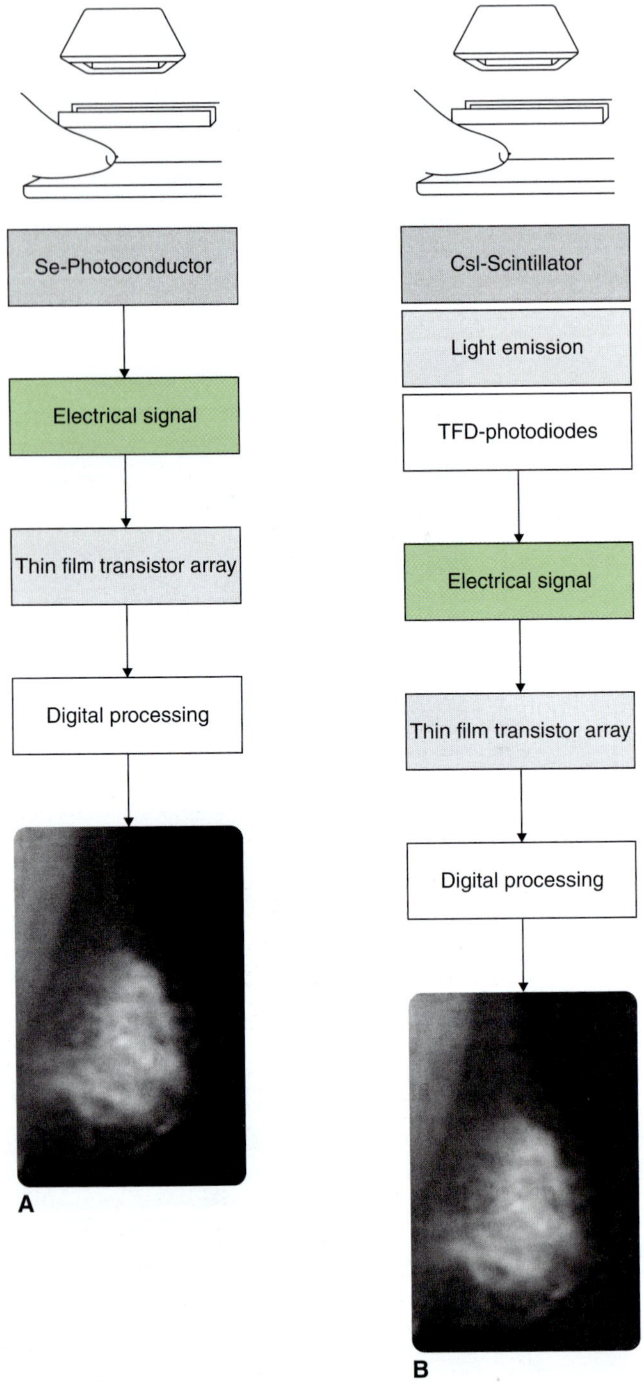

Figure 7-27. Flat-panel detector system (A) direct capture, (B) indirect capture. (Reproduced with permission from Peart O: Mammography and Breast Imaging PREP: Program Review and Exam Prep. New York, NY: McGraw-Hill Education; 2012.)

72. **(B)** Spot compression increases compression to the area of a suspected abnormality, allowing the tissue to spread more evenly, and eliminating pseudomasses. Because of the need to reduce extraneous light (increased visualization of breast tissue), coned collimated images

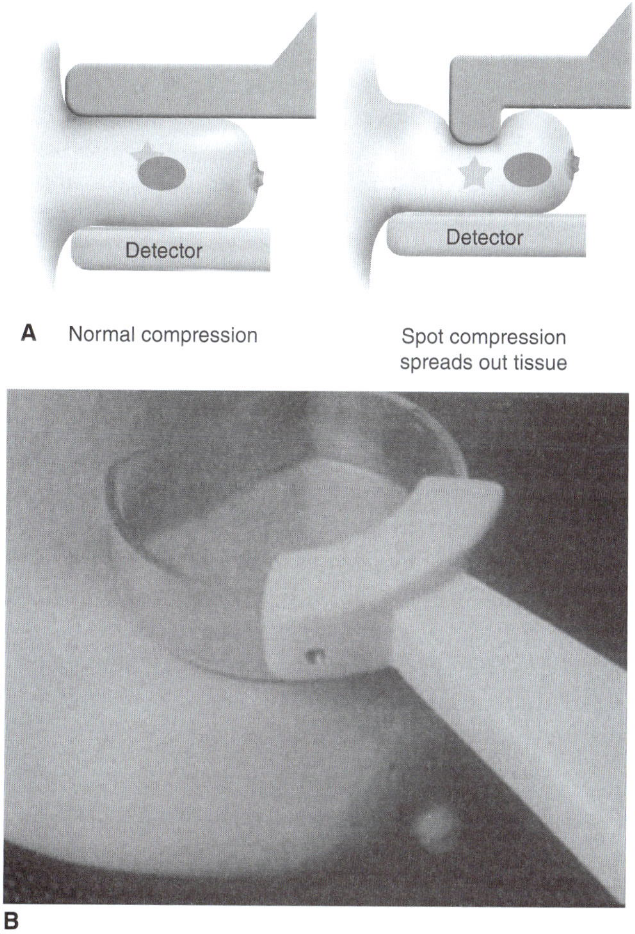

Figure 7-28. Spot compression device (A) schematic, (B) actual.

are not taken when imaging with spot compression (Figure 7-28).[9]

73. **(B)** This is a skin fold. Closed *Inframammary fold* is not visualized on the craniocaudal (CC) projection. The pectoralis muscle is seen at the far posterior aspect of the breast, and veins, when calcified, show as high density tubular structures.[9]

74. **(B)** If the patient stands away from the detector and bends forward, her chest will move forward and hopefully the protruding abdomen will project away from the imaging area. If this does not achieve the desired result, and the abdomen still protrudes on the inframammary fold, the mammographer cannot sacrifice posterior and lateral tissue to image the anterior breast. Two projections would be required—a lateral of the anterior breast and the mediolateral oblique (MLO) for the posterior and upper-outer quadrant (UOQ) of the breast. Take must be taken to get an open fold.[9]

75. **(B)** A halo around a lesion suggests that the lesion is circumscribed and could be a mammographically benign tumor. If the lesion is suspected to be benign, further testing is needed to assess the benign or suspicious nature of the lesion. An ultrasound would be the best next step to differentiate a solid versus a cystic lesion.[9,19]

76. **(B)** The specimen should always be compressed and radiographed to ensure that the lesion was completely removed. If there are calcifications present, the lesion should be magnified to ensure that all the calcifications were removed.[19]

77. **(A)** Analog receptors can produce an acceptable image within a range of 30% underexposure and 50% overexposure. In digital imaging, if a graph of the optical density (called the signal) and the relative exposure is plotted, the relationship is not the characteristic curve (also called Hurter and Driffield [H & D] or sensitometric curve); rather, it is a straight line (Figure 7-29). The digital image therefore has much wider latitude than analog mammography systems. This ability to adjust the final image (thus reducing the need for repeats) is 1 of the greatest advantages of digital imaging. Digital imaging can produce an acceptable image at 50% underexposure and 100% overexposure. This means that digital can correct exposure factors 100% greater than or 50% less than normal range. The disadvantage is that visual cues of over and under exposure not easily seen. Overexposure is seen as decreased contrast and underexposure is seen as quantum noise, an excessively noisy image.[7,8]

78. **(B)** Gynecomastia is a benign proliferation of tissue in the male breast. The condition usually has a high rate of spontaneous regression and can occur at birth, during teenage years

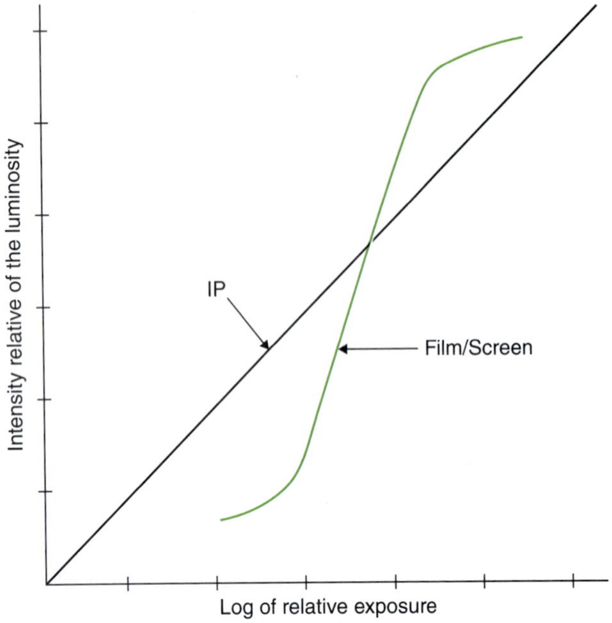

Figure 7-29. Characteristic curve (also called sensitometric curve or Hurter and Driffield [H & D] curve) from screen-film versus digital imaging. A graph of the optical density signal and the relative exposure for a digital detector has a linear response to x-ray. This is unlike the curvilinear response of a screen-film system. (Reproduced with permission from Peart O: Lange Q&A: Mammography Examination, 2nd ed. McGraw-Hill Medical; 2008.)

(can last up to 18 months), or in males above age 50. It is often seen bilaterally but can be unilateral. Gynecomastia is not associated with increased risk for breast cancer in males.[4,5]

79. **(C)** The Montgomery glands (glands of Montgomery) are seen as protrusions on the surface of the areola. They are actually specialized sebaceous glands that usually become more prominent during pregnancy and lactation.[4]

80. **(B)** Aluminum (Al) is used as the filtration in some digital tomosynthesis units and photon-counting imaging systems. Molybdenum (Mo) and rhodium (Rh) targets are often used as target material and filtration in analog units, where the filters used are often the same element as the x-ray tube target. Matching the filter to the same element as the x-ray tube target will allow the K-characteristic x-rays to pass while blocking the higher and lower energy Bremsstrahlung x-rays. In digital units, if the tube target is tungsten, Rh can be used for fatty breast and silver (Ag) for large or dense breast. Some tungsten targets use Mo for fatty breasts and Rh for dense breast.[18]

81. **(D)** With tungsten targets, Bremsstrahlung x-rays will predominate at energies above and below the 17-24 keV range. Although tungsten emits "harder" spectrum rays, the wider dynamic range can be utilized in digital imaging. Molybdenum targets produce characteristic x-rays in the 17-19 keV range after a photoelectric interaction. These are ideal when imaging fatty breast using an analog system. The characteristic x-ray produced using rhodium targets are similar to that from molybdenum, but because rhodium has a slightly higher atomic number, more Bremsstrahlung x-rays are produced and the K-characteristic x-rays will be 3-4 keV higher, which provides a better penetration of dense breast in the analog systems. Aluminum can be used as the filtration material in digital tomosynthesis and photon counting systems.[18,24]

82. **(A)** Above 40, it is recommended that a woman have a clinical breast examination (CBE) at about the same time as the annual mammogram, even if the woman has no symptoms and no significantly higher risk for breast cancer.[1,2]

83. **(D)** When imaging for the craniocaudal (CC) projection, the detector must be level with the entire length of the raised inframammary fold. If the detector is too high, the posterior and inferior breast will not be imaged. If the detector is too low the superior and posterior breast tissue is missed (Figure 7-30).[9]

84. **(A)** Capture elements function to collect or capture the x-rays. In mammography imaging these can include: Cesium iodide (CsI) used to releases light photons, gadolinium oxysulfide (GdOS) which is also a scintillator and amorphous selenium (a-Se) a photoconductor used in non-scintillator detectors. Photomultipliers are used in the computer reader. They collect the blue-purple light given off by the trapped electrons as they

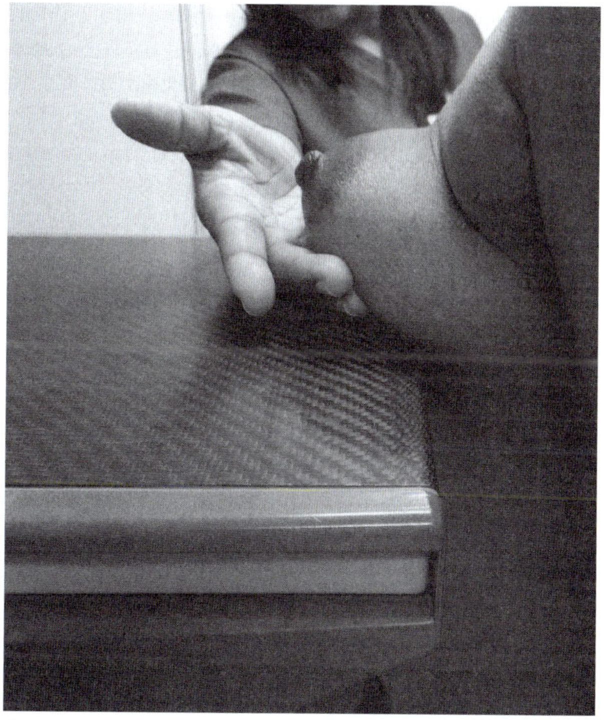

A

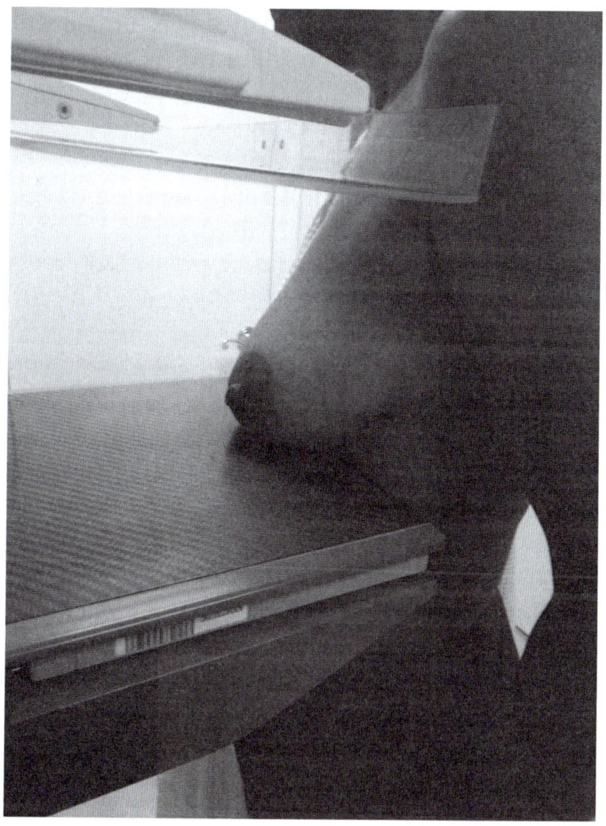

B

Figure 7-30. The detector position is important when imaging the CC. (A) Detector too high and (B) detector too low on CC positioning.

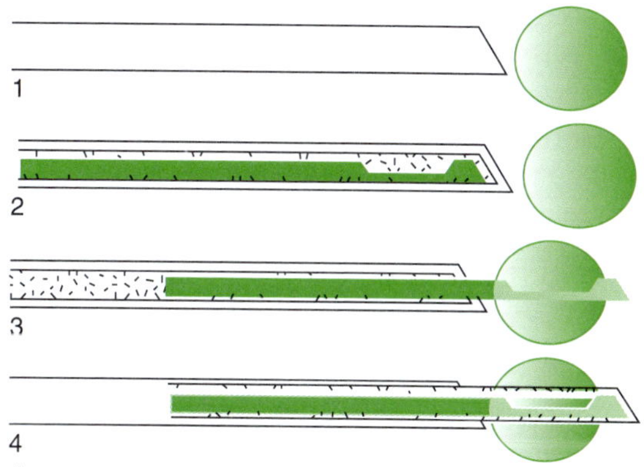

A

1. The trough without the needle approaching lesion - pre-fire.
2. Trough with needle - pre-fire
3. Post fire into the lesion.
4. The cut breast tissue remains in the trough and is slowly pulled into the needle

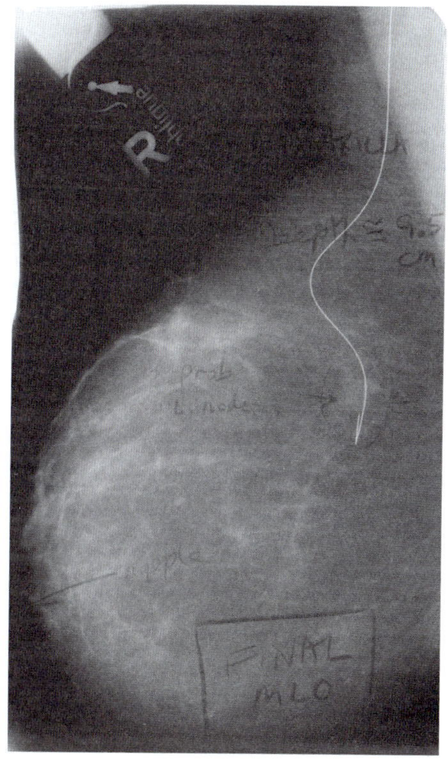

B

Figure 7-31. (A) The biopsy gun traverse the lesion to remove a sampling and (B) wire localization technique showing the hook wire in place in the lesion. (Reproduced with permission from Peart O: Mammography and Breast Imaging PREP: Program Review and Exam Prep. New York, NY: McGraw-Hill Education; 2012.)

return to their normal state and convert the light energy to an electrical signal. (See Figure 7-27.)[6,7]

85. (D) A core biopsy removes a cylinder of tissue using a 14 or higher gauge needle (Figure 7-31). The sample from a core biopsy is larger than that from fine-needle biopsy (FNB). Tissue samples from a core biopsy are assessed histologically. FNB or fine-needle biopsy is performed using a small-gauge, 20-23 gauge, needle to remove cellular material for cytological analysis. The accuracy of the procedure is dependent on the skills of the radiologist or surgeon performing the procedure. During the procedure, the presence of a cytotechnologist or cytopathologist is recommended to verify the adequacy of the cell samples and to prepare the slides. Excisional biopsy is a surgical biopsy where the entire lesion as well as surrounding margins of normal-appearing tissue is removed. Wire localization is a procedure during which the location of a nonpalpable lesion or calcifications in the breast is identified by placing a thin needle into the breast. The needle is guided through the lesion or calcifications using mammogram or ultrasound monitoring, and a small hook wire is left in placed to mark the site of the suspected abnormality before surgery (Figure 7-32).[19]

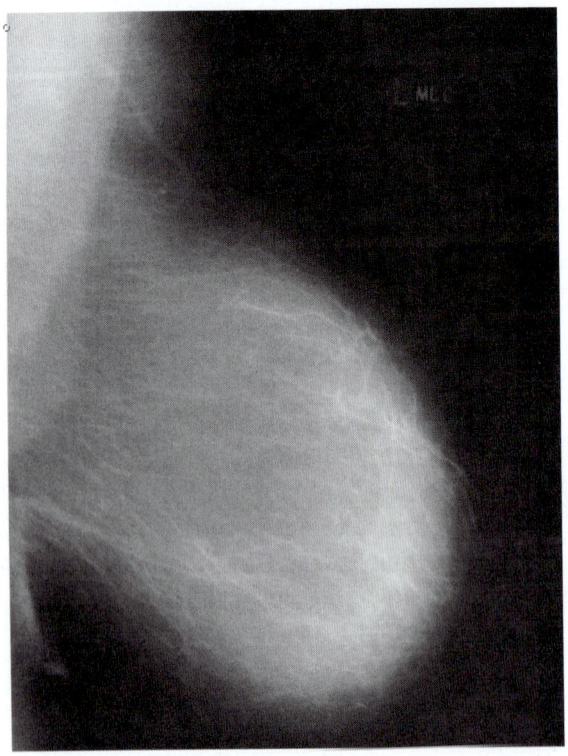

Figure 7-32. Radiograph showing drooping of the anterior breast on the MLO. (Reproduced with permission from Peart O: Lange Q&A: Mammography Examination, 2nd ed. New York, NY: McGraw-Hill Education; 2008.)

86. (D) The rolled medial or the rolled lateral (RM or RL) are both useful in separating glandular structures of the breast to resolve questions of superimposition. The implant-placed (ID) projection is used in imaging the augmented breast clear of the implants. The mediolateral oblique (MLO) is a routine projection and would not be used as an additional projection. The exaggerated craniocaudal (XCCL) is best for imaging the posterolateral parts of the breast with the x-ray traveling craniocaudal.[9,10]

87. (C) If too much shoulder muscle and axilla are allowed in the compression field, the axilla will be compressed but the thickness of the axilla will not allow for compression of the lower breast. The high placement of the detector unnecessarily elevates the shoulder, pulling breast tissue from the compression field. There will be poor pectoral muscle and possibly missed posterior breast but compression of the lower breast is not usually compromised. The pectoral muscle must be demonstrated to the level of the nipple. A horizontal inframammary fold is important for craniocaudal (CC) positioning but not for the mediolateral oblique (MLO) (Figure 7-32).[9,10]

88. (C) As a woman ages, declining hormone levels affect both the breast stroma and epithelium. The breast loses its supporting structure to fat, producing a smaller breast or a larger, more pendulous breast because of the loss of the epithelial structures and stroma and gain of fat. The duct system remains but the lobules shrink and collapse. This process generally speeds up at menopause and may continue for 3-5 years. It is referred to as atrophy or *involution*. Increased estrogen or hormone levels, which occur during menstruation, result in an increase in breast stroma and epithelium leading to denser breast tissue.[12,13]

89. (D) The arm position will help to minimize skin folds. The patient's ipsilateral arm should hang relaxed by her side with the humerus externally rotate. If there is a persistent fold the mammographer can slide a finger under the compression device to roll the folds posteriorly and laterally. Patient should face forward with head turned toward the contralateral breast. (A) will maximize visualization of the posterior lateral tissue. (B) and (C) will improve visualization of the medial breast (Figure 7-33).[9,10]

90. **(B)** Turbid phosphors have crystals distributed throughout the phosphor level. They produce lateral spreading of light which can reduce the spatial resolution of the image. Turbid phosphors include barium fluorobromide and europium, bariumfluoroiodide with europium, barium strontium-fluoride baromide-iodide, gadolinium oxysulfide and rubidium chloride. Needle phosphors have crystals growing in columns. They have less lateral spread of light and better spatial resolution. For example, cesium iodide. Amorphous selenium (a-Se) is a photoconductor. It is used to convert x-ray to electrons.[7]

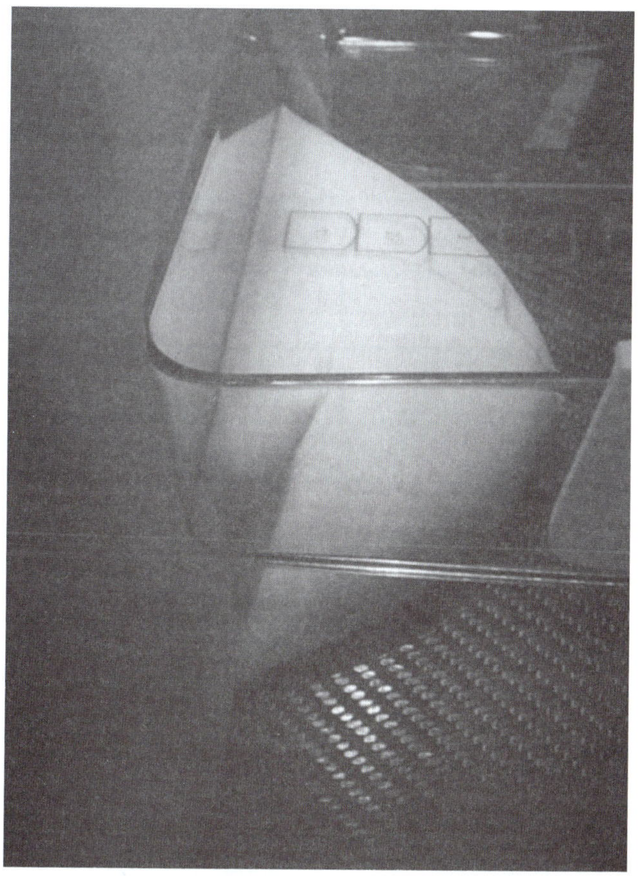

Figure 7-33. Lateral fold on the CC must be removed be sliding a finger under the compression and gently rolling the fold laterally. Do not sacrifice breast tissue by pulling the skin posteriorly.

91. **(B)** Grids are used to reduce scatter and increase subject contrast. However, grid use is contraindicated in magnification mammography because the large air gap acts as a grid in reducing scattered radiation. Grid use in magnification is therefore not necessary and would unnecessarily increase the exposure dose to the patient.[14]

92. **(D)** The from below (FB) best visualizes the central and medial abnormalities high on the chest wall and can be done for all these reasons. The beam is directed inferiorly to superiorly.[9]

93. **(D)** The image is missing the inframammary fold. There is sufficient pectoralis muscle and posterior breast because the pectoralis muscle extends below the posterior nipple line. The skin fold in the far posterior breast is minimal and does not obscure breast tissue. The fact that the skin marker does not fully cover the lesion is not a major problem. The mediolateral oblique (MLO) projection best demonstrates the posterior and upper-outer quadrant (UOQ) of the breast. Considerations when evaluating the MLO projection includes the pectoral muscle should be wide superiorly with a convex anterior border and should extend to or below the level of the posterior nipple line, the inframammary fold should be open, dense areas of the breast should be adequately penetrated, there should be no drooping of the anterior breast and distortion of the architectural structures and abdominal tissue should not overlap the breast tissue.[9]

94. **(A)** Parallel grid designs are common in mammography. Here the lead strips are aligned adjacent and parallel to each other and placed lengthwise in grid structure. Parallel grids allow central ray angulation in the direction of the lead strips only and will remove scatter in 1 direction. Option (B) describes the crossed (crosshatch or crisscross) grid design. This is similar to having 2 linear grids with their linear patterns at right angles to each other. Crossed grids do not permit any central ray angulation and will clean up scatter in both directions. Option (C) describes the focused grid where the lead strips are virtually parallel in the midsection but at the periphery they incline slightly toward the center of the grid. The focused grid must be used at its designed source-to-image receptor distance (SID) to avoid grid cutoff and work well with mammography units which are designed to operate at a fixed SID. Grid cutoff is the unwanted absorption of the primary beam by the lead strips of the grid. Option (D) describes the moving grid. Grids can be stationary or moving. The stationary grid will sometimes produce observable images of the grid lines. The moving grid "moves" during the exposure. In breast imaging, the grid is a reciprocating grid that moves back and forth versus the oscillating grid that moves in a circular pattern (Figure 7-34).[14]

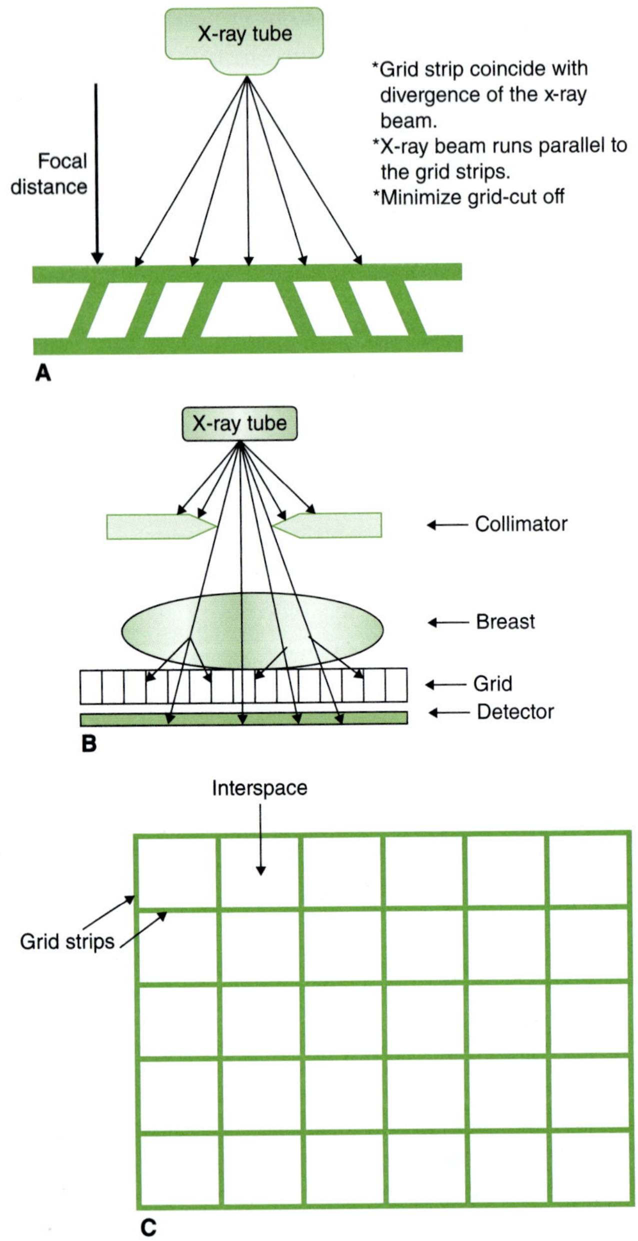

Figure 7-34. Types of grids (A) focus, (B) parallel ,(C) cross-hatched.

95. **(C)** The charge-coupled device (CCD) is a silicon-based semiconductor that is light sensitive. It can detect very low levels of visible light and has a linear response to radiation. When light from the scintillator material strikes the CCD the light is converted to an electrical charge that is directly proportional to the intensity of radiation absorbed by the scintillator. Instead of the CCD, some systems use complementary metal-oxide silicon (CMOS), which is used to convert light into an analog signal that is sent to the analog to digital converter (ADC). The CMOS is a semiconductor transistor similar to the CCD in that it has either a fiber optic coupling or a lens system. Each array of MOS capacitors represents a pixel. A CMOS is smaller than the CCD and will therefore take up less space.[7,8]

96. **(A)** When the x-ray beam strikes a scintillator such as cesium iodide, the cesium iodide converts x-rays to light. A charge-coupled device (CCD) converts light to electrons. When the x-ray beam strikes the photoconductor such as amorphous selenium (a-Se), the a-Se converts x-rays to electrons. Instead, of the CCD some systems use a complementary metal-oxide silicon (CMOS) which is used to convert light into an analog signal that is sent to the analog to digital converter (ADC). The CMOS is a semiconductor transistor similar to the CCD in that it has either a fiber optic coupling or a lens system. Each array of MOS capacitors represents a pixel. The CMOS is smaller than the CCD and will therefore take up less space.[7,8]

97. **(B)** When the x-ray beam strikes the photoconductor, e.g., amorphous selenium (a-Se), the a-Se converts x-ray to electrons. When the x-ray beam strikes the scintillator, e.g., cesium

iodide the Cesium iodide converts x-ray to light. A charge-coupled device (CCD) also converts light to electrons. Instead of the CCD some systems us a complementary metal-oxide silicon (CMOS) to converts light into an analog signal that is sent to the analog to digital converter (ADC). The CMOS is a semiconductor transistor similar to the CCD in that it has either a fibro optic coupling or a lens system. Each array of MOS capacitors represents a pixel. CMOS are smaller than CCD therefore will take up less space. (See Figure 7-27.)[7,8]

98. **(A)** The overall repeat rate should be approximately 2% or less, but a rate of 5% is adequate. If the repeat rate exceeds the acceptable level (2-5 percentage points) or if repeat or reject rates change from the previously measured rate by more than ±2 percentage point, the change should be investigated and corrective action taken.[16,17]

99. **(C)** Oil cysts show mammographically as high-density tumors with lucent centers and eggshell-like calcifications. They usually form as a result of fat necrosis or are slowly calcifying hematomas. Fat necrosis is death of fatty tissue in the breast that can occur spontaneously, but is usually the result of a biopsy or injury. When the fat tissue dies, it changes to oil. The body then forms a capsule around the oil to protect itself. The capsule generally has a thin layer of calcifications, which give an eggshell-like appearance on the mammogram. Oil cysts are benign. Ductal papillomas are benign masses associated with the ducts and are not seen mammographically. A fibroadenoma is a benign radiolucent mass that may or may not contain calcifications. A hematoma is seen as a circular-oval lesion with mixed density. It is a benign mass associated with injury or surgery. (See Figure 3-18.)[4,5]

100. **(C)** Thin-film transistor (TFT) in the flat-panel detector systems are used to collect electrons from the detector elements (DELs). The electrons are then extracted off the TFT array and sent to the ADC, which sends the digital signal to the computer as an image. The TFT is a device made of electrodes, photoconductor, storage capacitor, and other components. A common material is amorphous silicon (a-Si) or amorphous selenium (a-Se). a-Si is a photoconductor that can be deposited on thin films (hence the name thin-film diodes or transistors).[7,8]

101. **(C)** The implant-displaced (ID) projection is a method of imaging the augmented breast. The method displaces the implant posteriorly to exclude it from the compression area. ID projections are taken in addition to the routine projections. In general, the routine series of projections for a patient with breast augmentation would include the routine craniocaudal (CC) of both breasts, the routine mediolateral oblique (MLO) of both breasts, CC with ID of both breasts, and MLO with ID of both breasts (Figure 7-35).[9,10]

102. **(D)** Under the final regulations of the US Food and Drug Administration (FDA), all mammographers satisfying the interim regulations can still perform mammograms. All new mammographers must: complete at least 40 hours of documented training in mammography under the supervision of a qualified instructor or, before April 28, 1999, have satisfied the requirements of the interim regulation of the FDA. The 40 hours must include 27.5 hours of the mammography course and 12.5 hours of documented performance of a minimum of 25 examinations under direct supervision of a qualified mammographer. A least 8 of the 40 hours must document training in each mammography modality in which the mammographer intends to practice (e.g., digital or tomosynthesis) if the mammographer started working in the new modality after April 28, 1999. The mammography course must include breast anatomy and physiology, positioning and compression, quality assurance/quality control techniques and imaging of patients with breast implants.[17,25]

103. **(B)** Of the 2 routine projections the mediolateral oblique (MLO) offers the maximum amount of breast tissue on a single projection.

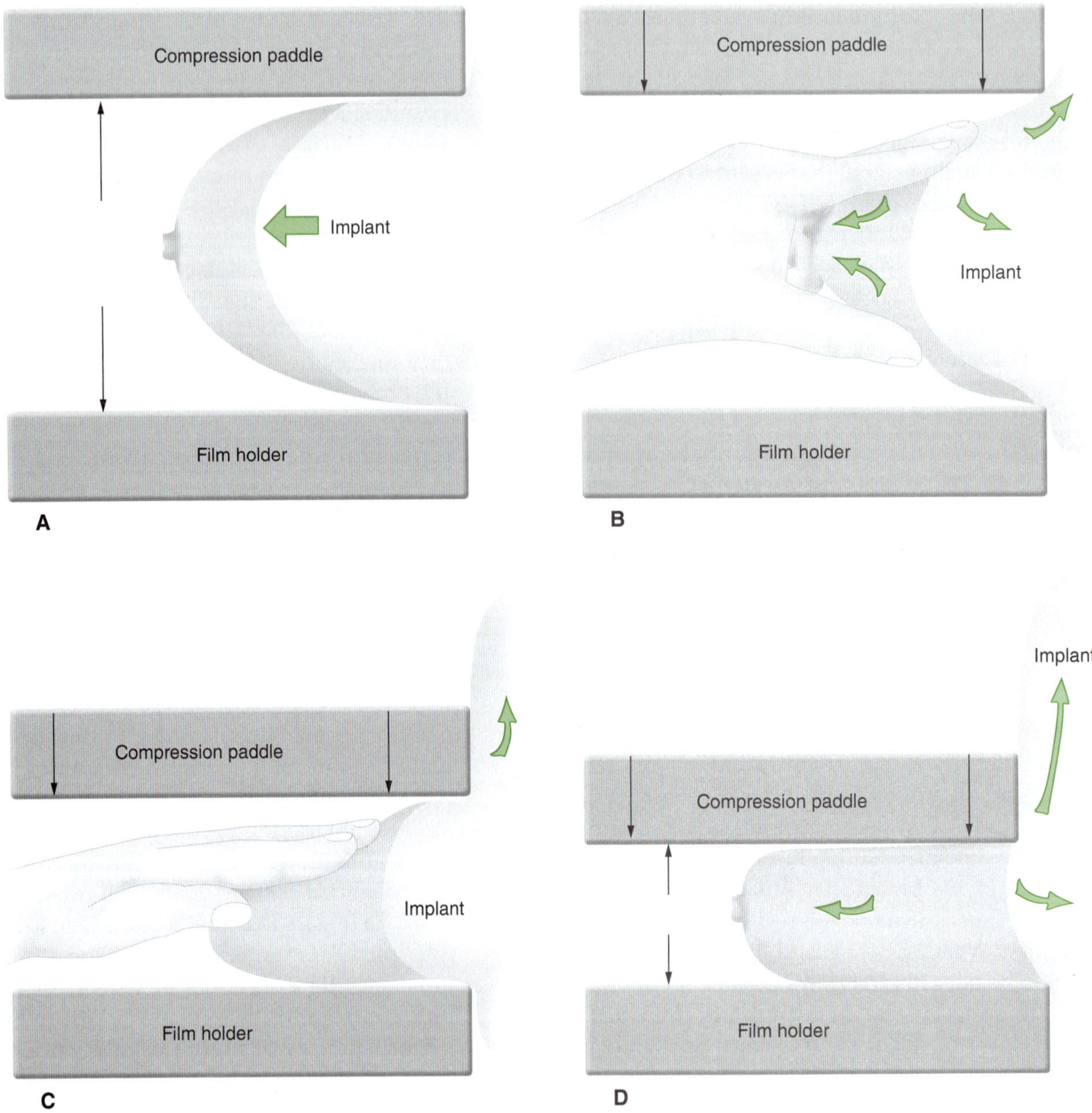

Figure 7-35. ID positioning. (Reproduced with permission from Peart O: Mammography and Breast Imaging PREP: Program Review and Exam Prep. New York, NY: McGraw-Hill Education; 2012.)

The MLO projection best demonstrates the posterior and upper-outer quadrant (UOQ) of the breast. Considerations when evaluating the MLO projection includes: the pectoral muscle should be wide superiorly with a convex anterior border and should extend to or below the level of the posterior nipple line; the inframammary fold should be open; dense areas of the breast should be adequately penetrated; there should be no drooping of the anterior breast and distortion of the architectural structures; the skin fold must be open and abdominal tissue should not overlap the breast tissue (Figure 7-36).[9]

104. (A) Ductal ectasia is a benign inflammatory condition of the ducts, which leads to nipple discharge, nipple inversion, or periareolar sepsis. The condition may resemble breast carcinoma. Paget disease of the breast is a special form of ductal carcinoma associated with changes of the nipple. *Peau d'orange* is a condition where the skin of the breast becomes thickened and dimpled, resembling

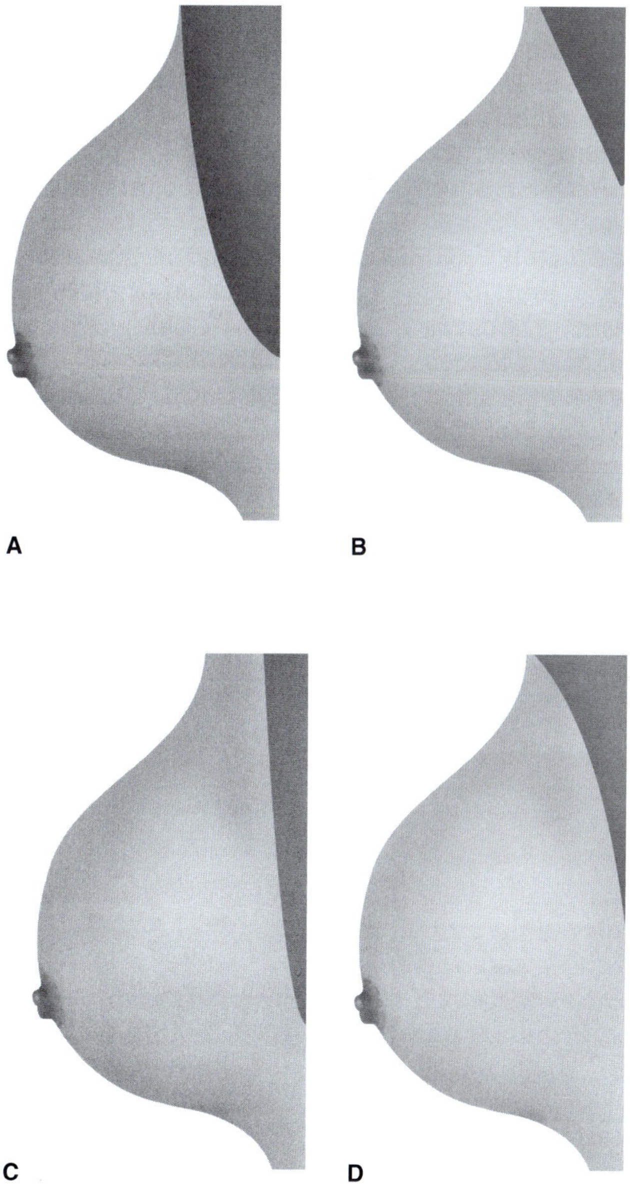

Figure 7-36. MLO (A) good convex pectoral muscle, (B) pectoral muscle does not reach the PNL. Image must be repeated, (C) vertical pectoral muscle. Suboptimal study, (D) concave pectoral muscle. Suboptimal study.

an orange; this may be the result of either benign or malignant conditions. Ductal papillomas are benign masses associated with the ducts and are not usually seen mammographically.[4,5]

105. **(A)** In the immature breast the ducts and alveoli in the lobule are lined by a 2-layer epithelium of cells. After puberty this epithelium proliferates, forming 3 alveolar cell types: superficial (luminal) A cells, basal B cells (chief cells), and myoepithelial cells forming the innermost layer or basal surface of the epithelium. Beneath the epithelium is connective tissue that helps to keep the epithelium in place. Between the epithelium and the connective tissue is a layer called the basement membrane. The basement membrane provides support and acts as a semipermeable filter under the epithelium (Figure 7-37).[12,13]

106. **(B)** Patients must have all the information that they need to make decisions about their healthcare in order to give consent. Information must be related in a language the patient

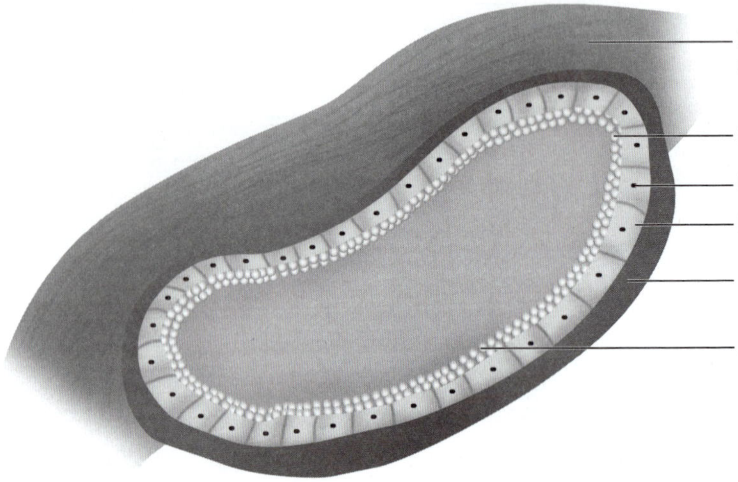

Figure 7-37. Multilayer epithelium.

can understand. This information includes: the nature of the procedure; purpose of the procedure; possible risks associated with the procedure including complications or side effects, the benefits and desired outcome; any alternative procedures that could be performed; the risks and benefits of alternative procedures.[22,25]

107. (B) Mammoplasty is the general term used when describing reshaping of the breast. The breast can be lifted to reduce a sagging breast, enlarged (augmented), or reconstructed after the removal of a tumor. Reduction mammoplasty is the term used to describe the reduction of the size of the breast by removing excess breast tissue. A breast biopsy is the removal of breast tissue for histological testing.[4,13]

108. (C) Each pixel contains *bits* of information and the number of *bits* per pixel determines the shade of gray demonstrated. A digital image can have between 25,000 and 1,000,000 pixels and the smaller the pixels, the greater the *spatial resolution*. The greater the number of pixels, the greater the *image resolution* and the number of bits per pixel determines the shade of gray demonstrated or the *bit depth*.The level of gray will determine the overall image quality or *contrast resolution*.[7,8]

109. (B) The detector elements (DELs or dexel) are located within the thin-film transistor (TFT). The DEL is a part of the complex circuit device of the TFT. The DEL is the sensitive component of the TFT which collects electrons emitted from either amorphous selenium (a-Se) or amorphous silicon (a-Si) that represent individual components of a digital image. Each square in the TFT matrix can have sensitive and nonsensitive areas. The *fill factor* is the ratio of the sensitive area to the entire detector area and is usually expressed as a percentage. Fill factor will affect the spatial resolution and signal-to-noise ratio. A typical fill factor is 80%. DEL size controls the recorded detail, or spatial resolution, for the flat-panel device. DEL size also contributes to the image blur present in a flat-panel detector receptor. The larger DELs in a flat-panel detector cause more image blur. The technologist cannot change the size of the DEL, which is fixed by the individual manufacturer.[7,8]

110. (C) In the superoinferior oblique (SIO) projection, the beam is directed from the superolateral to the inferomedial surface of the breast; therefore, the medial breast is closest to the detector (Figure 7-38).[9]

111. (D) In general, male breast imaging will present the same difficulty as imaging a small, female breast and the breast size of males is sometimes no different than that of females. However, chest hair on males can make imaging the craniocaudal (CC) difficult. With hairy chest the compression tends to slide off

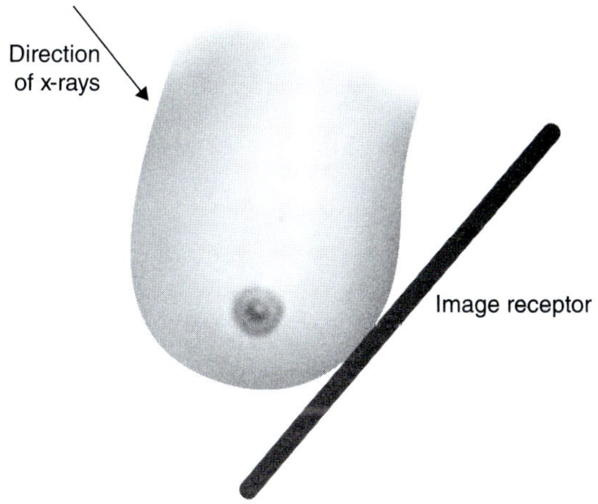

Figure 7-38. SIO. (Reproduced with permission from Peart O: Lange Q&A: Mammography Examination, 2nd ed. New York, NY: McGraw-Hill Education; 2008.)

and the breast tends to slip from under the compression. The pectoral muscles can present a problem on the mediolateral oblique (MLO) projection.[9]

112. (D) In the superoinferior oblique (SIO), the rays are directed from the lateral portion of the upper axilla to the lower medial portion of the breast, that is, superolateral to inferomedial. The superomedial to inferolateral is the routine mediolateral oblique (MLO) and the inferolateral to superomedial is the lateromedial oblique (LMO). The inferomedial to superolateral has no American College of Radiology (ACR) label.[9]

113. (B) Under current regulations, an accreditation body can be a private, nonprofit organization or state agency. Currently, the US Food and Drug Administration (FDA)-approved accreditation bodies are the American College of Radiology (ACR) and the states of Arkansas, Iowa, and Texas. Accreditation bodies established for individual states can accredit only those facilities located within their respective states.[26]

114. (B) The mediolateral oblique (MLO) is 1 of the routine imaging projections. The reverse of this is the lateromedial oblique (LMO). The LMO provides a true reverse of the MLO image and is useful in imaging patients with pacemakers. The LMO and also the LM are good alternatives to the routine images and both can also be used for patients with infusa-port (port-a-caths inserted for long-term chemotherapy treatment), the kyphotic patient, and patients with recent open-heart surgery. The ML is not a good replacement because it is poor at imaging the posterior and lateral aspects of the breast. The exaggerated craniocaudal (XCCL) best images the posterolateral breast tissue.[9]

115. (C) Ductal carcinoma occurs in 90% of all women with breast cancer. Lobular carcinoma affects 5%-10% of women with breast cancer. Other forms of breast carcinoma, including medullary carcinoma, account for less than 10% of the total breast cancer cases.[4]

116. (D) These are the Mammography Quality Standard Act (MQSA) requirements. The assessment of findings refers to the final result (e.g., benign). Additional patient identifiers could be the patient's age, date of birth, or medical record number. The report must also identify the interpreting radiologist.[26]

References

1. American Cancer Society: Early Detection, Diagnosis, and Staging. Can breast cancer be found early? http://www.cancer.org/cancer/breastcancer/detailedguide/breast-cancer-detection. Last Review 01/31/2014. Accessed March 14, 2014.
2. Peart O. Patient education and assessment. In: *Mammography and Breast Imaging: Prep*. New York, NY: McGraw-Hill; 2012:23-64.
3. U.S. Department of Health & Human Services. Health Information Privacy. http://www.hhs.gov/ocr/privacy/. Accessed March 22, 2014.
4. Peart O. Breast benign and malignant diseases of the breast. In: *Mammography and Breast Imaging: Prep*. New York, NY: McGraw-Hill; 2012:263-332.
5. Venes D, Biderman A, Adler E. *Taber's Cyclopedic Medical Dictionary*. 21st ed. Philadelphia, PA: F.A. Davis; 2005:1-2518.
6. Bushong SC. Advanced x-ray imaging. In: *Radiologic Science for Technologists—Physics, Biology and Protection*. 10th ed. St. Louis, MO: Mosby; 2004:371-384.
7. Fostbinder R, Orth D. Special imaging techniques. In: *Essentials of Radiologic Science*. Philadelphia, PA: Lippincott Williams & Wilkins; 2012:204-252.
8. Bushong SC. The digital radiographic image. In: *Radiologic Science for Technologists—Physics, Biology*

and Protection. 10th ed. St. Louis, MO: Mosby; 2004: 265-332.

9. Peart O. Breast imaging mammography. In: *Mammography and Breast Imaging: Prep*. New York, NY: McGraw-Hill; 2012:213-262.
10. Andolina VF, Lille SL, Willison KM. The mammogram. In: *Mammographic Imaging: A Practical Guide*. 3rd ed. Philadelphia, PA: Lippincott Williams & Wilkins; 2010:119-274.
11. American Cancer Society: Early Detection, Diagnosis, and Staging. Can breast cancer be found early? http://www.cancer.org/cancer/breastcancer/detailedguide/breast-cancer-detection. Last Review 01/31/2014. Accessed March 14, 2014.
12. Peart O. Breast anatomy, physiology and pathology of the breast. In: *Mammography and Breast Imaging: Prep*. New York, NY: McGraw-Hill; 2012:263-332.
13. Tortora GJ, Derrickson B. The reproductive systems. In: *Principles of Anatomy and Physiology*. 12th ed. New York, NY: John Wiley & Sons; 2009:1110-1112.
14. Bushong SC. The radiographic image. In: *Radiologic Science for Technologists—Physics, Biology and Protection*. 10th ed. St. Louis, MO: Mosby; 2004:161-264.
15. Fostbinder R, Orth D. Special imaging techniques. In: *Essentials of Radiologic Science*. Philadelphia, PA: Lippincott Williams & Wilkins; 2012:92-183.
16. Papp J. Mammography quality standards. In: *Quality Management in the Imaging Sciences*. 3rd ed. St. Louis, MO: Mosby; 2006:195-229.
17. Peart O. The US Mammography Quality Standard Act (MQSA). In: *Mammography and Breast Imaging: Prep*. New York, NY: McGraw-Hill; 2012:437-500.
18. Bushberg JT, Seibert JA, Meidholdt EM, Boone JM. Mammography. In: The Essential Physics of Medical Imaging 3rd ed. Philadelphia, PA: Lippincott Williams & Wilkins; 2012:238-281.
19. Peart O. Interventional procedures. In: *Mammography and Breast Imaging: Prep*. New York, NY: McGraw-Hill; 2012:363-396.
20. American Cancer Society: Causes, Risk Factors and Prevention. What are the risk factors for breast cancer? http://www.cancer.org/cancer/breastcancer/detailedguide/breast-cancer-risk-factors. Last Medical Review: 01/14/2014. Accessed March 14, 2014.
21. Peart O. Mammography equipment. In: *Mammography and Breast Imaging: Prep*. New York, NY: McGraw-Hill; 2012:117-156.
22. Adler A, Carlton R. Health records and health information management. In: Galocy LC, Skurka MA, eds. *Introduction to Radiologic Science and Patient Care*. 5th ed. St. Louis, MO. Elsevier Saunders; 2012:317-328.
23. Tabár L, Dean PB. Calcifications on mammogram. In: *Teaching Atlas of Mammography*. 4th ed. New York, NY: Thieme; 2011:149-238.
24. MicroDose Mammography. http://www.healthcare.philips.com/us_en/clinicalspecialities/womenshealthcare/imaging/mammography/microdose/features.wpd#Full-fielddigitalmammographysystem%28FFDM%29Section.
25. Adler A, Carlton R. History taking. In: *Introduction to radiologic Science and Patient Care*. 5th ed. St. Louis, MO. Elsevier Saunders; 2012:141-145.
26. FDA U.S. Food And Drug Administration. Policy Guidance Help System. http://www.fda.gov/Radiation-EmittingProducts/MammographyQualityStandardsActandProgram/Guidance/PolicyGuidanceHelpSystem/default.htm#Quality. Last Update March 20, 2013. Accessed March 22, 2014.

Index

Note: Page numbers followed by *f* and *t* denote figures and tables.